CONCEPTS
IN
FITNESS
PROGRAMMING

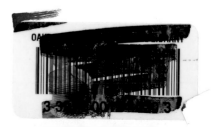

CRC Series in Exercise Physiology

Series Editor
Ira Wolinsky

Titles included in the Series

CONCEPTS in FITNESS PROGRAMMING
Robert G. McMurray

EXERCISE THROUGHOUT the LIFE CYCLE:
A Comprehensive Handbook
Richard R. Suminski and Jie Kang

PHYSICAL ACTIVITY and CANCER
Laurie Hoffman-Goetz

EXERCISE and DISEASE MANAGEMENT
Brian C. Leutholtz

CONCEPTS IN FITNESS PROGRAMMING

Robert G. McMurray

CRC Press

Boca Raton   London   New York   Washington, D.C.

Acquiring Editor:	Norina Frabotta
Project Editor:	Michelle Davidson
Cover Design:	Denise Craig

Library of Congress Cataloging-in-Publication Data

McMurray, Robert G.
    Concepts in fitness programming / by Robert G. McMurray.
       p. cm.
    Includes bibliographical references and index.
    ISBN 0-8493-8714-0
    1. Exercise.   2. Physical fitness.   3. Nutrition. I. Title.
QP301.M3754   1998
613.7'1--dc21
                                             98-31113
                                              CIP

© 1999 by CRC Press LLC

No claim to original U.S. Government works
International Standard Book Number 0-8493-8714-0
Library of Congress Card Number 98-31113
Printed in the United States of America 1 2 3 4 5 6 7 8 9 0
Printed on acid-free paper

Preface

Concepts in Fitness Programming was written to serve as a resource for exercisers and fitness instructors. Experience has shown that those individuals can benefit from a variety of knowledge beyond the simple how tos of fitness programming. Exercisers typically ask three types of questions: How do I exercise properly? What are the best foods for me to eat? How do I treat this injury? Hence, there is a need to have some background not only in fitness but also in exercise-related injuries and nutrition. For safety, the exerciser and instructor need to know which medical problems limit exercise capacity, what problems can eliminate a person from safely exercising, and what drugs used for those medical problems can affect exercise. Along with those areas of expertise, there is a need to have a background in medical terminology and the interrelationships of diseases and exercise to be able to understand the exercise literature.

The book contains 19 chapters and three appendices, covering a diversity of topics. The book is divided into four sections, each with a specific purpose. Section I contains a summary of exercise physiology. That section provides the background as to how the body responds to exercise and training. The emphases are on the important concepts with regard to the cardiovascular, muscular, and metabolic systems, as well as environmental concerns. Section II is the primary focus of the text, examining fitness assessment and program issues. That section, the largest in the manual, starts with a discussion of screening potential participants and includes fitness testing, ways to develop safe exercise prescriptions, information about fitness equipment, and a short discussion of motivation. Section III discusses medical and legal implications. It contains information on exercising diseased populations, injuries, medications, and liability issues of which instructors need to be cognizant. The section contains considerable terminology and may serve more as a reference or resource. The final section, Section IV, discusses the issues of nutrition, weight control, cardiovascular disease, and stress management. That section is an elementary discussion of the topics and should serve as a quick reference. The appendices were developed to give an assortment of methods and tables so that fitness assessments/testing can be easily interpreted. All sections are referenced for further information.

Because the book is not an exhaustive treatise on fitness-related topics, readers should examine the references listed at the end of each chapter and throughout the appendices to develop their own professional library.

Author

Dr. Robert McMurray is currently Professor of Physical Education, Exercise & Sports Science, Professor of Nutrition, Professor of Physical Therapy, and Director of the Applied Physiology Laboratory at the University of North Carolina at Chapel Hill. Dr. McMurray has been with the university for 20 years. He teaches a number of undergraduate and graduate human physiology, exercise physiology, and sports nutrition courses. Before coming to UNC, he worked as a swimming, soccer and lacrosse coach at Union College in Schenectady, NY, and at State University of New York at Oneonta, NY. He completed his undergraduate education at the State University of New York at Cortland, received his master's degree at Ball State University in Muncie, IN, and his doctorate at Indiana University in Bloomington. In addition, he has completed postdoctoral experiences at the Institute of Environmental Stress in Santa Barbara, CA, and St. Bartholomew's Hospital in London. He has been widely published in the scientific literature, has served as a reviewer for a wide variety of exercise and medical journals, and is presently serving on the Editorial Board of Medicine and Science in Sports and Exercise. He is past president of the Southeast Chapter of the American College of Sports Medicine and is a Fellow in the American College of Sports Medicine.

Dr. McMurray's research career has incorporated many areas of interest, which has resulted in collaborations with other faculty in the UNC Medical School, School of Nursing, Dental School and School of Public Health, studying the effects of exercise in various populations. His past research on exercise during pregnancy was partially instrumental in the revisions of the Guideline for Exercise during Pregnancy by American College of Obstetrics and Gynecology. He is presently part of a research team that has been funded for eight years by the National Center for Nursing Research and the National Institute of Health, to develop strategies for implementing cardiovascular disease risk-reduction programs in the youth. The results of this project have already produced changes to the State of North Carolina elementary school curriculum requirements for physical education. He has also examined the effect of exercise on insulin in obese children and the effect of physical activity on obesity in children. At the same time, Dr. McMurray has been involved in a project to reduce cardiovascular disease risk factors in North Carolina Public Safety Officers. His research has also focused on endocrine system responses to exercise and the role of nutrition in optimizing exercise performance. His research has resulted in over 90 refereed publications, 130 research abstracts, and 7 book chapters. In addition to his professional life, Dr. McMurray is an avid photographer, swimmer, cyclist, backpacker, and white-water kayaker.

Acknowledgments

The author of this manuscript would like to acknowledge the following organizations and individuals for their help in developing this manual:

Elizabeth E. Wright, M.A., and Lawrence F. Johnston, M.A., who worked on the initial concept and development of a similar manuscript as a resource for the North Carolina Department of Justice.

Centers for Disease Control for the financial assistance, grant #5-38334-0-110-4985.

University of North Carolina Center for Health Promotion and Disease Prevention for its financial and editorial assistance.

The Public Safety Officers Project of the UNC Center for Health Promotion and Disease Prevention.

The following individuals were consulted in preparing specific chapters in the text:

Dr. Barbara Ainsworth, Ph.D., MPH, exercise physiologist, Department of Epidemiology, University of South Carolina, Columbia, SC.

Dr. Carlton Bessinger, Ph.D., Nutrition and Dietetics Department, Marywood College, Scranton, PA.

Dr. Thomas Griggs, M.D., cardiologist, School of Medicine, University of North Carolina, Chapel Hill, NC.

Dr. Charles J. Hardy, Ph.D., sport psychologist, Department of Exercise and Sport Science, Georgia Southern University, Statesboro, GA.

Dr. Joanne Harrell, Ph.D., RN, School of Nursing, University of North Carolina, Chapel Hill, NC.

Ms. Deborah Murray, MA, AT, Sports Medicine Program, Department of Physical Education, Exercise and Sport Science, University of North Carolina, Chapel Hill, NC.

Dr. James H. Patterson, Ph.D., School of Pharmacy, University of North Carolina, Chapel Hill, NC.

Ms. Peggy Schaefer, MS, Instructor/Coordinator, North Carolina Justice Academy, Salemburg, NC.

Mr. Reece Trimmer, attorney, legal agency specialist, North Carolina Justice Academy, Salemburg, NC.

Mr. Jeremy Bailey, MA, Exercise Physiology, University of North Carolina, Chapel Hill, NC.

Table of Contents

SECTION III: MEDICAL & LEGAL IMPLICATIONS

SECTION IV: LIFESTYLE CONSIDERATIONS

APPENDICES

Section I

The Physiology

1 Basic Physiological Concepts

PART I: CARDIOVASCULAR PHYSIOLOGY

Purpose: To provide the reader with a basic background in the cardiovascular system so that he can begin to understand how the system works and adapts to exercise.

Objectives: At the end of this section, the reader will be able to understand the following:

1. The basic anatomical organization of the cardiovascular system and how it works.
2. The concepts of heart rate, stroke volume, cardiac output, and blood pressure.
3. How exercise modifies heart rate, stroke volume, cardiac output, and blood pressure.
4. How physical training modifies heart rate, stroke volume, cardiac output, and blood pressure.
5. Diseases of the heart, as well as the difference between the heart of an endurance athlete "athletic heart" and the heart of a person with hypertension.

BASIC CARDIOVASCULAR PHYSIOLOGY

The cardiovascular system consists of three parts: the blood, which carries the oxygen and metabolites to and from the cells of the body; the vessels (arteries, capillaries, veins), which carry the blood to all parts of the body; and the heart, which pumps the blood through the system. The major purpose of the system is to transport substances to and from different parts of the body. As such, the cardiovascular system serves six major functions:

1. Supplies the tissues with nutrients.
2. Removes wastes or toxic substances from tissues.
3. Circulates hormones and antibodies.
4. Distributes and balances water and electrolytes.
5. Distributes and dissipates body heat, thermoregulation.
6. Causes coagulation and clotting.

Blood

There are two main parts of the blood: specialized cells and a liquid, plasma, in which the cells are suspended. The plasma is composed of mostly water, but it is responsible for carrying all the nutrients, proteins, electrolytes, hormones, and waste. The cellular portion of the blood includes red blood cells (RBCs), white blood cells (leucocytes), and platelets. The RBCs are responsible for carrying oxygen to the cells of the body and removing carbon dioxide. Those functions make them extremely important for exercise. Anything that reduces the ability of the RBCs to carry oxygen, such as anemia, will therefore affect the ability to exercise. The leucocytes are important for defense against foreign cells and matter. The platelets, which are actually cell fragments, play a crucial role in blood clotting.

Hematocrit is the percentage of RBCs in the blood. The hematocrit is easily obtained from a finger prick blood sample. The blood is then separated into cells and plasma by high-speed centrifugation. Normally, the hematocrit of men is higher than women: men 38 to 45%, women 37 to 42%.[1] *Hemoglobin* is the substance found in the red blood cell that carries the oxygen and carbon dioxide. Hemoglobin concentration is another typical measurement that is obtained in addition to measuring hematocrit. Normal hemoglobin levels are 12.5 to 15.5 mg/dl for men and 12 to 14.5 for women. Low hematocrit and hemoglobin are crude indicators of anemia.[1] Some highly trained endurance athletes appear to have marginally low hematocrits and hemoglobin but actually are not anemic. That is because their endurance training has caused the plasma volume to increase more than their RBCs, thus lowering the hematocrit and hemoglobin concentrations. Those individuals are probably not truly anemic; however, other clinical tests will be necessary to confirm a diagnosis.

Vessels

Blood pumped out of the heart leaves through the aorta. It is then passed from the aorta through the arteries into arterioles, or small arteries that serve as control points for blood distribution. The distribution of the blood is important because the body only has about 4 to 5 liters of blood, but the vascular system has well over 100 sq. meters of space. Thus, if all the blood vessels were to open simultaneously, blood pressure would drop from about 100 mmHg to <10 mmHg and the individual would not be able to remain conscious. The arterioles have specialized muscle cells that can adjust blood flow to areas that need extra blood and away from areas requiring little blood. Thus, when muscles need blood for exercise, arterioles in the working muscles dilate, which allows more blood to flow into the muscles. At the same time, arterioles in the digestive system constrict, reducing blood flow to that area. Conversely, after eating a big meal the vessels in the stomach and intestine dilate to aid digestion while the vessels in the muscles may constrict.

Arterioles branch into a huge number of very small, very thin vessels called capillaries. Capillaries are the working units of the system in that they are the site for the exchanges of fluids, oxygen, carbon dioxide, and nutrients between blood and tissues. From the capillaries, the blood flows back to the heart through venules and veins, finally entering the heart via the vena cavae. The pressures in the veins and venules is very low such that a nearly contracting muscle can cause them to collapse, forcing the blood into other parts of the veins. However, to keep the blood flowing back to the heart, these veins have one-way valves. These one-way valves have an important role in maintaining blood flow back to the heart during exercise. The effect of those valves has been called the *muscle pump* and is discussed in more detail later in this chapter.

The blood first enters the right side of the heart and is pumped to the lungs for oxygenation and removal of carbon dioxide. That is called the pulmonary circulation. The blood then circulates back to the left side of the heart from which it is pumped to all other parts of the body. That portion of the system is referred to as the systemic circulation. Pulmonary circulation is a low pressure system (about 30 mmHg) in comparison to systemic circulation (about 100 mmHg). That means that the right side of the heart does not have to work as hard to pump blood to the lungs as the left side of the heart has to work to pump blood to the rest of the body.[1]

The Heart

The primary pump for the circulation of blood is the heart. It is actually a double pump (Figure 1.1), with the right side concerned with pulmonary (lungs) circulation and the left side concerned with systemic circulation. Each side of the heart as an atrium into which blood enters and a ventricle out of which blood exits for circulation. There are one-way valves between atrias and ventricles, as well as between ventricles and the pulmonary artery or aorta. Those valves function to stop "leak back," which means that the blood being pumped travels in only one direction. Those valves can become damaged or may not close properly. If that happens, the heart will not be able to pump sufficient blood. In these cases, surgery is usually required to correct or replace the valve with a "synthetic" model.

The heart muscle takes on specific characteristics depending upon its location because of the differences in pressure loads within different parts of the heart. The muscles of atriums are usually very thin because they normally work against a low pressure, with gravity directing most of the blood flow. In contrast, muscles of the ventricles are usually thicker because they work against a high-pressure load and also against gravity. In addition, the muscles of the left ventricle are normally thicker than the muscles of the right ventricle because the pressure needed for systemic circulation is greater than the pressure required for pulmonary circulation.

Heart muscle also contains specialized tissues that allow nervous impulses to be easily transmitted through the heart.[1] Those nervous impulses are measured by an electrocardiogram to determine if the heart is working properly. The impulses travel through a specific pathway within the heart to cause the muscle to contract (see Figure 1.2). The impulses start in the right atrium near the vena cava at a specialized bundle of nerve tissue called the sino-atrial node (SA node). They are then transmitted throughout the atriums and down to the bottom of the atria to the atrio-ventricular node (AV node). As the impulses travel from the SA node to the AV node, the atrias contract and force the blood into the ventricles. The AV node consists of specialized nervous tissue that slows the progress of the nervous impulse through

HEAD and UPPER EXTREMITY

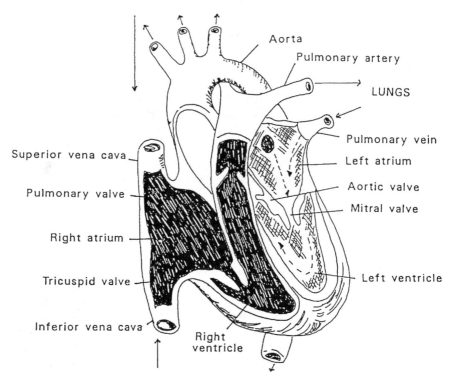

FIGURE 1.1 The anatomy of the heart. Based on Guyton, A.C., *Textbook of Medical Physiology*, W.B. Saunders, Philadelphia, 1981.

the heart. That is done so that blood will have time to enter the ventricle before it contracts. Without this time delay, the ventricles would be contracting at the same time as the atriums and would pump little blood.[5]

The nervous impulses leave the AV node and travel through the muscle wall between the two ventricles using the Common Bundle and the Right and Left Bundle Branches, which go their respective ventricles. The impulses are then transmitted throughout the muscle cells of the ventricles by specialized Purkinje fibers. That results in contraction of the ventricles, which forces blood out of the heart and into the lungs and systemic circulation. The electrocardiogram (ECG) is a graphic representation of the electrical conduction pathways through the heart. Thus, looking at an ECG and knowing the pathway, interpretations can be made regarding diseased parts of the heart.[1]

The arteries that supply blood to the heart are located at the base of the aorta, the main artery leaving the left side of the heart. Those coronary vessels are closed off when blood is being pumped out of the heart and receive their blood between contractions of the heart via "back flow." Therefore, a lower heart rate usually results in better blood flow to the coronary vessels, while a very high heart rate (above

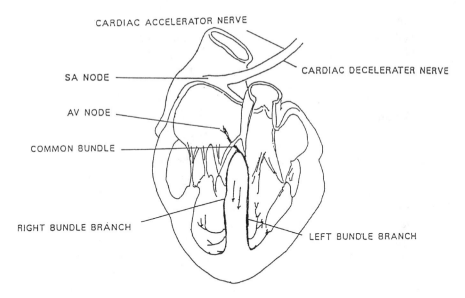

CARDIAC ACCELERATOR NERVE

CARDIAC DECELERATER NERVE

SA NODE

AV NODE

COMMON BUNDLE

RIGHT BUNDLE BRANCH

LEFT BUNDLE BRANCH

FIGURE 1.2   Pathway of the nervous impulses through the heart. Based on Langley, L.L., Telford, I.R., and Christensen, J.B., *Dynamic Anatomy & Physiology*, McGraw-Hill, New York, 1974.

200 bt/min) will usually cause reduced blood flow to the heart muscle.[1] Individuals that exercise with very high heart rates (above 200 bt/min) have a potential problem of inadequate oxygenation for the heart because there is not sufficient time between beats for the heart to receive adequate blood.

Key Concepts

There are five key concepts to understanding basic cardiovascular physiology: heart rate (beat/minute), stroke volume (volume pumped/beat), cardiac output (blood pumped/minute), blood pressure, and the muscle pump.

Heart Rate

This refers to the number of times the heart beats each minute. Normal resting rates can vary between 60 and 100 bt/min. A rate below 60 bt/min is referred to as bradycardia and is common in well-conditioned endurance athletes or individuals with certain types of heart disease.[2] A resting rate of over 100 bt/min is considered tachycardia and should be checked out by a physician.[3] Of course, during exercise heart rates can rise to over 200 bt/min, particularly in youths and younger adults. The heart rate is controlled by the nervous system and catecholamines (adrenaline). As an individual grows older, maximal heart rate will decrease.[1,4] A typical 20-year-old has a maximal heart rate of about 200 bt/min, while a 40-year-old has a maximal rate of about 180 bt/min.[2,4] That needs to be considered when developing exercise prescriptions.

Prolonged aerobic or endurance training improves the efficiency of the heart by lowering the resting heart rate.[2,5] The heart is most efficient pumping a larger volume of blood a fewer number of times. Thus, lowering the heart rate allows time for more blood to empty into the heart, giving it a larger volume to pump. Conversely, the heart is least efficient pumping a small amount of blood numerous times.

Stroke Volume

This is the amount of blood pumped out of the heart with each beat. In a normal, healthy heart, this amount is the same for left and right sides of the heart, approximately 70 ml, or about 2.5 oz.[1] The stroke volume is controlled by the nervous system, hormones (catecholamines), and the amount of blood returning to the heart. During exercise, the muscle pump also helps to maintain stroke volume. Exercise can cause the stroke volume to increase twofold.[2,5] Aerobic training increases stroke volume at rest.[2,5] The increased stroke volume is related to a slower heart rate, which allows for more time for blood to fill the heart. It is also related to an increase in blood volume (the total amount of blood in the body), which occurs with aerobic training. Aerobic training may also increase the size of the ventricle of the heart — a larger cavity will hold more blood.[2,4] Maximal stroke volume will also increase with training as a result of improved blood flow back to the heart.[2] Anaerobic training, such as weight lifting, may not cause those changes in stroke volume to occur.[4]

Cardiac Output

Cardiac output is the amount of blood pumped per minute. It is the product of the number of times the heart beats and the amount of blood pumped each beat: heart rate times stroke volume. At rest, it is usually 4 to 5 liters per minute.[1] Small people have a lower cardiac output than larger individuals.[1] During exercise, cardiac output can increase to 25 or more liters per minute.[2,4,5] Aerobic training does not alter resting cardiac output; the amount of blood to maintain the organism remains constant. However, aerobic training can cause the maximal cardiac output to almost double that of an untrained individual. That is a result of training increasing stroke volume. Anaerobic training and weight lifting do not appear to have as much of an effect on cardiac output as aerobic training.

Blood Pressure

This is the force at which the blood moves through the systemic circulation. Maximal pressure is reached during ventricular ejection of the blood (systolic pressure) and minimum pressure occurs when the ventricles are not contracting and are filling with blood (diastolic pressure). Blood pressure is generally dependent upon cardiac output and resistance to blood flow caused by the small arterioles.[3] Resting blood pressure can vary. Systolic pressure normally ranges from 100 to 140 mmHg, while diastolic pressure ranges from 60 to 90 mmHg.[3] Readings above these numbers (140/90) are considered hypertension and should be checked out by a physician. Aerobic training does not appear to lower normal resting blood pressure.[3] However, it will help to reduce resting pressure of individuals with mild to moderate hypertension.[3] Aerobic training may also lower maximal blood pressure because training reduces the resistance to blood flow.

Muscle Pump

The small veins throughout the body have one-way valves.[1] The valves open only in the direction that forces blood back to the heart. When muscles contract, they squeeze the veins thus pushing blood forward, back to the heart. When the veins are relaxed, the blood tends to back-flow, which causes the valves to close so that blood cannot move away from the heart. Aerobic exercise, which is rhythmic in nature, causes a pumping action on the veins that enhances blood flow back to the heart. That pumping action helps to maintain cardiac output.[1,2,4] But when the muscles are still, there is no pumping action and blood flow is difficult to maintain. That situation can happen two ways. First, during an isometric contraction, when the muscle contraction is maintained for 10 to 15 seconds. The isometric contraction squeezes or collapses the vein such that blood flow through the muscle is reduced or even stopped and therefore, blood flow back to the heart is also compromised. Compromised venous return can lead to syncope. Second, exercise may cause the person to become hot and sweaty. To remove the heat, the body dilates the blood vessels in the skin, causing more blood flow to the skin and compromising venous return. After exercising, this hot and sweaty person stands stationary in a hot shower; thus, the muscle pump is inactivated. The combination of too much blood in the periphery with little returning to the heart can cause a person to become light-headed and pass out. That is why it is always best to cool down after exercise before taking a shower.

As Figure 1.3 shows, the heart rate and stroke volume combine to produce cardiac output. The cardiac output and the resistance to blood flow (total peripheral resistance) combine to produce the blood pressure. It is the blood pressure that the body monitors and tries to maintain so that adequate blood flow can occur, especially to the brain. A simple example may help to understand how the system works. If a major hemorrhage occurs, blood volume is lost. That results in less blood returning to the heart and a lower stroke volume. If stroke volume is lost then cardiac output is reduced, causing blood pressure to decline. The body senses the loss of pressure and causes the heart rate to increase and the blood vessels to constrict. The increased heart rate helps to maintain the cardiac output, and the constriction causes the peripheral resistance to increase. Those two results combine to attempt to return blood pressure back to normal.

CIRCULATION DURING EXERCISE

Exercise results in an increase in systolic blood pressure and cardiac output. During exercise diastolic pressure remains relatively stable.[3] However, systolic blood pressure increases with increased exercise intensity. In fact, there is a direct relationship between exercise intensity and systolic blood pressure: that is to say as exercise intensity increases, so does systolic pressure. The reason systolic pressure increases

mean system arterial pressure = cardiac output x total peripheral resistance

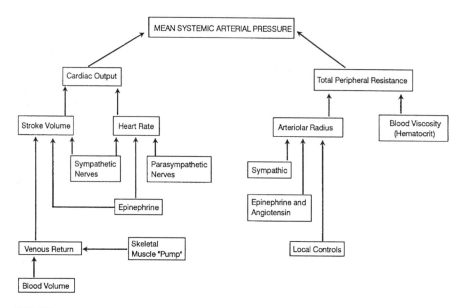

FIGURE 1.3 A schematic of the interrelationship of heart rate, stroke volume, cardiac output, peripheral resistance, and blood pressure.

is somewhat complicated. Cardiac output increases during exercise to deliver more blood to the working muscles. The blood flow is directed to the working muscles by having some blood vessels not involved with exercise constrict (reduce flow), while others in the active muscle dilate (increase flow). This ultimately reduces resistance to blood flow. One would think that the reduced resistance would lower blood pressure. However, the decrease in resistance is less than the increase in cardiac output, and blood pressure rises.[1,4] For example, during moderate intensity exercise resistance will decline by 30 to 50%, whereas cardiac output will more than double.

The elevation of cardiac output during exercise is related to changes in both the stroke volume and heart rate. During exercise, the heart rate increases in proportion to the intensity.[1,2,4] Thus, the heart rate has been used as an indicator of how hard the exerciser is working. Normally, the relationship between heart rate and exercise intensity is fairly straightforward, e.g., a 10% increase in exercise intensity causes roughly a 10% increase in heart rate. However, during some forms of exercise, the heart rate increases more than expected and is not truly representative of intensity.[2,4] This dissociation of heart rate and intensity occurs in exercise that has a significant isometric component, high muscle tension without much movement. The high muscle tension blocks blood flow through the muscle, reducing the flow back to the heart. To compensate, the heart rate increases to elevate blood pressure in an attempt to increase blood flow through the muscle. That is why extremely high heart rates occur during weight lifting, yet, overall metabolic rates are moderate. The dissociation also occurs during exercise in the heat, when the body is trying to provide for muscle blood flow and blood flow to the skin to reduce body heat.

Stroke volume increase with increased exercise intensity up to about 60 to 70% of maximal aerobic capacity.[2] Above this point, only small changes of stroke volume can occur.[1,5] Above 70%, the heart appears not to be able to obtain any more blood to increase the volume and increase contractility any further so it cannot squeeze any more blood out.[1] Therefore, as the person exercises harder and harder, above 60 to 70%, cardiac output is increased due to increases in heart rate and no further changes in cardiac output.

During exercise, blood is usually directed toward active muscles and away from the digestive system, kidneys, and other organs that are not actively involved with exercise. However, the brain always gets the amount of blood it needs. This balance between brain, organs, and muscle blood flow can be disrupted when the body starts to overheat. As the body starts to heat up, more blood is transferred to the skin to dissipate heat. This increased blood flow to the skin is countered by a further shutdown of blood flow to the digestive and renal systems.[2,5] As exercise continues and further heat is built up, more blood is shunted to the skin. Some of this blood comes from supplies that could be going to active muscles. At some point, too much blood will be diverted to the skin and working muscles, causing circulatory compromise. Blood pressure will then start to decline because too much blood will be in the periphery (skin and muscles) and not enough will be returning to the heart to maintain cardiac output and brain blood supply. If this response continues, the individual may pass out. Typically, warning signs precede the fainting. First, heart rate will rise more than expected, maximal heart rate may even be obtained.[2,4,5] Second, the individual will feel fatigued from what is normally an easy workout.[4] Third, if the blood pressure is taken, it will not be as high as expected.[4,5] Because the maintenance of cardiac output is primarily related to heart rate, the use of target heart rates during exercise in the heat can be extremely useful. The amount of exercise needed to bring about a given heart rate will be reduced in the heat. Thus, to stay in the target range, the individual will have to reduce the intensity and duration of the exercise. The reduced intensity will cause less heat production, allow the body to better thermoregulate, and help to avoid circulatory compromise.

Aerobic exercise training results in an increase in total blood volume.[2,5] That change can occur in as little as one week of training. Increased blood volume is beneficial to the athlete because more blood will be available to maintain the supply to the exercising muscles and at the same time to go to the skin for heat dissipation. Thus, the increased blood volume reduces the risk of circulatory compromise during prolonged exercise in the heat.

CONCEPTS REGARDING CARDIOVASCULAR DISEASE

Left ventricular hypertrophy (LVH) is an increase in the size of the left ventricle of the heart, either cavity or muscle thickness.[3] The increased size of the ventricle can be a result of either hypertension or exercise training. Exercise-induced LVH results from aerobic training, which places more of a "volume load" on the heart; exercise increases the amount of blood the heart needs to pump. Training causes the left ventricular cavity to increase in size to pump more blood, and like any muscle, some muscle hypertrophy can be expected. However, improvement in circulation does occur in an athlete's heart. Thus, LVH induced by aerobic training is not hazardous to the health of the individual but aids blood flow.[3] In contrast, anaerobic training and weight lifting increase the arterial blood pressure the heart must pump against. There may be considerable cardiac muscle hypertrophy, usually without any improvement in coronary circulation, similar to hypertension. Thus, there may be an increased health risk. Further research may be needed to fully understand this issue.

Hypertension-induced LVH is usually considered dangerous. With hypertension, the left ventricle must pump harder against the increased blood pressure in the systemic circulation. To increase the strength to overcome the resistance, the heart muscle increases in size (hypertrophy). With hypertension, there is usually an increase in the muscle thickness of the heart, but there may not be any compensatory increase in cardiac blood supply. Thus, the same amount of blood must now supply a larger muscle mass. Ultimately that means less available blood to the heart muscle for emergencies or exercise. Any narrowing or constricting of blood flow to the area can result in a heart problem.

Angina Pectoris is severe suffocating chest pain caused by a lack of oxygen supply to the heart muscle.[3] It may result from a stress-induced coronary artery spasm (constriction) or an increased physical demand on the heart. The heart muscle cells are weakened by the temporary lack of oxygen but the cells do not die. Exercise increases the demand of the heart for oxygen. If the coronary arteries are narrowed by atherosclerosis or spasm, sufficient oxygen may not be able to get to the muscle and pain will occur.

Myocardial Infarction (MI), commonly referred to as a heart attack, is death of heart muscle cells.[3] The cell death is attributed to a prolonged insufficient blood supply. The cells die and are replaced with scar tissue that is a noncontractile tissue and therefore does not help in pumping blood. Most MIs occur in the left ventricle, which pumps the blood into the systemic circulation. MIs also can be due to a disturbance in the electrical rhythm of the heart, which interferes with the heart's ability to pump blood. MIs can be brought about by exercise, but that is rare.

Stroke is a condition in which the brain tissue is deprived of blood supply and oxygen.[3] It can be caused by either a blockage of a blood vessel in the brain due to a clot or by a hemorrhage of a blood vessel in the brain. In either case, the result is death to that tissue that receives its blood supply from the damaged vessel and possibly loss of the functions that the specific part of the brain controls.

Congestive Heart Failure is a condition in which the heart is weakened and is physically unable to deliver adequate blood to satisfy the needs of the heart.[3] A chronic reduction in cardiac output causes fluids to accumulate in the lungs and lower body. The condition usually worsens and is disabling and life-threatening.

CONCLUSION

Aerobic exercise conditioning causes changes to the cardiovascular system that improve its efficiency to pump blood and to get nutrients to and waste from the cell.

Those changes are directly related to the exercise training and are of considerable health benefit to the average person. Aerobic training also has the hidden benefit of improving heat tolerance. Those positive circulatory adaptations may not occur with anaerobic training or weight lifting.

PART II: METABOLISM

Objectives: At the end of this section the reader will be able to understand the following:

1. The basic aerobic and anaerobic metabolic pathways and their sources of energy.
2. When carbohydrates, fats, and proteins are used as sources of energy.
3. How exercise affects substrate utilization.
4. The concept of oxygen uptake and maximal oxygen uptake.
5. Different types of exercise.
6. Muscle fiber types.
7. The effects of aerobic and anaerobic training on muscle fibers.
8. The concepts of hypertrophy and hyperplasia.
9. How ergogenic aids affect muscle.
10. What exercise-induced muscle soreness is and how to reduce it.

Metabolism is the sum of all chemical reactions that occur within the living organism, the processes by which compounds are built up or broken down.[5] Building muscle by exercise is a metabolic function, as is breaking down carbohydrates and fats to form energy to be used during exercise. Most discussions of metabolism focus on energy production because energy keeps the body alive. The source of energy during exercise is adenosine triphosphate (ATP). ATP is a high energy compound that is stored within muscle cells and other tissues. Under specific conditions, ATP breaks down, and energy for muscle contraction is liberated. The energy liberated is commonly measured in kilocalories or kcal.[6] The rate at which that energy is used is referred to as the metabolic rate. The amount of energy used at rest is referred to as the resting metabolic rate (RMR). Energy used for exercise is over and above the RMR. For most individuals, the RMR accounts for the majority of calories used each day, whereas exercise accounts for only a small portion. For example, a 60 kg woman has an RMR of roughly 1350 kcal/d, whereas 30 minutes of exercise uses about 300 kcal.

ENERGY PRODUCTION

The quantity of ATP found within muscle cells is quite limited. In total, there is only enough for a few contractions. However, the cells do contain another high-energy compound, phosphocreatine (PC), that can also serve as an immediate source of energy.[1,2,5,6] The combined effect of the ATP plus the PC gives the individual enough energy to run about 100 meters. Although that is small in amount, it is immediately available and can be used at a very fast rate. Thus, ATP and PC serve

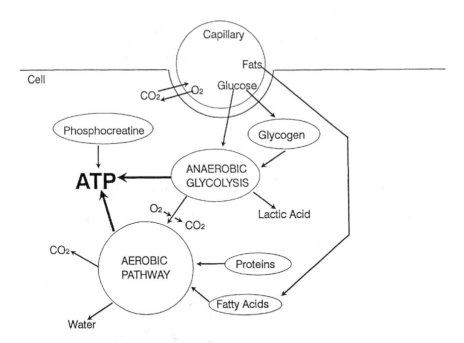

FIGURE 1.4   Schematic representation of the metabolic pathways for energy production.

as the source of energy for short bursts of exercise, such as sprinting or lifting a weight.[1,2,5,6] Since the body has relatively little ATP directly available for use, it has to generate ATP by anaerobic or aerobic metabolic pathways using various energy substrates, or sources. [1,2,5,6] Those pathways are summarized in Figure 1.4. *Anaerobic* pathways require no oxygen while *aerobic* pathways need oxygen to fully metabolize the substrate (carbohydrates, fats, and proteins).

Anaerobic pathways are used for high-intensity exercise that lasts less than 3 to 4 minutes.[1,2,5,6] These pathways have three sources for the production of ATP. One, the system can use phosphocreatine. When PC is broken down, it liberates energy that can be used to form ATP. Two, the system can use glucose. Glucose goes through an 11-step process called glycolysis, which produces pyruvic acid. The pyruvic acid is then converted to lactic acid if oxygen is not sufficiently available. Typically, the pain felt in the muscles at the end of a hard sprint is related to lactic acid. [1,2,5,6] Three, the anaerobic system also can use glycogen. Glycogen is the muscle cellular store of glucose.[1] Glycogen uses the same metabolic pathways as glucose, but it produces energy more efficiently. Glycolysis does not produce large amounts of energy but the production rate is fairly fast. Anaerobic glycolysis can provide sufficient energy for about 3 to 5 minutes of hard exercise.[1,2,5,6] Typically, when glycogen stores run low, the ability to exercise hard is diminished and the person fatigues.

Aerobic pathways can use any of four sources of fuel to produce energy: carbohydrates such as glucose and glycogen, fats, and proteins. The body prefers to use carbohydrates and fats, while conserving proteins for other use. In addition, the proportions of fats or carbohydrates is based on the exercise intensity, as discussed below.

Carbohydrates include both blood glucose and muscle and liver stores of glycogen. Since the body has minimal stores of circulating glucose, only about 20 grams, or 80 kcals, muscle glycogen becomes the preferred substrate. The body has sufficient glycogen to allow an untrained person to exercise for at least 90 minutes. Of course that assumes that an untrained person would not fatigue for other reasons. A trained person could exercise longer because training increases glycogen stores.[2,5]

After glucose or glycogen in the muscle goes through glycolysis and oxygen is present, the pyruvic acid continues to be metabolized to form carbon dioxide and water. In this process, about eight times as much energy is produced as in anaerobic glycolysis.[1,2,5,6] The glycogen stores in the liver are converted back to glucose under hormonal control and released back into circulation, where they can be picked up by the muscle cells to be metabolized for energy production. Thus, the liver stores supplement the blood glucose levels.

Fats are the second most important source of energy. For fats to be used as a source of energy, they first must be broken down into free fatty acids and glycerol.[1,5] Free fatty acids go through a process that converts them to small molecules that can then use the same intermediate aerobic pathway as glucose or glycogen. Glycerol also can be metabolized to form energy. It takes more oxygen to metabolize fats than carbohydrates. Thus, fats are predominantly used during low- to moderate-intensity exercise when oxygen is not at a premium.

The third choice of the exercising muscle is proteins. For proteins to become a source of energy, they first must be broken down into amino acids.[5] Amino acids have their nitrogens removed, then the remaining carbon structure produces energy by undergoing processes that allow proteins to enter the same aerobic pathway as glucose. Proteins are typically conserved during exercise and not used to any major extent to produce energy. However, a caloric-deficient state, as in dieting, the resting body initially will choose to use protein over fat.

The total amount of energy formed by glucose, fats, and proteins is considerably different. Metabolism of 1 g of glucose will produce approximately 4 kcals of energy and about 3 ml of water.[5] Protein will metabolize to form a similar number of kcal (4 kcal/g), but the water production is greatly enhanced, 15 ml/g of protein.[5] Fats form the most energy, about 9 kcal/g, and also form the least water, less than 0.1 ml/g of fat.[5] The relationship between water and carbohydrate or protein will become important during weight-loss regimens.

The question then becomes: With all these substrates, how does the body choose which is the most appropriate metabolic system to use to produce energy? This is a complicated process. At rest, when the body's stores of energy are filled, the body will choose a combination of carbohydrates and fats. Should the glucose stores be low, the body will choose to burn fats and proteins.[1,2,5,6] Actually, the proteins may not only be used directly for energy but can also go to the liver where they form glucose. The formation of glucose from protein is important because fats can be utilized as a source of energy when some glucose is present. That is the origin of the comment that "fats burn in a carbohydrate glow." Thus, when dieting and carbohydrate stores are low, considerable protein as well as fats will be used for energy production.[5] Aerobically trained individuals will modify their metabolism to

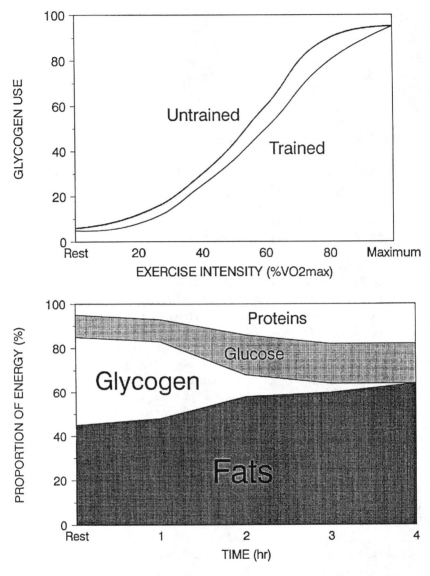

FIGURE 1.5 The effect of exercise intensity on the proportions of fats and carbohydrates used for energy. Part A shows the effect of exercise intensity, and Part B shows the effect of duration of steady-state exercise.

use more fats and less carbohydrates. Although that occurs at rest, the response is particularly true during exercise.[2,3,5,6]

At the onset of exercise, the body will utilize mostly carbohydrate sources of energy. If the exercise is long enough to obtain a steady state (at least 5 minutes), the body will then burn a combination of carbohydrates and fats depending on the intensity of the exercise. Thus, during moderate-intensity exercise, it takes only about

5 minutes to start to use fats. During steady-state exercise, the choice of substrate will depend on the intensity of the exercise (see Figure 1.5). At low intensities (<50% maximal capacity) the body will use more fats than carbohydrates because more oxygen is available.[2,3,5] As the intensity of exercise increases, the amount of fats burned will be reduced and the carbohydrate contribution will increase until at maximal exertion less than 10% of the energy comes from fats.[2,5] Supra-maximal high-intensity exercise will use mainly glycogen because oxygen availability is low yet the rate of energy demand is very high. Proteins are minimally used as a source of energy during exercise (<10%).[2,5] That is because the body attempts to conserve protein during exercise. Thus, using exercise to lose weight usually results in greater fat use and conservation of protein. If the exercise progresses in duration, blood glucose and glycogen stores will diminish and the body will utilize more fats. At the same time, more proteins will be diverted to the liver where they will be converted to glucose to help sustain blood glucose levels. Keep in mind that the brain uses only glucose as its source of energy. Thus, low blood glucose affects brain functioning. On another point, it is important to note that as aerobic conditioning improves, more fats (than carbohydrates) will be utilized during exercise.

ANAEROBIC THRESHOLD

Both the aerobic and anaerobic energy systems operate during exercise. The dominance of one system over the other is dependent upon the intensity. Thus, as indicated above, the aerobic pathways supply most of the energy during low- to moderate-intensity exercise while the anaerobic system is relatively unimportant. As the intensity of the exercise increases the aerobic pathways increase their rate of energy production. But at some point, those aerobic pathways cannot keep up with the rate of energy demand. To meet the increased energy demand beyond this point, the anaerobic pathways must increase their energy output. This is not to say that at this point the body switches from aerobic to anaerobic metabolism; the anaerobic pathways become super-imposed on the aerobic pathways. The aerobic pathways are still working to their potential to produce energy, but the anaerobic pathways start to contribute significantly to the energy production and lactic acid production increases. The point at which an anaerobic system starts to contribute significantly is called the *anaerobic threshold* (AT).[2,4,5] In an untrained individual, the AT is about 50 to 70% of maximal capacity. Highly trained aerobic athletes have ATs upwards of 80 to 90% of maximal capacity, while sprint and strength trained athletes have about the same ATs as untrained individuals.[5]

The anaerobic threshold has been used as an exercise training tool. Exercise completed at an intensity below the threshold is aerobic, or steady-state, and can theoretically be continued until the exerciser runs out of energy. Exercise training completed just below the threshold has the potential to cause the greatest increase in endurance capacity. That occurs because the athlete can train for long periods of time using predominantly the aerobic systems. Exercise above the threshold causes an abrupt increase in lactic acid that is disproportionate to any increase in exercise intensity. As significant lactic acid accumulates, fatigue follows closely. Thus, the accumulation of lactate reduces the duration an individual may exercise. For example, an exerciser working at 50% of maximal capacity could work for 90 minutes.

If the same exerciser works just above the anaerobic threshold, he may be able to exercise for only 20 to 30 minutes. Similarly, if the exerciser works at 90% of maximal capacity, well above the AT, he may be able to work for only 5 to 10 minutes.

Endurance athletes will have their AT measured and their heart rate at AT determined. They then monitor heart rate during training, keeping at a rate just below the AT, which allows them to train for long durations at the highest intensity without lactic acid accumulation. Thus, they have maximal aerobic and minimal anaerobic involvement. This form of training also causes an elevation of AT as a proportion (percentage) of maximal capacity. The higher the AT, the closer to maximal capacity that an athlete can compete. If two athletes have a similar maximal capacity but one has an AT of 65% of maximal capacity and the other has an AT of 80%, the athlete with the 80% AT will be able to run faster for longer periods of time without lactic acid accumulation. That is a benefit for long-distance runners.

The measurement of AT is not simple. Typically, the person completes a graded exercise test on a treadmill or cycle ergometer. During this test, respiration, heart rate, and metabolic rate (oxygen uptake) are monitored. Blood samples are obtained every 30 seconds or at least every minute of exercise, and lactic acid content is measured. Typically, the AT is the point at which the lactic acid measures 4 mmol/L. The athlete then finds the heart rate at which the lactic acid is 4 mmol/L and uses that heart rate for training. Some researchers say the AT can be determined by simply measuring respiration and finding the point where respiration increases abruptly compared to the metabolic rate.[2,5] Basically, the theory is that when lactic acid is produced and enters the circulatory system, signals are sent back to increase respiration.[2,5] Therefore, the point that respiration increases abruptly, more than expected, represents the AT. Although that method is not accurate, it does provide a rough estimate. Determining AT for training is discussed in more detail in Chapter 6.

ENERGY EXPENDITURE

At rest, the body's energy expenditure is related to the gender and size of the individual.[1] At rest, women generally expend about 0.8 kcal per kilogram per hour (kcal/kg/h) while men expend about 1.0 kcal/kg/h.[1] Persons with larger muscle mass usually have higher metabolic rates than those with smaller muscle mass. Individuals with very little body fat may also have higher metabolic rates. Aerobic training appears to have little effect on RMR. However, strength training, which increases muscle mass, will increase RMR. Finally, many endocrine abnormalities may increase or decrease metabolic rates.

Energy expenditure during exercise can increase 12- to 20-fold, depending upon the condition of the individual. Thus, a typical 160-lb (72.5 kg) male will burn about 10 kcal/min when running, or about 100 kcal/mile. A larger than average person uses more calories and a smaller person burns fewer calories. The energy expenditure is not the same for all activities. Some, such as volleyball, leisure cycling, walking, or baseball, will use only about 200 kcal in 30 minutes. Others, such as running, swimming, ski machines, competitive basketball, or squash, may use upwards of 450 kcal in 30 minutes.

Oxygen Uptake

To determine the metabolic rate, exercise physiologists and researchers usually measure the oxygen needed to create energy. That can be easily accomplished by measuring inspired and expired oxygen percentages and how much air a person breathes. Knowing the oxygen uptake, caloric cost can then be computed because there is about 5 kcal per liter of oxygen. Thus, an activity such as running that uses 1.5 l of oxygen per minute will use 7.5 kcal each minute or 225 kcal in 30 minutes.

Maximal oxygen uptake (VO_2max), or aerobic power, is the greatest amount of oxygen that one can utilize under the most strenuous exercise — the highest metabolic rate attainable.[2,5] VO_2max defines the maximal capacity of the oxygen transport system and correlates very highly with maximal cardiac output. As such, it presently represents the best estimate of cardio-respiratory fitness. The correlation is so exact that a formula can be written:

$$VO_2max = Cardiac\ Output \times Cellular\ Oxygen\ Extraction$$

Larger individuals with more muscle mass usually have a larger capacity to use oxygen (liters of oxygen per minute). Thus, their VO_2max, expressed in liters/minute, is usually higher than that of a smaller person. To account for the difference in VO_2max that is related to size, the units of VO_2max are best described in terms of milliliters of oxygen per kilogram body weight per minute (ml/kg/min).[1-3,5,6] An automobile engine makes a good analogy. A car with a large engine has more power than a car with a small engine. Similarly, a person that has a large muscle mass has a larger oxygen uptake in terms of l/min. Continuing the analogy in terms of the efficiency of the engine, using the term "miles per gallon," the more miles per gallon the more efficient the engine. Thus a smaller person, because of less weight or less fat, may have a higher VO_2max than a larger person expressed as ml/kg body weight/min. VO_2max increases with physical training or loss of body weight.

VO_2max is usually measured using a treadmill or cycle ergometer. The person exercises at increasing work loads until he can no longer work.[3,5] It is quite stressful and can be hazardous to the health of some individuals. Another approach is to estimate VO_2max by using, submaximal testing and a normogram. That can be accomplished using a cycle ergometer, a treadmill, or a step test in which the heart rate is elevated to approximately 140 to 160 bt/min. The work load and heart rate are then put into a normogram to estimate VO_2max. That form of testing is not as accurate as maximal testing, but there is less risk to the participant.

Types of Exercise

Aerobic exercises are those that are of a repetitive nature and are completed over a relatively long period of time.[3] They include jogging, walking, bicycling, swimming, rowing, skating, cross-country skiing, and aerobic dance. The exercise is usually completed at heart rates of less than 160 or at a level of exertion at which a conversation can take place (Talk Test). This type of exercise utilizes mostly fats and some carbohydrates (usually glycogen). If the exercise is carried out long enough, the body will use its glucose stores. That would take about 90 minutes in an unconditioned individual.[2]

Anaerobic exercises are high-intensity activities of relatively short or intermittent duration.[2,6] They include sprinting, racquetball, tennis, football, weight lifting, softball or baseball, and even basketball. Those types of activities use ATP-PC stores, as well as cell stores of glycogen or glucose, as their sources of energy. The fatigue from those exercises results from a buildup of lactic acid.

CONCLUSION

The body has three choices for energy to use during exercise: carbohydrates, fats, and proteins. Exercise of an aerobic nature causes the body to utilize fats rather than carbohydrates as its main source of energy and at the same time conserve proteins. As the intensity of the exercise increases, the body shifts more toward carbohydrate sources. As the duration of the exercise increases, the body shifts more toward fat utilization. In addition, the use of fats will increase as the person becomes better aerobically trained. During anaerobic exercise, the body will use its carbohydrate stores and not fats or proteins. Thus if an individual wishes to lose weight, aerobic exercise will burn more fat calories.

PART III: MUSCLE PHYSIOLOGY

There are two major types of muscle fibers: *slow twitch* and *fast twitch*.[1,2] *Slow twitch* fibers (ST) are characterized by a well-developed aerobic capacity, many capillaries, and a limited anaerobic capacity. As such, they generate little lactic acid and do not have the capacity to generate high power. However, ST fibers are considered fatigue-resistant. This muscle fiber type dominates the muscles of posture, which are located in the back, abdomen, and lower legs. ST fibers are predominantly used during steady state (aerobic) exercise. Furthermore, they are the first fibers to be activated during any muscular contraction. ST fibers also have the ability to use lactic acid as a source of energy.[1,2] This ability serves as the basis for "active recovery," in which an exerciser after finishing high-intensity exercise continues to exercise at a moderate to low rate to help remove lactic acid.

Fast twitch fibers (FT) can generate high levels of power. They have well-developed anaerobic capacity (produces lactic acid) but a poorly developed aerobic system, so they fatigue easily.[2,5,6] FT fibers are called upon only when large amounts of force are needed or when the activity calls for fast action. There are actually two subtypes of FT fibers. One, the fast twitch glycolytic (FG) has a well-developed anaerobic system and a poorly developed aerobic system, but it generates the most force of all muscle fiber types. Two, the fast twitch oxidative-glycolytic fibers (FOG), which have fairly well-developed aerobic and anaerobic systems, cannot generate as much force as the FG fibers. FOG muscle fibers are like a chameleon in that they respond to training by taking on the characteristics of the type of training. That is to say sprint training will cause changes in the FOG fibers that mimic the FG fibers (increased anaerobic capacity), while long-distance running will cause changes that mimic the ST fibers (increased aerobic capacity).[2,5]

Training Effects

The effect of training on muscle is dependent upon the type of training.[1-3,5,6] Aerobic training will cause an increase in the number of capillaries in the muscle. It will also cause the ST and FOG fibers to enhance their aerobic capacity. Conversely, the anaerobic capacity of the muscle will decline. Aerobic training will not result in much muscular hypertrophy (enlargement). There will also be a reduction in the overall power of the muscle.[2,4,5]

Anaerobic training will result in an increased anaerobic capacity of all muscle fibers. Aerobic capacity of the muscles may or may not decline, depending upon the training methods. The overall ability of the muscle to increase power output will increase. In general, power is related to the cross-sectional area of the muscle.[1-3,5,6] However, the increase in power during the early phases of training (the first 2 to 4 weeks) will be related to neurological training, as the muscle learns to improve the efficiency of movement.[2,4,5] The increased power thereafter will be a result of muscle hypertrophy.

Increased muscle size can be a result of either *hypertrophy*, which is enlargement of the muscle fibers, or *hyperplasia*, which is an increase in the number of muscle fibers.[2,4,5] Hypertrophy is caused by an increase in muscle proteins and muscle water; for every gram of protein retained, 15 ml of water is retained. Hyperplasia is caused by the need of the muscle to perform fast contractions with significant power output. It is known that a large cell cannot contract as quickly as a small cell. Thus, if the muscle cells became too large, the speed of contraction would be slowed. Hyperplasia may also be due to the inability of the fiber to get nutrients into the center of the cell and waste products removed. Although the reasons are presently speculative, new fibers develop or existing fibers can split and cause the hyperplasia.

As an individual ages, there may be some loss of fast twitch fibers. That may be a result of lack of use or it could be a degenerative process of aging. Whatever the reason, it means that older individuals may not have the ability to hypertrophy as much as younger exercisers.[3,5,6] But that does not mean they cannot improve their strength, just that more of the gains in strength can be accounted for by neurological adaptations.

Some individuals will try to increase muscle size faster than expected by taking drugs or using ergogenic aids. Anabolic steroids have been used by a number of strength athletes.[2,5-7] Anabolic steroids do increase muscle strength and size, but they are not without their drawbacks. They are usually illegal. Their use can result in possible liver dysfunction and tumors. They can cause impotence in males because steroids stop the production of testosterone. And they lower HDL (good cholesterol) levels. They may cause increased aggression. They will cause the masculinization in females (facial hair, deepened voice, enlarged clitoris).

Since anabolic steroids have major side effects, another drug, growth hormone, is widely used.[2,5] This drug is extremely expensive. Although growth hormone does increase muscle mass in older individuals, it has not had the same effects on muscle as steroids have had on younger people. Growth hormone does increase fat use and can therefore cause a reduction in body fat. Other than giantism, there do not seem to be too many other adverse effects.

Since steroids and hormones are expensive and illegal, many weight lifters have turned to foods that are supposed to have the same muscle-building effects.[7] An increased intake of protein and amino acids is thought to increase muscle mass. Also, some amino acids are thought to stimulate growth hormone (arginine, orni- thine, methionine, leucine). However, scientific data does not bear this out. Most of the data suggests that based on the typical American diet, additional protein is not needed.

DELAYED-ONSET MUSCLE SORENESS

The muscle soreness that usually occurs during exercise is mainly due to a buildup of waste products (lactic acid). This type of soreness is usually alleviated within a short time after exercise stops. Sometimes soreness is not noticed during exercise, but the intensity of the pain tends to increase for the next 24 to 48 hours, particularly during movements. This type of soreness is called delayed-onset muscle soreness (DOMS).[2,4-6] The exact cause of DOMS is not known. However, lactic acid is not the cause.[2,4-6] There are two theories: One suggests that exercise causes micro-tears in the tissue, which results in pain. The second theory suggests that exercise causes the release of a pain substance (substance P), which causes the pain-sensing nerves in the muscles to respond. This is then followed by a reflex muscle spasm, which reduces the range of motion of the muscle, thus the tightness in the muscle that is noticed when the muscle is used.

Regardless of the cause, exercises that produce DOMS have several things in common. They are of higher intensity than normal, involve fast movements in many directions, and involve muscles that are used in a relatively "new" pattern. With these facts in mind, the following are suggested to reduce DOMS:

1. Stretching will not only help prevent soreness, but it will also relieve it. Static stretching is best, no bouncing or jerking.
2. Exercise intensity should gradually increase. That will allow muscles to adapt to exertion. Slow progression refers not only to the overall program but also to the daily routine.
3. Increased intake of vitamin C and E may help. Several articles, as sum- marized in References 3 and 7, have shown that 100 mg of vitamin C and 400 IU of vitamin E for 30 days may reduce the soreness. That suggestion warrants further investigation.

Keep in mind that any time activities are changed, muscle soreness can be expected. A jogger beginning biking, a swimmer taking up racquetball, or a tennis player starting weight lifting can all expect soreness. Sometimes a significant increase in routine training induces soreness, but gradual progression should minimize this.

CONCLUSION

There are two types of skeletal muscle cells: slow twitch and fast twitch. The slow twitch fibers are called upon for most activities but dominate during aerobic exercise.

These have good aerobic capacities and do not fatigue easily. Fast twitch fibers are used mainly for anaerobic activities, including weight lifting. Fast twitch fibers generate more force but fatigue quickly. Doing activities that involve heavy resistance will result in increased strength, causing muscle hypertrophy and possibly DOMS. Activities that involve more FT fibers usually result in more muscle soreness than aerobic exercise which relies on ST fibers.

PART IV: ENVIRONMENTAL CONSIDERATIONS

Objectives: At the end of this section, the reader will be able to understand the following:

1. The ways in which the body gains and loses heat.
2. The effects of exercise training on the ability to exercise in the heat.
3. How to dress properly for hot and cold environments.
4. The effects of dehydration on exercise and heat loss capacity and how to reduce the possibility of dehydration.

Human beings are homeotherms because we have a relatively narrow range of body temperature in which we can survive. The normal core temperature of humans ranges from about 97 to 99°F (~36 to 37.3°C).[1] Body temperatures lower than 97°F can result in *hypothermia*, while body temperatures over 100°F (37.5°C) result in *hyperthermia* and those over 105°F (40.5°C) can lead to death.[1] The body likes to keep a relatively narrow heat balance: heat gain = heat loss. When heat gain is greater than heat loss, body temperature rises. Conversely, when heat loss outstrips gain, body temperature falls. In fact, maintenance of proper core temperature is so important that thermoregulation will take precedence over other bodily functions. Because exercise produces a considerable amount of heat, it is important for the exerciser to understand how to maximize heat loss. Conversely, because man does not always exist in a comfortable environment, it is important for the exerciser to understand how to protect the body from cold as well as heat.

METHODS OF HEAT EXCHANGE

The body has three means of both gaining and losing heat: radiation, convection, and evaporation.[1,2,5] The body can also lose heat by means of conduction from one surface to another. But during exercise this is not important unless the skin is in direct contact with an object (e.g., bare feet on the floor).

Radiation refers to heat taken up or given off by electromagnetic waves. For example, the sun and electric lights radiate heat. Heat can also be radiated off the surface of water or sand. That is why individuals on the beaches or in the water seem to burn more easily than sunbathers on a grassy surface. At rest, humans lose about 60% of their heat through radiation. During exercise, radiant heat loss makes up only a small percentage of all heat lost.

Convection is the transfer of heat from one place to another by the movement of a fluid or air. For example, a fan blowing across the body removes heat from the body via convection. Water wicks heat away from the body 25 times faster than air due to its convective abilities. Convection also occurs when blood carries heat from the muscles to the surface of the body. Convective heat loss can account for as much as 20 to 30% of the heat loss during exercise on land and as much as 80% during exercise in water. Convective heat loss is the underlying principle for the Wind Chill Factor during exposures to cold temperatures.

Evaporation is heat lost when a liquid becomes a vapor. At rest, evaporation accounts for only a small amount of heat loss. This evaporation comes from respiration and the insensible sweating that occurs at the skin even when the individual is not hot. Evaporation is the major means of heat loss during exercise. Evaporative heat loss during exercise can account for up to 500 to 600 kcal in one hour. The ability to evaporate sweat is inversely related to the relative humidity: as humidity increases, sweat evaporation decreases.

Conduction is the transfer of heat directly from one surface to another. For example, touching ice results in heat being transferred from the fingers to the ice causing the ice to melt. Conductive heat loss is not of significance in modern society due to the layers of clothing we normally wear.

In summary, at rest in a thermoneutral climate, radiation accounts for the majority of heat loss. Some evaporation does occur through respiration, and a very minor amount of heat is lost through sweating. Convection becomes important if a wind is blowing across the body or the body is immersed in the water. During exercise, evaporation (via sweating) accounts for the majority of heat loss, with radiation and convection having only a minor impact.

PHYSICAL TRAINING AND HEAT EXPOSURE

When an individual exercises in a hot environment, the body responds by vasodilating to increase heat flux from the core to the skin in an attempt to dissipate heat. Vasodilation increases the amount of blood in the periphery (skin) and reduces the amount of blood flowing back to the heart (venous return). As peripheral blood flow increases, blood vessels in the gut constrict to maintain adequate blood flow to the active muscle and skin. If the body heats up too much, central vasoconstriction cannot compensate for the amount of blood in the periphery and venous return decreases, causing stroke volume to decline. To maintain cardiac output, the heart rate increases disproportionately to the exercise requirement. The demands of exercise and heat dissipation can become greater than the ability of the body to compensate. In such cases, the heart rate will be maximized, stroke volume diminished to the point that cardiac output cannot be maintained, blood pressure will fall, and syncope may ensue.[2,4,5] At the same time that those circulatory adjustments occur, sweating increases to evaporate the heat. Blood, extra and intracellular water are the sources for sweat. Thus, prolonged sweating can lead to loss of cellular and intracellular water, as well as blood volume (dehydration), which further contributes to circulatory compromise. Dehydration ultimately decreases sweating, reducing the body's ability to dissipate the heat. Thus dehydration during heat exposure exacerbates heat-related maladies.[1,2,4,5]

Aerobic training improves heat tolerance. The improved tolerance is a result of adaptations that occur in the cardiovascular system and improvements in sweating. [2,4,5] Aerobic training increases blood volume. Increased blood volume enhances the ability to maintain blood flow to the skin and muscle, thus it preserves stroke volume, cardiac output, and blood pressure. Heart rate is maintained at more normal levels. The increased blood volume will also mean greater water reserves for sweating. Aerobic training causes an earlier onset of sweating, which allows the body to start eliminating heat before too much is stored. At the same time, training increases sweat rate, which means that the body is better able to dissipate heat. Those training effects are not the equivalent to complete heat acclimatization (which takes at least two weeks) but can have considerable impact on the body's ability to exercise in warm environments. Those training effects have allowed athletes to train in relatively mild climates and compete in very hot climates with minimal heat-related problems.

Exercising in the Heat and Humidity

There are several considerations or precautions that should be followed when some-one exercises in the heat. [2,4-6]

1. Breathable fabrics should be worn. These fabrics, such as cotton or poly-propylene, wick moisture away from the body and allow evaporation to occur. Shirts should be short-sleeved, loose fitting, and light in color. Expose as much skin as possible to the air. Thick, heavy clothing that insulate the body and impede sweat loss should be avoided. If exposure to the sun is prolonged, the use of sunscreen is advised. But avoid the heavy creams because they may limit sweating, and apply the screens often because sweating will wash them away. There are some sunscreens that advertise that they will not wear off with sweating or in water. But if sweating or exposure to water is prolonged and profuse, it is best to re-apply the sunscreen regularly.

2. Reduce the training level. Sometimes it will be necessary to reduce dura-tion or intensity of exercise to avoid heat-related illness. Also, consider exercising during a cooler part of the day to avoid the heat. This is a situation during which heart rate monitoring can be helpful. Monitoring heart rate will alert the individual to impending danger. In addition, as indicated above, when the body heats up, heart rate usually increases. Thus, the heat rate during exercise in the heat is higher at a given amount of work. Likewise, exercise in the heat at a given heart rate will occur at a lower metabolic rate. The lower metabolic rate will reduce heat produc-tion. Less heat production, less chance of heat problems.

3. Check the temperature and relative humidity before starting exercise. If they are high (temperature above 80°F (26.5°C) and humidity above 70%), reduce the intensity or duration of the exercise session. [2] Extreme condi-tions may require reductions in both intensity and duration or even can-celing the exercise session.

4. Drink plenty of fluid before exercising (8 to 10 oz.) and at 15 minute intervals during exercise (3 to 7 oz.).[2,5,6] Avoid caffeinated beverages because they can enhance dehydration by causing increased urination (diuresis). [6]

5. Training throughout the change in seasons will help to acclimatize to the heat. It takes about two weeks for the average adult to acclimatize to a hot environment. Start with 20 minutes of light exercise, and increase the duration and intensity over the next 10 days. The exerciser needs to be exposed to the heat in order to acclimatize. Thus, liberal use of air conditioning may prolong the process. However, air conditioning can help to cool down after an exercise session in the heat.

6. Check body weight frequently, and keep a record of daily weight before and after exercise. The differences recorded will represent water loss, not fat loss. Repeated days of heavy sweating can lead to progressive dehydration and major heat illness. In a typical fitness program, about 4 lb. of weight loss occurs daily. The individual should be back within a pound of the previous day's weight before exercising.

7. Exercise with a partner and share the responsibility for each other's well-being.

8. Know the initial signs and symptoms of heat-related illness: fast heartbeat, light-headedness, flushed appearance, muscle cramps, syncope (fainting).

Dehydration

Dehydration is the loss of body fluids. It can occur through diseases that cause vomiting or loss of skin (burns). But more frequently it is a result of prolonged sweating. Dehydration causes a reduction in sweating and heat transfer to the skin, increasing the likelihood of heat maladies.[2,4,5] Dehydration can also cause electrolyte imbalances, which can lead to muscle cramps or even cardiac arrhythmias.[1] The key to avoiding dehydration is to ingest fluid — hydrate. *Water should not be restricted.*

SPORTS DRINKS

Many exercisers use commercially available *sport drinks* or solutions. These solutions usually contain some sugar (for energy) and small quantities of electrolytes. Although the body needs water, these solutions can be of benefit, particularly if exercise is over 90 minutes. The best commercial solutions have several characteristics in common. The drinks are low in sugar, usually less than 8%. If they contain a glucose polymer, the concentration is less than 10%. Small amounts of sugar may help water uptake, whereas higher quantities of sugar or polymer will slow water uptake.[6] The solutions should be low in potassium, less than 75 mEq per serving. Research has shown that large amounts of potassium are not lost in sweat unless the sweating is very prolonged. Furthermore, a high amount of potassium slows water uptake. The drinks should contain some sodium to replace what is lost by sweating; sodium also enhances water uptake. The osmolarity of the solutions should be less than 300 milliosmoles. Above this amount, water uptake will be significantly

---

TABLE 1.1

Fluid Replacement Guidelines for Exercise. Based on Reference Numbers 5,6

Condition	Pre-exercise	During Exercise	Post-exercise
< 1 hour	3–500 ml H_2O 30–50 g CHO	0.5–1.0 L H_2O	Forced H_2O
1–3 hours	3–500 ml H_2O 30–50 g CHO 0.75 g glycerol	0.5–1.0 L/h H_2O 6–8% CHO 10–20 mEq Na^+ 10–20 mEq Cl^-	Forced H_2O 50 g/h CHO 30–40 mEq Na^+ 30–40 mEq Cl^- 3–5 mEq/L K^+
3 hours	3–500 ml H_2O 30–50 g CHO 0.75 g glycerol	0.5–1.0 L/h H_2O 6–8% CHO 20–30 mEq Na^+ 20–30 mEq Cl^-	Forced H_2O 50 g/h CHO 30–40 mEq Na^+ 30–40 mEq Cl^- 3–5 mEq/L K^+

CHO = carbohydrate: glucose, sucrose, starch or glucose polymer
Na^+ = sodium, K^+ = potassium, Cl^- = chloride

---

slowed. Some experts recommend that glycerol be added to the mixture, as glycerol has been shown to cause the body to retain more fluids.[8] It may not be recommended to mix the solution unless the exerciser is very familiar with glycerol because too much glycerol can cause GI distress (nausea or upset stomach). Table 1.1 provides a summary of the recommended hydration procedures, dependent upon the duration of exercise. And Table 1.2 shows the composition of some of the sports drinks that are presently on the market, compared with some standard drinks. Note that many of the standard drinks do not provide the optimal sugar, sodium, potassium, and osmolarity.

THE COLD ENVIRONMENT

Physical activities in cold climates fall under two general headings: sporting events and wilderness experiences. Sporting events, such as skiing, football, and running, rarely presents serious problems to the exerciser because the exposure time is somewhat limited, shelter is available, protective clothing can be worn, and the exercise generates heat. Frostbite may be the most likely consideration. Conversely, wilderness experiences such as backpacking, hiking, mountain climbing, and cross-country ski touring can lead to cold-related injuries, hypothermia, or even death.

One question asked frequently of exercisers is whether their lungs will freeze in the cold. Cold can produce some irritation in the throat, but it will not cause the lungs to freeze.[2] Studies have shown that even when exposed to temperatures of –65°F, the lungs do not freeze.

The body's first response to cold is a generalized constriction of the blood vessels to conserve heat.[1] The vasoconstriction causes an increased urine output (diuresis).

TABLE 1.2
Composition of Some Marketed Sports Drinks and Some Other Familiar Drinks

Product Manufacturers	Flavors Tested	Carbonated	CHO (%)	CHO Source	Sodium (mg)	Potassium (mg)	Nutrients**	Osmolality
Gatorade The Gatorade Co.	Citrus Cooler Lemon Lime	no	6	Sucrose, Glucose, Fructose	110	30		347–351
All Sport Pepsi-Cola Co.	Orange Fruit Punch	yes	8.6	Fructose	55	50	Thiamine, Niacin, Vit B_6, Vit B_{12}, Folate, Pantothenic Acid	526–529
Powerade Coca-Cola Co.	Fruit Punch Lemon Lime	no	8.2	Fructose, Maltodextrose	55	30		410 397
Hy-5 Grey Eagle Enterprises	Orange Grape	no	5.6	Fructose, Maltodextrose	40	70	Niacin, Vit B_6, pantothenic Acid, Zinc	320–327
Pedialyte Ross Products Division	Fruit	no	<1	Glucose, Fructose	236	179	Chloride	293
Gookinaid Gookinaid E.R.G.	Fruit Punch Orange Competition	no	5.2	Glucose, Fructose	64	100	Vit C	271 247 287

	Flavor			Sugars			Other	
Endura Unipro	Lemon Lime	no	6.5	Fructose, Glucose, Polymers	46	190	Calcium, Niacin, Magnesium, Phosphorus, Vit E, Riboflavin, Pantothenic Acid, Vit B$_6$	367
Cytomax Champion Nutrition	Citrus	no	6.5	Fructose, Glucose, Dextrose, Complex CHO	70	110	Chromium	338
	Orange		6.9		64	120		357
Crystal Light General Foods Corp.	Lemonade Iced Tea	no	0	Maltodextrose	0	0	Vit C	55 23
Exceed Ross Laboratories	Orange	no	7.4	Fructose, Glucose	50	54		307
Minute Maid Orange Juice Coca-Cola Co.		no	11.7	Sucrose, Fructose	25	480	Vit C, Thiamin	612
Coca-Cola Coca-Cola Co.		yes	11.7	Fructose, Sucrose	35	trace		705
Sprite Coca-Cola Co.		yes	11.2	Fructose, Sucrose	45	trace		685

* Serving size = 8 fluid ounces
** Has equal to or greater than 5% RDA

That is usually not too important during limited cold exposure but may exacerbate hypothermia during prolonged exposure. If vasoconstriction does not cause heat balance to be attained, the body will respond with goose bumps.[1] This reaction serves no real purpose in humans but can serve as a visible sign that the body is cooling down. The most dramatic response to cold is shivering.[1,5] That causes the metabolic rate to increase, thus heat production is doubled. Shivering also serves as an indicator of impending danger.

Tolerance to cold is dependent upon several factors:[2]

1. Body surface area: A smaller person is required to produce more heat to maintain body temperature than a larger person.
2. Age: Young adults tolerate cold better than children or the elderly.
3. Gender: Females tolerate cold better than males because of their thicker layer of subcutaneous fat.
4. Physical fitness: Fit individuals have lower thresholds for feeling cold and delayed onsets of shivering.

Exercising in the Cold

Exercising in the cold can be easily completed by taking some extra precautions. The exerciser should check the temperature and wind chill factor before exercising. Generally, a wind chill factor of −22°F (−30°C) is well-tolerated. The key to exercising in the cold is to dress properly.

1. Wear multiple light layers so that as the body heats up a layer can be removed. Wear cotton or polypropylene next to the body to wick away moisture. As a middle layer of insulation, wear fabrics such as wool, synthetics (Holofil® or Quilofil®), or down. On the outside wear a windbreaker that actually keeps the wind out. Avoid nylon shorts, shirts, and warm-up pants because they typically will not retain heat.
2. Do not wear clothing that constricts or binds. Areas in which blood circulation is reduced are prime targets for frostbite: fingers, toes, ears, nose, and other distal parts of appendages.
3. Wear a hat. Considerable heat is lost through the head, but not 40 to 50% as suggested in the popular press.
4. Wear gloves. Cloth gloves are better than leather gloves because they allow sweat to evaporate. Unevaportaed sweat that drips or wet gloves actually wick heat away, increasing cooling.
5. Normally multiple layers of socks are not necessary. That is because the feet usually produce heat and remain warm. However, if multiple layers are worn, then the inside should be of lighter material and the outside of wool or a synthetic insulative material.
6. Exercisers should also know the early signs of frostbite and hypothermia, such as localized hot spots, numbness, loss of fine coordination or excessive shivering.

POLLUTANTS

Any discussion of exercise in the environment would be remiss without a reference to air pollution. Airborne chemicals can reduce exercise capacity. The major pollutants include carbon monoxide, ozone, and sulfur dioxide. Car and factory emissions account for the majority of these. When exercising in a polluted area, check the levels. If a pollution alert has been issued and the exerciser tends to be allergic to pollutants, he should not exercise. In addition, if the exerciser is not used to exercising in a polluted area and a pollution alert has been issued, he should consider not exercising or at least cutting back on the training intensity or time.

CONCLUSION

Exercise in either hot or cold conditions can be successfully completed with minimal risk to the participant. During exercise in the heat, evaporation should be maximized by wearing appropriate clothing. Also, fluids need to be ingested. When exercising in the cold, once again the clothing becomes important. Multiple layers allow the exerciser to adjust to his own heat production. Finally, the body should be given the opportunity to adapt to either heat or cold by exercising through the change of seasons.

REFERENCES

1. Vander, A.J., Sherman, J.H., and Luciano, D.S., *Human Physiology: The Mechanism of Body Function*, McGraw-Hill Book Company, New York, 1985.
2. Fox, E., Bowers, R., and Foss, M., *The Physiological Basis for Exercise and Sport*, Brown & Benchmark, Dubuque, 1993.
3. Pollock, M.L. and Wilmore, J.H., *Exercise in Health and Disease*, W.B. Saunders, Philadelphia, 1990.
4. Noble, B.J., *Physiology of Exercise and Sport*, Times Mirror/Mosby College Publishing, St. Louis, 1986.
5. Powers, S.K. and Howley, E.T., *Exercise Physiology: Theory and Application to Fitness and Performance*, Brown & Benchmark Publishers, Madison, 1997.
6. Lamb, D.R. and Williams, M.H., *Ergogenics*, Brown & Benchmark, Dubuque, 1991.
7. Williams, M.H., *Nutrition for Fitness and Sport,* Brown & Benchmark Publishers, Madison, 1995.
8. Gisloﬁ, C.V. and Duchman, S.M., Guidelines for optimal replacement beverages for different athletic events, *Med. Sci. Sports Exer.,* 24, 679, 1992.

Section II

Exercise & Fitness

2 Health Risks and Exercise

Purpose: To familiarize individuals with preprogram medical screening and exclusion criteria, and to make fitness instructors aware of medically related factors that could limit a participant's exercise abilities.

Objectives: To obtain a basic understanding of the screening procedures needed both to ensure the safety of and reduce the risk of injury to participants of exercise programs. In addition, to become acquainted with criteria that would require the temporary or complete suspension of exercise.

INTRODUCTION

One of the primary considerations for all exercise programs is to ensure the safety of the participant. As such, specific policies, procedures, and guidelines regarding who should and should not participate in an exercise program, as well as when an exercise program should be suspended, should be developed to reduce the risk of injury. One must keep in mind that there is no way to completely eliminate the risk of injury during exercise. Exercise by its very nature involves risk. No one, not even the most highly trained athlete, is immune to injuries from exercise or even sudden death during exercise. Although in general the risk of serious medical complication is low during exercise, it is still higher than during sedentary activities. The American College of Sports Medicine (ACSM) points out that the death rate during vigorous exercise for individuals without cardiovascular disease is about one death per 187,500 hours of exercise.[1] In addition, the rate of having a heart attack for male joggers is about one a year for every 18,000 joggers.[1] The incidence of death is approximately doubled for those with cardiovascular disease.[2] Thus, for the protection of the potential participant, screening guidelines need to be developed. Screening guidelines also reduce the risk of legal liability for a fitness instructor.

Screening should be completed to identify and exclude those individuals with medical contraindications to exercise, identify persons that should receive further medical evaluation before starting an exercise program, identify persons with significant diseases that should be referred to a medically supervised program, and identify the special needs of a participant.[2] The first step in the screening process is to stratify individuals by potential risk category. Those individuals deemed apparently healthy can be included in a nonmedically supervised or nonsupervised program. Those deemed to be at "high risk" or "diseased" are better served by programs that provide medical supervision.

THE SCREENING PROCESS

The screening process determines a candidate's ability to participate in the exercise program.[2] For the fitness instructor this process should result in either accepting the candidate into the program, referring the candidate for further medical testing and evaluation prior to acceptance into the exercise program, or referring the candidate to a more appropriate exercise program.

RISK STRATIFICATION

The first step is to obtain a medical history that will allow for stratification based on risk of cardiovascular disease. The American College of Sports Medicine (ACSM) suggests three risk strata:[1,2]

1. *Apparently Healthy*: Those individuals who are less than 40 years of age, have symptoms or known heart disease, and have no more than one major cardiovascular disease (CVD) risk factor. The American College of Sports Medicine defines major risk factors to include:

    A. Diagnosed hypertension: $BP_{systolic} \geq 140$, $BP_{diastolic} \geq 90$ mmHg
    B. Serum total cholesterol of >200 mg/dl or HDL level < 35 mg/dl
    C. Cigarette smoking
    D. Family history of CVD in parents or siblings prior to age 55
    E. Diabetes mellitus, particularly adult onset
    F. Completely sedentary

These apparently healthy individuals can begin *moderate* intensity exercise programs without the need for exercise testing or medical examination. But for women above age 50 and men above age 40, it is highly recommended that these individuals have a medical examination and a graded exercise test before starting a *vigorous* exercise program.

2. *High Risk*: These are individuals that have two or more CVD risk factors, or symptoms suggestive of cardiovascular, metabolic or pulmonary disease. Besides the CVD risk factors listed above, individuals with the following signs or symptoms fall into this category:

    A. Pain or discomfort in the chest or surrounding areas
    B. Unusual shortness of breath or shortness of breath during mild exertion
    C. Dizziness or syncope
    D. Dyspnea — labored or painful breathing
    E. Ankle edema — swelling
    F. Palpations or tachycardia — resting heart rate over 100 bt/min
    G. Claudications — lameness or pain during walking
    H. Known heart murmur

A medical examination, as well as a physician-monitored, graded exercise test, prior to beginning a vigorous exercise program is highly recommended. The liability of having these individuals in a medically unsupervised program is increased dramatically. So, for their own safety, a medically supervised program may be in their best interest.

3. *Individuals with Disease*: These are persons with known cardiac, pulmonary or metabolic diseases. These individuals should not participate in an unsupervised, vigorous exercise program. These individuals should be referred to a medically supervised, structured program.

EXERCISE READINESS

Another way of determining readiness of an individual to participate in an exercise program is to obtain health information other than the specific CVD risk factors. The following questionnaire has been developed to identify adults who should receive medical advice before exercising or for whom exercise may not be appropriate. It was developed by the British Columbia Department of Health in June 1975. The questionnaire has been found to be 100% sensitive for the detection of medical contraindications to exercise. But because it is not very sensitive to ECG abnormalities, it is recommended only as a minimum for prescreening. (Copies can be obtained from: Government of Canada, Fitness and Amateur Sports, 365 Laurier Ave. West, Ottawa, Ontario, Canada K1A OX6.) An answer of yes to any of the following questions indicates the need for a candidate to obtain medical clearance before taking part in exercise testing or an exercise program.

A. Has your doctor ever said you have heart trouble?
B. Do you frequently suffer from pains in your chest?
C. Do you often feel faint or have dizzy spells?
D. Has your doctor ever told you that you have a bone or joint problem such as arthritis that is aggravated by exercise or might be made worse with exercise?
E. Is there a good physical reason not mentioned here why you should not follow an activity program even if you wanted to?
F. Are you over age 65 and not accustomed to vigorous exercise?

The exerciser should also complete a self-administered health questionnaire. This questionnaire is used to obtain more in-depth information concerning the health of the candidate. The information can be used not only to screen the candidate but also to determine if limitations exist that need to be considered in the development of a customized exercise program for the candidate. As the title indicates, it is self-administered and should be signed by the participant. The following histories should be included.[2] Some of this information overlaps with the above questions and need not be obtained more than once. However, asking about the same information using a different question format could bring about a different answer. A candidate's responses to this questionnaire will indicate to the instructor whether or not physician approval should be sought before the candidate begins an unsupervised exercise program.

1. Heart attack, coronary bypass surgery, angioplasty, or other cardiac surgery, including family histories
2. Chest discomfort during exercise
3. Light-headedness or faintness during exercise
4. Shortness of breath during exercise
5. Tachycardia or palpations
6. Heart murmurs or unusual cardiac findings
7. High blood pressure
8. Stroke
9. Ankle swelling other than that related to a sprain
10. Peripheral vascular disease — claudications
11. Phlebitis
12. Pulmonary disease, including asthma, emphysema, bronchitis, and chronic obstructive pulmonary disease
13. Abnormal blood lipids. Include family histories
14. Anemia
15. Diabetes
16. Orthopedic problems, including arthritis
17. Drug use, including present medications, allergy medications, and recreational use (alcohol, caffeine)
18. Emotional disorders, including eating disorders
19. A recent illness, hospitalization, or surgery
20. Tobacco use
21. Exercise history — habitual level (intensity, duration, frequency) and type of exercise
22. Name, address and phone number of the person's physician

PHYSICAL EXAMINATION

Once the questionnaire information has been obtained and the decision as to risk category has been made, the logical follow-up for some individuals is the physical examination. For individuals participating in an exercise program, the following information could be obtained by the fitness instructor before the exercise evaluation. However, other information must be obtained by a physician.[1,2]

Standard information usually obtained by fitness instructors:

1. Height, weight, and percentage of body fat
2. Resting pulse rate and regularity
3. Blood pressure — supine, sitting and standing
4. Total cholesterol (if available)

The following should be performed, determined, or obtained by a physician:[1,2]

1. Auscultation of the lungs
2. Auscultation of the heart for murmurs, gallops, clicks, and rubs
3. Palpation and auscultation of the carotid, abdominal, femoral, and pedal pulses
4. Palpation and inspection of the extremities for edema
5. Presence or absence of xanthoma or xanthelasma
6. Presence of orthopedic or other medical conditions that would limit exercise
7. Blood measures such as lipid profile, fasting blood glucose, hemoglobin
8. Any cardiac or pulmonary diagnostics — ECG, X-rays, spirometry
9. Interpretation of medical history questionnaires with respect to above exam

CONTRAINDICATIONS FOR EXERCISE

There are persons for which the risk of exercise is greater than the benefits of participation. The following is a long list of these contraindications for exercise. These guidelines have been developed by the American College of Sports Medicine and should be strictly followed.[1] Although it is appropriate for instructors to understand that individuals with these conditions should not participate in an exercise program, it may not be necessary for instructors to possess a complete knowledge of these medical conditions. The first 14 are considered *absolute* contraindications. That is to say, it is not in the best interest of the individual to participate in an exercise program. Items 15 through 25 are considered *relative* contraindications in that there may be some situations, on a case-by-case basis, in which the benefits of exercise may outweigh the risks. Individuals with relative contraindications are best suited for medically supervised exercise programs. If there is any doubt as to the risk/benefit to the individual, an exercise program should not be prescribed and medical advice should be sought.

Absolute Contraindications

1. A recent significant change in the resting ECG suggesting infarction or other acute cardiac events
2. Recent myocardial infarction — heart attack
3. Unstable angina
4. Uncontrolled ventricular arrhythmia — abnormal rhythm
5. Uncontrolled atrial arrhythmia that compromises cardiac function
6. Third-degree A-V block — uncoordinated contractions between the atriums and ventricles of the heart
7. Acute congestive heart failure
8. Severe aortic stenosis — narrowing of the aorta

9. Suspected or known dissecting aneurysm — weakening or hole in the wall of the heart or aorta
10. Active or suspected myocarditis or pericarditis — inflammation of the heart
11. Thrombophlebitis or intracardiac thrombi — blood clot
12. Recent systemic or pulmonary embolism — a plug occluding a blood vessel
13. Acute infection
14. Significant emotional distress or psychosis

Relative Contraindications

15. Resting diastolic blood pressure greater than 115 mmHg *or* resting systolic blood pressure greater than 200 mmHg
16. Moderate valvular heart disease
17. Known electrolyte abnormalities: hypokalemia, hypomagnesemia — low plasma potassium or magnesium
18. Fixed-rate pacemaker (rarely used)
19. Frequent or complex ventricular ectopy — unusual heart beats
20. Ventricular aneurysm — weakness in the wall of the heart
21. Cardiomyopathy, including hypertrophic cardiomyopathy — disease of the heart walls
22. Uncontrolled metabolic disease: e.g., diabetes, thyrotoxicosis (excess thyroxine), or myxedema (low thyroxine production)
23. Chronic infectious disease (e.g., mononucleosis, hepatitis, AIDS)
24. Neuromuscular, musculoskeletal, or rheumatoid disorders exacerbated by exercise
25. Advanced or complicated pregnancy

DISCONTINUING EXERCISE PROGRAMS

The instructor should keep in mind that screening reduces the risk to the participant, but it does not eliminate the possibility of complications. Therefore, reasons exist to stop an individual from exercising even though the person has been cleared. The following lists have been compiled by Painter and Haskell and published in the *Resource Manual for Guidelines for Exercise Testing and Prescription* and should be used as guidelines to temporarily or permanently suspend exercise.[2]

INDICATIONS TO STOP EXERCISE:

1. Orthopedic problems aggravated by activity
2. Progression of cardiac illness unresponsive to medical therapy
3. Development of new systemic disease aggravated by exercise
4. Major surgery
5. Psychiatric decompensation
6. Acute alcoholism

Reasons to Temporarily Stop Exercise

1. Recurrent illness
2. Progression of cardiac disease
3. Abnormally elevated blood pressure
4. Recent changes in symptoms
5. Orthopedic problem
6. Emotional turmoil
7. Severe sunburn
8. Cerebral dysfunction — dizziness or vertigo
9. Sodium retention — edema (swelling) or weight gain
10. Dehydration
11. Environmental factors: weather (excessive heat or humidity) or air pollution (smog or carbon monoxide)
12. Overindulgence: heavy, large meal within two hours; alcohol (hangover); coffee; tea; soda; or other stimulating beverages
13. Drug use: decongestants, bronchodilators, atropine, weight-reduction agents
14. Any signs or symptoms of excessive effort
    A. During and/or immediately after exercise:
       1. Anginal discomfort
       2. Ataxia (unstable gait), light-headedness or confusion
       3. Nausea or vomiting
       4. Leg claudication
       5. Pallor or cyanosis
       6. Dyspnea persisting for more than 10 minutes
       7. Any heart arrhythmia, inappropriate bradycardia
       8. Decrease in systolic blood pressure
    B. Delayed signs or symptoms:
       1. Prolonged fatigue (24 hours or more)
       2. Insomnia
       3. Weight gain due to fluid retention — salt and water overload
       4. Excessive weight loss due to dehydration
       5. Persistent tachycardia
       6. Persistent pain lasting longer than four days

CONCLUSION

A person that exercises has a risk of a medical complication occurring during exercise. Although the risk is small, it can be reduced with proper screening prior to commencement of an exercise program. In addition, the risk of complication during exercise can be further reduced if the instructor follows prudent guidelines that stipulate when to temporarily or permanently suspend exercise. The above guidelines should be followed to reduce the risk of injury and, at the same time, to reduce the instructors' risk of liability.

REFERENCES

1. American College of Sports Medicine, *Guidelines for Exercise Testing and Prescription*, Williams & Wilkins, Baltimore, 1995.
2. American College of Sports Medicine, *Resource Manual for Guidelines for Exercise Testing and Prescription*, Williams & Wilkins, Baltimore, 1998.
3. Pollock, M.L. and Wilmore, J.H., *Exercise in Health and Disease*, W.B. Saunders, Philadelphia, 1990.

3 Methods of Exercise Testing

Purpose: To review assessment techniques and introduce some alternatives.

Objectives: Upon completion, the reader should understand the following:

1. How to measure blood pressure using a sphygmomanometer and stethoscope.
2. The theory and rationale of aerobic fitness assessment.
3. Simple methods of monitoring heart rate.
4. The purpose and procedures for assessing aerobic fitness with a submaximal step test and a submaximal cycle ergometer test.
5. The purpose and procedures for assessing aerobic fitness with the following maximal tests: 12-minute run test, 1.5-mile run test, shuttle run test, and graded treadmill test.
6. The purpose and procedures for assessing strength using a bench press test and a leg press test.
7. The purpose and procedures for assessing muscle endurance using a timed sit-up test and a timed push-up test.
8. The purpose and procedures for assessing flexibility using a sit-and-reach test.

INTRODUCTION

Assessment of physical capabilities is the cornerstone of any physical training program and is a prerequisite to tailoring an appropriate training regimen. Feedback from testing often can be an important motivational factor for the participant. Further, comparisons of original results with future assessments of the same fitness parameters permit an evaluation of the effectiveness of the program and also the individual's progress within the training program.

Four key components comprise fitness assessment: aerobic power (cardiorespiratory capacity), flexibility, muscular endurance, and strength. Once medical screening has taken place, those four components should be evaluated. (The medical screening can determine which tests may or may not be appropriate for the potential exerciser as well as the need for medical supervision of testing.) There appears to be no optimal order for assessment, but it seems easiest if the flexibility testing occurs first, followed by muscular endurance, then strength, and finally aerobic power testing. If submaximal tests are used to predict aerobic power, then the test of aerobic power should come before the muscular endurance and strength to avoid any residual effect of the exercise on heart rate response. This will be discussed later in the chapter. The following discussion is focused on measures needed to make a good overall fitness assessment.

BLOOD PRESSURE

Blood pressure is measured using a sphygmomanometer, which consists of an inflatable compression bladder enclosed within a cuff, an inflation bulb that increases the cuff pressure, a manometer or gauge that indicates the cuff pressure, and a controllable valve on the inflation bulb that permits steady deflation of the cuff.[1] By placing the cuff over the brachial artery and increasing the pressure until it exceeds the pressure within the brachial artery, the artery becomes compressed so that blood cannot flow through it from above and the pulse below the cuff can no longer be palpated (no sounds can be heard through the stethoscope). When the valve of the inflation bulb is released, the cuff pressure falls. When the pressure has fallen to the level of peak pressure generated by left ventricular contraction, blood begins to squirt through the brachial artery, producing sharp, rhythmic, knocking sounds with each cardiac beat. As the cuff pressure is gradually decreased, the sounds change in quality and intensity, may become transiently inaudible, and finally disappear when the cuff pressure is less than the pressure in the artery throughout the full cardiac cycle. Those sounds are described in five phases.[1] At rest, usually only two, and sometimes three, phases can be heard.

Phase 1 is the *systolic pressure*, or the pressure level at which the first faint, clear tapping sounds are heard. The sounds gradually increase in intensity as the cuff is deflated. The sound then may become a "muffled" sound. The point at which the muffling occurs is Phase 4, or the true *diastolic pressure*. The pressure level when the last sound is heard and after which all sound disappears is considered Phase 5. Phase 2 and Phase 3 cannot be measured with a typical blood pressure cuff and stethoscope. Since it is very often difficult to differentiate Phase 4 and Phase 5, Phase 5 is usually used to represent the diastolic pressure. Three things are needed to obtain a good blood pressure reading: a sphygmomanometer with appropriate sized cuffs to accommodate the range of arm sizes, a stethoscope, and a quiet environment to obtain the reading.

BLOOD PRESSURE TESTING TECHNIQUES AND PROCEDURES[1,2]

1. The person taking the blood pressure (BP) measurement must be able to hear well enough to recognize faint blood pressure sounds, see well enough to read calibration marks on the manometer, and coordinate eye, hand, and listening skills.
2. Observations must be recorded accurately.
3. The measurement should be taken after the person has been seated or lying supine for five minutes and in a quiet room in which the optimal temperature is 70 to 74°F.
4. The subject should be dressed in a T-shirt or sleeveless shirt for easy adjustment of the cuff. He should be seated in a comfortable chair or in a supine position.

5. Blood pressure should be taken from both the left and the right arms. (Because of arterial obstructions, sometimes the pressure in one arm is different from the pressure in the other.) In subsequent blood pressure evaluations, measure the BP in the arm found to have the higher pressure initially.
6. A cuff of proper size must be used. A large cuff on a small arm will cause the readings to be too low and vice versa. Frequently used adult cuffs are the 17 to 26 cm cuff and the 32 to 42 cm cuff. To select the proper cuff size measure the upper arm circumference at the midpoint between the elbow and the shoulder.
7. The cuff should be applied directly over the compressible artery, approximately 2.5 cm above the antecubital space (the inside of the elbow).
8. The stethoscope should be positioned over the palpated brachial artery below the cuff near the inside of the elbow.
9. Ear pieces on the stethoscope should point forward. The bell head of the stethoscope should be applied with light pressure, ensuring skin contact at all points.
10. With the stethoscope in place, the pressure cuff should be inflated rapidly to approximately 30 mmHg above the point at which the pulse disappears and then deflated at a rate of 2 to 4 mmHg per second. A slower speed should be used for persons with very low heart rates.
11. Leave the cuff deflated for approximately one to two minutes between determinations.
12. Persons with a resting systolic BP of more than 150 mmHg or a diastolic BP of higher than 95 mmHg should be referred to a physician before further testing or training.

Sphygmomanometers should be calibrated at least once a year. The mercury gravity manometer and the aneroid manometer are the two most widely used blood pressure measuring instruments. The aneroid type is the most popular. The aneroid manometer can be calibrated using a mercury manometer or other pressure standard. That is done by connecting a Y connector to the inflation bulb and attaching the tube from the aneroid gauge to one branch of the connector and a tube from the mercury gauge to the other branch of the connector. The inflation bulb is then squeezed to increase the pressure so that several points over the entire pressure range can be observed simultaneously in both gauges as the pressure is released. This simulates an actual BP measurement. If you are unable to obtain the equipment for calibrating the manometer, you should contact the manufacturer.

AEROBIC POWER/FITNESS ASSESSMENTS

Aerobic capacity tests are used by physicians to develop preventive and rehabilitative programs for patients, by exercise physiologists for research purposes, and by physical educators to develop and monitor aerobic fitness programs for individuals. Maximal oxygen uptake, maximal aerobic power, aerobic capacity, and VO_2max are all terms that refer to an individual's capacity for the aerobic (oxygen requiring)

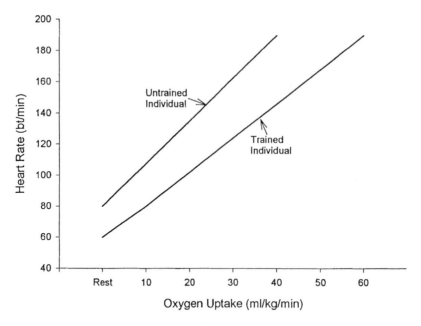

FIGURE 3.1   The effect of aerobic fitness on the relationship between heart rate and oxygen uptake.

production of ATP (adenosine triphosphate, the molecule that supplies all the energy-requiring processes of the cell).[3,4] Maximal oxygen uptake (VO_2max) is a measure of the maximum amount of oxygen that can be absorbed by the blood and delivered to the cells under the most strenuous exercise.[3,4] Since VO_2max summarizes what is going on in the oxygen transport system, the VO_2max test is used as the measure most representative of cardiorespiratory fitness.

Direct measurement of VO_2max is used in research that requires a very precise appraisal of aerobic power. It involves analysis of expired air samples collected as the subject performs graded, maximal exercise. Direct measurement of VO_2max is often not feasible due to equipment and personnel requirement; potential health risks to subjects; the high degree of motivation required to perform exercise to exhaustion; and the length of the test.[2,5] Consequently, other tests have been developed for estimating VO_2max from physiologic responses during submaximal exercise or from performance tests.

SUBMAXIMAL EXERCISE TESTING

Submaximal exercise testing is probably the safest means of estimating VO_2max for a wide variety of individuals regardless of age, fitness levels, or disabilities. This form of testing requires minimal equipment, staffing, budget, and time compared to maximal testing. It presents relatively low health risks to the person being tested. The variety of protocols and ergometers used for the exercise allow for individualization of

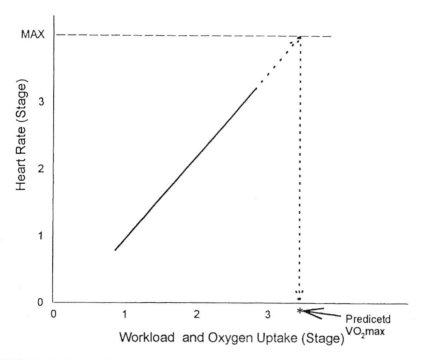

FIGURE 3.2 Schematic representation of the relationship between submaximal heart rates and at least two work loads with extrapolation to age-predicted maximal heart rate to estimate maximal aerobic power, VO₂max.

the test dependent upon the person's capabilities and limitations. Although not as accurate as maximal testing, it does provide a good estimate of aerobic power. Furthermore, this form of testing works well in test/retest situations.

The underlying principle of the submaximal test is that a relationship exists among heart rate, work load, and oxygen uptake.[3,5] Under normal conditions there is a linear relationship between increased oxygen uptake and heart rate during submaximal work. The slope of the line changes relative to an individual's state of physical training or physical fitness;[6] a fit person is able to transport a given amount of oxygen at a lower heart rate than an unfit person (see Figure 3.1). In other words, the heart of a fit person is more efficient and will beat slower than the heart of an unfit person when doing the same amount of work. Based on this relationship, VO₂max can be estimated by projecting the steady-state heart rate at a specified work load or resistance to an estimated age-adjusted maximal heart rate (HR_{max}) (see Figure 3.2). There are several assumptions that are the basis for submaximal testing.[7] One, the work load is reproducible. That is to say that everyone using the test can accurately reproduce the work load in any setting. Two, a steady-state heart rate is obtained during each stage. Three, the maximal heart rate for a given age is the same for all individuals. Four, mechanical efficiency is constant. Five, the heart rate/oxygen uptake relationship is related to fitness and not other factors.

GENERAL PROCEDURES FOR MEASURING HEART RATE

Heart rate (HR) can be measured by ECG monitoring, telemetry (an electrical apparatus that measures the HR and transmits the result to a receiver), or palpation. Palpation of the radial pulse is a suitable method when assessing large groups. Palpation can be performed by any of the three following techniques: 1) Place the tips of the first two fingers on the radial artery, inside of the wrist below the base of the thumb and count the pulsations for 10 seconds. 2) Place the heel of the hand over the left side of the chest, at the apex of the heart, and count the pulsations for 10 seconds. 3) Place the tips of the first two fingers on the carotid artery, located slightly to the left or right of the Adam's apple, and count the pulsations for 10 seconds. Multiply the count by 6 to obtain heart rate per minute. Care should be taken when using the carotid pulse because excessive pressure applied to the carotid artery may slow the heart rate by reflex action. Normally pulsations at the apex of the heart can be only felt after an individual has engaged in vigorous exercise. If an accurate count cannot be made using any of the aforementioned sites, then a stethoscope can be used to listen to the pulse.

Resting Heart Rate: Resting heart rate is assessed during medical examinations. It serves as the baseline for some tests of aerobic fitness. Because resting heart rate is lowered by aerobic conditioning, it is important for monitoring progress in training programs. Resting heart rate is influenced by age, cardiorespiratory fitness, and environmental factors. It ranges from extremes of 40 bt/min in highly trained athletes to 100 bt/min in normal, sedentary adults. Resting heart rate is usually higher in older individuals. It also increases in the heat or when an individual is shivering from the cold. Counting pulse for a full minute prior to rising from bed is an ideal way for an individual to measure his resting heart rate. A 10- or 15-second count after sitting or lying down for at least five minutes is an alternative. When making comparisons between individuals' resting heart rates, it is important to be consistent in the method used for obtaining the heart rate (sitting, lying in bed, time of day, counting method).

Post Exercise Heart Rate: Sometimes it is necessary to obtain an accurate heart rate for the minute immediately following the cessation of exercise (e.g., at the completion of the 3-minute step test to obtain the test result or at the completion of a training bout to obtain a recovery heart rate). It is imperative to begin the count as soon as possible because heart rate will begin to decelerate soon after cessation of exercise (usually after only 15 seconds). A wristwatch, wall clock, or stopwatch can be used. A stopwatch will be the most accurate. One should count the pulse for 10 seconds and multiply by 6 to estimate a minute pulse rate. Only 2 to 4 seconds are needed to position the hand or fingers properly and to feel the heartbeat rhythm. The count starts on a full beat with the first count being zero. If the 10 seconds do not end with a full beat, 1/2 beat is added to the count. That is an important detail because each one-beat error results in a 6 bt/min total error. A 15-second counting procedure can also be used. This technique is easier for beginners. By counting the beats over a longer time span, counting errors can be reduced. It is also easy to multiply the 15-second count by 4 to obtain the heart rate per minute. (See Appendix A, Table A-1 for transforming 10- or 15-second counts to bt/min.)

STEP TESTS

Step tests in general range from 3 to 5 minutes in duration and can use benches as high as 24 inches. However, these longer tests and higher bench heights can be extremely difficult for short stature individuals, people in poor physical condition, people with coordination problems, and the elderly. Thus, a three-minute test that uses a relatively low bench is a good all-around choice. The underlying assumption of many of these tests is that the rate of recovery after exercise is related to the fitness level: faster recovery, the better aerobic fitness.[7] Step tests in general are not very accurate, having an error of about 16%.[7] However, these easily administered tests work well for monitor progress — test/retest.

Three-Minute Step Test

Based on the linear relationship between heart rate and oxygen uptake in response to work, this simple test allows the prediction of VO_2max.[2,3] The subject performs a given amount of work, stepping up and down onto a bench at the same rate for three minutes. The subject whose heart rate is low at the completion of the test is in good physical condition and will have a high VO_2max. This test can be easily administered with minimal equipment to a group of subjects in a short period of time. This field test can be used for classification purposes when a high degree of accuracy is not required. For some individuals, this test may be difficult or impossible.

Equipment needed:

1. A bench for stepping that is 12 in. high
2. A clock with sweep second hand or stopwatch for timing test and counting HR
3. A metronome to maintain step rate
4. A stethoscope to count HR (optional)

Procedures:[3]

1. The subject steps up and down off the 12-in. bench for three minutes in cadence to a metronome set at 96 bt/min (24 steps/min). Because it is very easy for the subject to make an incomplete step, it is necessary for the instructor to demonstrate and monitor the correct stepping technique (placing the feet fully on the bench and floor with the leg fully extended with each step as opposed to landing lightly on the toes only without full leg extension). Since the amount of work performed is dependent on the stepping rate, the subject must step in beat with the metronome.
2. Immediately following three minutes of stepping, the subject sits down and the instructor counts his heart beats for one minute. Counting must begin within five seconds of the completion of the stepping.
3. The instructor should then refer to the norms tables in Appendix A, Table A-6 to find percentile rankings based on the heart rate obtained from the 60-second count.

SUBMAXIMAL CYCLE ERGOMETER TEST

Modified Astrand and Rhyming Protocol

Astrand and Rhyming Submaximal Cycle Ergometer Work Test is administered for the purpose of predicting maximal oxygen uptake expressed in milliliters per kilogram of body weight (VO_2max ml/kg/min) and for the determination of physical classification score.[6,8,9] Thus, the test is of value for screening and classification purposes. The heart rate/oxygen uptake relationship is the basis for the nomogram to predict maximal oxygen uptake which was developed by Astrand and Rhyming.[6,8] The validity of the Astrand and Rhyming Work Test has been studied by several investigators and found to correlate with measured values ($r = 0.69$).[3,8] The correlation is increased to 0.92 (very high) when the estimated maximum oxygen uptake values were corrected for age.[6]

Equipment needed:

1. A cycle ergometer that is calibrated in kpms or watts
2. An electrical rpm counter or metronome
3. A stethoscope or heart rate monitor (optional)
4. A stopwatch
5. A Borg or Rating of Perceived Exertion (RPE) Scale (optional)

Procedures: The general protocol of the test requires that the subject pedal a cycle ergometer at 50 rpm until a steady-state heart rate is attained. Maximum oxygen uptake is then estimated on the basis of the work rate using tables established by Astrand and Rhyming. Trained personnel are required for administration of the test. The general procedures are as follows.

The subject should:

1. Not participate in physical activity prior to the test on the day of the assessment. (Aerobic fitness testing should be done before other strenuous fitness tests, e.g., bench press, sit-ups, 1.5-mile run).
2. Abstain from food or drink for an hour before the test, but water is allowable. (If a heavy meal has been eaten, more time should be allowed before testing.)
3. Abstain from tobacco products for at least two hours prior to testing.
4. Be dressed in gym clothes.

The instructor should:

1. Record the subject's name (Sample form Appendix A, Table A-2).
2. Record the subject's birth date.
3. Record the date of the test.
4. Record to the nearest half-pound the weight of the subject without shoes but dressed in gym apparel.

5. Record the subject's pre-exercise heart rate.
6. Adjust the height of the seat so that there is a very slight bend in the knee joint when the ball of the foot is on the pedal when the pedal is in its lowest position.
7. Explain the test protocol to the subject.

The test administrator begins a countdown, at which time the subject begins pedaling and the stopwatch is started. Pedaling rate should be brought to 50 rpm as quickly as possible and maintained at a constant rate. The rpm is monitored on the display on the ergometer or by having the subject pedal in cadence to a metronome set at 100 bt/min. Subjects may need immediate coaching to reach and maintain 50 rpm; most tend to pedal at too rapid a rate initially. Pedal rate must remain constant during the work phase of the test. As soon as the subject begins to pedal, the resistance is added. Female subjects perform the test at an initial work load of 300 kpm/min (100 watts or 2 KP at 50 rpm) and males at 600 kpm/min (150 watts or 3 KP at 50 rpm). Work loads may be set in watts or kpm/min (watts = kpm/min divided by 6). The resistance and rpms should be closely monitored throughout the test to assure that the subject performs at a constant work load and work rate. Once the work load is initially set, the timing begins. Heart rate is monitored during the last 10 seconds of each minute. As a rule, exercise of about five minutes is sufficient to adapt the heart rate to the task being performed. By the end of the fifth minute of exercise, the subject's heart rate generally reaches steady-state. Provided that the fourth and fifth minute heart rates differ by no more than 5 bt/min, the heart rate at the end of the fifth minute is designated as the working heart rate for the submaximal test.

If the difference between the fourth and fifth minute heart rates exceeds 5 bt/min, the working time is prolonged one or more minutes until a constant level is achieved. If the working heart rate exceeds 130 bt/min, the load can be considered adequate and the test can be discontinued after five minutes. If the heart rate is less than 130 bt/min at the end of the fifth minute, then the load should be increased by 150 kpm/min (25 watts or 0.5 KP) for women and by 300 kpm/min (50 watts or 1 KP) for men for an additional five minutes. Each additional work period should be continued for the entire five minutes even if the heart rate should exceed 150 bt/min to a maximum of 175 bt/min, at which time the test is automatically terminated.

If during the first two minutes of the test, the heart rate exceeds 150 bt/min or the subject complains of pain, the work load is decreased by 150 kpm/min (25 watts) for women and 300 kpm/min (50 watts) for men. (At 50 rpm, that would be a decrease of 0.5 KP for women and 1 KP for men. Instructors should change the pendulum setting from 2 to 1.5 for women and from 3 to 2 for men.) Conversely, some highly fit individuals will not increase their HRs sufficiently at these initial work loads to enable an accurate prediction of VO_2max. If an individual's HR does not increase to 120 bt/min during the first two minutes of the test, then the work load should be increased from 3 KP to 4 KP (from 900 to 1200 kpm/min) for men and from 2 KP to 2.5 KP (from 600 to 750 kpm/min) for women. This increase should be made only if the individual is physically able to tolerate the higher work load for an additional five minutes. Note: When using an ergometer that has a friction belt around the flywheel, belt friction heats up as the test progresses and may increase, which increases work load. In that case, adjust to the resistance as needed.

POST-EXERCISE PERIOD

At the end of the exercise period, the work load is eliminated and the subject is instructed to continue pedaling at a comfortable rate. The subject should not pedal rapidly because this is the recovery phase of the test. The subject's heart rate is monitored during the last 10 seconds of this one minute of active recovery. The subject then rests quietly on the cycle ergometer for at least one minute. If the subject's heart rate declines to 120 bt/min or less during the last 10 seconds of rest, the subject is instructed to dismount the cycle and the test is concluded. If the resting heart rate remains above 120 bt/min, the subject remains on the cycle or moves to a chair until the heart rate declines to less than 120 bt/min. The test administrator should record heart rates for each minute of the exercise and recovery period. Following the exercise period, it is important that the observer maintain communication with the subject due to the possibility of syncope. The subject may wish to assume a supine position.

The rating of perceived exertion (RPE) scale developed by Borg is useful to the test administrator for monitoring the subject during exercise because perceived exertion and HR are linearly related to each other, to work intensity and to factors indicating relative fatigue (see Appendix A, Table A-5 for scale).   ·

Scoring

Maximal oxygen uptake in liters per minute (VO_2max l/min) is estimated from average exercise heart rate (HR) at a given work load in kilogram meters ($WKLD_{kgm}$) using the following gender specific formulas:

Men: VO_2max (l/min) = $6.98 + (WKLD_{kgm} \times 0.0035) - (HR \times 0.0459)$
Women: VO_2max (l/min) = $7.01 + (WKLD_{kgm} \times 0.0038) - (HR \times 0.045)$

The estimated maximal oxygen uptake in l/min is corrected for age by multiplying the VO_2max by the appropriate age correction factor (Appendix A, Table A-3). The relative maximal oxygen uptake in milliliters per kilogram of body weight per minute (VO_2max ml/kg/min) is obtained by dividing the estimated VO_2 in ml/min by the subject's body weight in kilograms. (See Appendix A, Tables A-4 and A-6 for examples and norms, respectively.)

SUMMARY OF MODIFICATIONS

The above test protocol includes several modifications to the original Astrand and Rhyming Submaximal Cycle Ergometer Test. A five-minute exercise period is used instead of a six-minute exercise period, since steady-state is generally achieved within five minutes. This has been implemented to decrease overall testing time.

Initial work loads for both men and women have been increased. These work loads generally elevate heart rates to desired levels within a five-minute period.

YMCA Protocol[10]

The YMCA protocol is in some ways very similar to the Astrand and Rhyming cycle ergometer test. It requires the same equipment and has three stages. However, the steady-state heart rates from for all three stages are used to predict VO_2max.

Protocol[10]

The protocol is different based on the gender of the subject and heart rate responses. Women start the test at a work load of 150 kgm (0.5 KP at 50 rpm). Men initiate the test at a work load of 300 kpm (1.0 KP at 50 rpm).

Procedures:

1. The person starts pedaling at 50 rpm, and the first work load is introduced.
2. Heart rates are obtained the last 10 seconds of each minute (multiplied by 6 = bt/min).
3. The person pedals at the work load for three minutes.
4. Heart rate during the third minute is obtained and used to determine the work load of the second stage based on Tables 3.1 or 3.2. For example, if the heart rate for a woman during the first stage is 115 then work load for the second stage would be 300 kgm (1.0 KP).
5. The person pedals the second stage (three minutes) following the same procedure as stage one but at the higher intensity. The heart rate from the third minute of stage two is then used to determine the work load for stage three.
6. If during stage two the heart rate reaches or exceeds 150 bt/min, the test can be terminated in two stages rather than three. Typically, if the heart rate exceeds 110 bt/min during stage one, then the heart rate will be greater than or equal to 150 bt/min during stage two.
7. The same post-exercise procedures are used as in the Astrand and Rhyming Test.

Scoring: The heart rate during the final minute of each stage is plotted on the y axis of a graph against the work load on the x axis (see Figure 3.3). The straight line of best fit is drawn through the three heart rates extended to the age-predicted maximal heart rate. A line is then dropped back to the x axis from the point of the intersection between the age predicted maximal heart rate and work load. The work load is then converted to oxygen uptake in liters per minute using the constant of 2 ml/min of oxygen per kgm of work load, and a resting oxygen uptake of 300 ml/min is then added. The result is then divided by the person's weight in kilograms to obtain VO_2max in units of ml/kg/min.

TABLE 3.1
Guide to Setting Work Loads for Men Using 50 rpm

Stage 1 Work Load	Heart Rate Response	Stage 2 Work Load	Heart Rate Response	Stage 3 Work Load
			>135	750 kg 2.5 KP
	>105	600 kg 2.0 KP	120–135	900 kg 3.0 KP
			<120	1050 kg 3.5 KP
			>135	900 kg 3.0 KP
300 kg 1.0 KP	90–105	750 kg 2.5 KP	120–135	1050 kg 3.5 KP
			<120	1200 kg 4.0 KP
			>135	1050 kg 3.5 KP
	<90	900 kg 3.0 KP	120–135	1200 kg 4.0 KP
			<120	1350 kg 4.5 KP

TABLE 3.2
Guide to Setting Work Loads for Women Using 50 rpm

Stage 1 Work Load	Heart Rate Response	Stage 2 Work Load	Heart Rate Response	Stage 3 Work Load
	>103	300 kg 1.0 KP	>123	450 kg 1.5 KP
			<123	600 kg 2.0 KP
150 kg 0.5 KP				
	<103	450 kg 1.5 KP	>123	600 kg 2.0 KP
			<123	750 kg 2.5 KP

MAXIMAL TESTS

12-MINUTE RUN[2]

The principle behind the 12-minute run test is simple: the farther a person can run or walk in 12 minutes, the better his aerobic power.[4] Thus, the subjects run as far as possible on a level course for 12 minutes. VO_2max is determined from the distance covered.

Equipment needed:

1. A stopwatch or clock with a sweep second hand.
2. A level indoor or outdoor track with markers placed at every 1/20 mile (every 88 yd — only five required on a 440-yd track). Tracks are preferred for administration of this test because they are level, less hazardous, and allow easy monitoring of the subjects.
3. A test form for recording results.

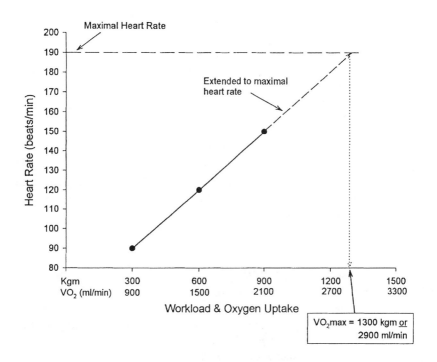

FIGURE 3.3   Example of the prediction of VO$_2$max using the results of the YMCA protocol.

Procedures:[2,4]

1. Prior to testing day, the subjects should have some practice in pacing the course to avoid starting the run at too fast a pace, which results in early fatigue.
2. Subjects should be instructed to refrain from smoking or eating for two hours prior to the test.
3. Prior to the test, subjects should warm up and stretch.
4. Following the run, subjects should cool down for at least five minutes. Standing around immediately following the run may induce syncope (faintness due to inadequate cerebral blood flow caused by venous pooling). Simply walking will aid recovery and enhance venous return.
5. Instructors should multiply the markers passed by .05 to obtain the distance run by the subject (e.g.,: 25 markers passed × .05 = 1.25 mile). Refer to Appendix A, Table A-6 for norms. VO$_2$max can also be predicted using the following equation:[7]

VO$_2$max (ml/kg/min) = 3.126 × (meters covered in 12 minutes) − 11.3

1.5-Mile Run[4]

The 1.5 mile run is similar to the 12-minute run and is best suited for active individuals because it requires maximal effort. Subjects run 1.5 miles as fast as possible on a level course. VO_2max is estimated from performance time.

Equipment needed:

1. Stopwatch or clock with a sweep second hand.
2. A level indoor or outdoor track measured to 1.5 miles. Tracks are preferred for administration of this test because they are level, less hazardous and allow easy monitoring of the subjects.
3. A test form for recording results.

Procedures:[2,4]

1. Prior to the testing day, the subjects should have some practice in pacing the course to avoid starting the run at too fast a pace, which results in early fatigue.
2. Subjects should be instructed to refrain from smoking or eating for two hours prior to the test.
3. Prior to the test, subjects should warm up and stretch.
4. If possible, individual lap times should be given.
5. Following the run, subjects should cool down for at least five minutes. Standing around immediately following the run may induce syncope. Simply walking will aid recovery and enhance venous return.
6. The instructor should record the 1.5-mile run time and refer to Appendix A, Table A-6 for norms.

One-Mile Run

The equipment and procedures are the same as for the 1.5-mile run. The only difference is that the predicted VO_2max is determined from an equation.[7] The equation works for both men and women and requires, mile run or walk time in minutes, age in years, and body mass index (BMI); weight divided by height (kg/m²), and gender (women = 0 and men = 1).

$$VO_2max = -8.41(time) + 0.34 \, (time)^2 + 0.21(age \times gender) - 0.84(BMI) + 108.94$$

Shuttle Run Test

Leger and Lambert developed the shuttle-run test for the prediction of VO_2max.[11] The test was adopted by the Council of Europe for assessing the physical development of school children. Work on the specificity and validity of the test for active adults has been undertaken by the Department of Physical Education and Sports Science at Loughborough University, England. Researchers there have developed a table for the prediction of VO_2max based on test results (1987). However, the table currently does not provide age- and sex-specific values. For most purposes, this simple, progressive, maximal field test is an accurate estimate of VO_2max. Individuals can use it to check their own fitness, or it can be used easily with large groups.

Equipment needed:

1. A flat, nonslippery surface at least 20 meters in length
2. A cassette player
3. A shuttle run audio cassette
4. Suitable footwear
5. A measuring tape to measure 20-meter track
6. Marker cones

Procedures: During this test, the subject runs back and forth between markers placed 20 meters apart on a level track. Running speed is progressively increased at approximately one minute intervals for up to 21 stages (levels). Running speed is monitored by the subject's arrival at one end of the shuttle at the same time the cassette tape emits a bleep sound. The number of shuttles run in the level at which the subject withdraws from the test is the score. A detailed procedures booklet is provided with the test cassette. To obtain the test cassette, contact White Line Press, 60 Bradford Road, Stanningley, Leeds LS28 6EF or National Coaching Foundation, 4 College Close, Beckett Park, Leeds LS6 3QH. The official reference is: J. Brewer, R. Ramsbottom, and C. Williams, Multistage Fitness Test: a Progressive Shuttle-run for the Prediction of Maximum Oxygen Uptake, Copyright @ Loughborough University, 1988, ISBN 0-947850-53-8.

GRADED TREADMILL TEST

In the laboratory, the treadmill is the apparatus of choice for determining VO_2max.[2,4] Work output is easily determined and regulated by varying either the speed or grade or both. A variety of protocols have been designed that start the subject at low work loads and proceed through short, two- to three-minute stages that progress in intensity until the subject is brought to VO_2max, ideally within 15 to 20 minutes. The choice of the protocol is based on the subject's health status, age, and fitness status. Cardiologists perform graded treadmill tests to detect ECG abnormalities in patients. They also use these tests to monitor rehabilitation in patients. Exercise physiologists administer maximal treadmill tests to directly measure VO_2max in athletes. To be reasonably sure that a person has achieved "true" VO_2max, the exercise physiologist looks for a leveling off or peaking-over (slight decrease) in oxygen uptake, blood lactic acid levels of 8 mm/l of blood or higher, attainment of age-predicted maximum heart rate, and a respiratory exchange ratio in excess of 1.08.[4,5] (The respiratory exchange ratio is the ratio of carbon dioxide produced to oxygen consumed when the exchange of oxygen and carbon dioxide in the lungs no longer reflects the oxidation of specific foods in the cells.) These tests are impractical for testing the general population because they require trained personnel and elaborate laboratory equipment, present a high risk to the subject, require high motivation on the part of the subject, and are time-consuming.

VO$_2$max can also be predicted from the maximal grade and speed the subject attains on graded maximal test.[2] That type of testing is routinely completed by physicians and exercise rehabilitation programs. This is referred to as "MET Capacity." One MET equals 3.5 ml O$_2$/kg/min. Normal individuals have a 10 to 14 MET capacity. Although this test does not require quite as much sophisticated equipment, it is less accurate and presents many of the same problems as tests measuring VO$_2$max directly (e.g., considerable liability).

ABSOLUTE STRENGTH TESTING

Strength refers to the ability of a muscle or muscle group to produce force. Estimates of upper and lower body strength can be obtained using the one-repetition maximum (1-RM) bench press and/or leg press tests.

BENCH PRESS

Equipment needed:

1. A bench press machine or
2. A barbell set with bench (collars are recommended)

Procedures:[2]

1. The machine or barbell is loaded with 50% of the maximum weight the subject is expected to lift, or use the following as the initial weight: males = 2/3 body weight; females = 1/2 body weight.
2. Subjects using the machine should assume a comfortable position on the machine with the bar grips set even with the chest. Subjects using free weights should lie on the bench with eyes directly under the bar and grip the bar at shoulder width or slightly wider, being sure that each hand is equidistant from the center of the bar. If help is not available to lift the bar off the stand, then the bar height must be set so the subject does not have to raise his body from the bench to lift the bar from its stand. When doing the bench press, subjects should place their feet on the bench to prevent lower back strain. However, certain individuals may feel uncomfortable in this position due to size of the bench, balance, or the amount of weight being pressed. They should be permitted to perform the test with feet flat on the floor. Subjects are not permitted to allow their lower back to come off the bench when performing the lift.
3. The bench press is performed by fully extending the arms and making a controlled return to the starting position. With free weights, the subject lowers the bar to chest level and then makes a full arm extension (elbows locked) before returning the bar to the racked position. Spotters should be positioned at both ends of the barbell. If the subject wishes, the spotters

may lift the bar to the starting height and release it on the subject's command. For the lift to be counted, the spotters cannot touch the bar during the extension phase. They may assist with racking the bar.

4. The 1 RM should be achieved within five to six lifts. Weight for successive lifts should be increased by 10 lbs (4 kg) or more. As the subject approaches 1 RM, increases should be no greater than 5 lbs (2 kg) with the free weights or the smallest increment allowed by the machine. Experienced weight lifters may wish to start at weights greater than those previously recommended. That is fine as long as they do not overshoot their 1 RM with the initial lift.

5. The instructor is responsible for monitoring and recording the lift. Spotters should load and unload the bar.

6. Because this is a maximal test, each subject should be encouraged to give maximal effort.

7. The score is obtained by dividing the weight lifted by the subject's body weight (see Appendix A, Table A-6 for norms).

LEG PRESS

Equipment needed: A leg press machine or similar apparatus

Procedures:[2,4]

1. Load the machine with the subject's body weight.
2. Subjects should assume a comfortable position on the machine with the seat adjusted so that the knee is flexed at 90° when the feet are placed in position on the lower foot plates.
3. The Universal leg press is performed by fully extending the legs and making a controlled return to the starting position.
4. The 1 RM should be completed within five to six lifts. As the subject approaches 1 RM, increases should be no greater than a single plate. Experienced weight lifters may wish to start at weights greater than those previously recommended. That is fine as long as they do not overshoot their 1 RM with the initial lift.
5. The instructor is responsible for monitoring and recording the lift.
6. Because this is a maximal test, each subject should be encouraged to give maximal effort.
7. The score is obtained by dividing the weight pushed by the subject's body weight (see Appendix A, Table A-6 for norms).

MUSCULAR ENDURANCE TESTING

Muscular endurance refers to the ability of a muscle or group of muscles to sustain contractions over time. Timed sit-ups are used to evaluate the endurance of abdominal muscles. Timed push-ups assess upper body muscular endurance (triceps, anterior deltoids and pectoralis major). Subjects should warm up prior to taking these tests.

Sit-ups per Minute

Equipment needed: A clock with sweep second hand or stopwatch and a soft surface or mat

Procedures:[2-4]

1. The subject lies on his back with knees bent and arms crossed over the chest. Feet are held firmly on the floor by a partner who will also count the number of sit-ups performed in one minute.
2. When told to start by the instructor, the subject raises his body so that the elbows come forward to touch the knees while the arms remain folded across the chest. The shoulder blades must touch the floor each time the subject lies back. Only correctly performed sit-ups are counted. If the subject stops before the minute is over then he should be encouraged to keep going until time is called.
3. Because this is a maximal test, each subject should be encouraged to give maximal effort.
4. The score is the total number of correctly performed sit-ups (see Appendix A, Table A-6 for norms).

Push-ups per Minute

Equipment needed: A clock with sweep second hand or stopwatch and a flat surface or mat

Procedures:[2]

1. The subject lies on his stomach with hands flat on the floor and positioned shoulder width apart.
2. When told to start by the instructor, the subject pushes his entire body except feet and hands off the floor until arms are straight. The subject then lowers the body until his chest touches the floor. Returning to the raised position he completes the push-up. Only correctly performed push-ups are counted. If the subject stops before the minute is over, he should be encouraged to keep going until time is called.
3. Because this is a maximal test, each subject should be encouraged to give maximal effort.
4. The score is the total number of correctly performed push-ups (see Appendix A, Table A-6 for norms).

FLEXIBILITY TESTING

Flexibility refers to the looseness or suppleness of the body or specific joints and involves the interrelationships between bones, muscles, fascia, tendons, ligaments, adipose tissue, and the joint capsule.

Sɪᴛ-ᴀɴᴅ-Rᴇᴀᴄʜ Tᴇsᴛ

The sit-and-reach test is a simple test to evaluate the flexibility of the muscles of the back of the legs (hamstrings), hips, and lower back. The sit-and-reach test is influenced by the subject's arm and leg lengths. A person with long arms and short legs will seem to have better than normal flexibility. Thus, instructors might need to qualify their interpretation of the test results. This test is particularly useful in monitoring changes in an individual's flexibility.

Equipment needed: A box (height: 10–12 in.; length: minimum 24 in.; width: minimum 16 in.) and a yardstick taped perpendicular to the box with the 15-in. mark aligned at the center of the near edge of the box.

Procedures:[2]

1. The subject sits on the floor or mat with shoes off, legs extended and heels placed firmly against the near side of the box. The subjects heels are spaced 4 to 8 in. apart straddling the yardstick.
2. The subject slowly reaches forward with extended arms, one hand on top of the other, palms down, and middle fingers aligned. The backs of the subject's knees must remain flat on the floor throughout the reach. The subject reaches as far forward as possible without bouncing.
3. The best distance reached as measured at middle fingertip placement on the yardstick during three trials is considered the flexibility score (see Appendix A, Table A-6 for norms).
4. The subject should warm up slowly by practicing the test.

GENERAL CONCLUSION

It is mandatory that the physical fitness instructor has knowledge of the purpose of and correct procedures for performing fitness assessments. The determination of an initial fitness level is a prerequisite for beginning a training program. With follow-up assessments, the fitness instructor is able to monitor progress toward training objectives. Learning and practicing correct assessment techniques will enable the fitness instructor to develop the skills to competently assess physical fitness components.

REFERENCES

1. Frolich, E.D., Grim, C., LaBarthe, D.R., Maxwell, M.H., Perloff, D., and Weidman, W.H., Recommendations for human blood pressure determination by sphygmomanometers, *Hypertension*, 11, 210A-222A, 1988.
2. Pollock, M.L. and Wilmore, J.H., *Exercise in Health and Disease*, W.B. Saunders, Philadelphia, 1990.
3. deVries, H.A. and Housh, T.J., *Physiology of Exercise for Physical Education and Athletics*, 5th ed., Brown and Benchmark, Madison, 1994.

4. Wilmore, J.H., and Costill, D.L., *Training for Sport and Activity*, Wm. C. Brown, Dubuque, 1988.

5. McArdle, W.D., Katch, F.I., and Katch, V.L., *Exercise Physiology: Energy, Nutrition, and Human Performance*, Williams & Wilkins, Baltimore, 1996.

6. Astrand, I., A method for prediction of aerobic work capacity for females and males of different ages. *Acta Physiologica Scandinavica*, 49(Suppl. 169), 45-60, 1960.

7. American College of Sports Medicine, *ACSM's Resource Manual for Guidelines for Exercise Testing and Prescription*, Williams & Wilkins, Baltimore, 1998, chaps. 41,43,44.

8. Astrand, P.O. and Rodahl, K., *Textbook of Work Physiology*, McGraw-Hill, New York, 1970.

9. Teraslinna, P., Ismail, A.H., and MacLeod, D.F., Nomogram by Astrand and Ryhming as a predictor of maximum oxygen intake. *J. Appl. Physiol.*, 21, 513-515, 1966.

10. Golding, L.A., Myers, C.R., and Sinning, W.E., *The Y's Way to Physical Fitness: The Complete Guide to Fitness Testing and Instruction*, YMCA Program Store, Champaign, IL, 1989.

11. Leger, L.A. and Lambert, J., A maximal multistage 20 m shuttle run test to predict VO_2max. *Eur. J. Appl. Physiol.*, 49, 1-5, 1982.

4 Measurements of Body Composition

Purpose: To enhance the reader's knowledge of the techniques for measuring body fat.

Objectives:

1. To be able to compare the accuracy of the various methods of body fat measurement.
2. To be able to measure body fat using skinfold calipers or body circumferences.
3. To understand the intricacies of the hydrostatic weighing technique.
4. To understand the problems of all the methods of body fat analysis.

INTRODUCTION

An analysis of body composition is important for any complete fitness program. Medical and fitness professionals have said a great deal about the relationships among body fat, physical fitness, and health. Numerous studies have found a significant inverse relationship between fat content and cardiovascular fitness. That is to say, that as body fat content increased, cardiovascular fitness declined. More important than fitness, a high percentage of body fat is also related to hypertension, diabetes, and a whole myriad of other diseases.[1,2] Furthermore, recent reports have indicated that the U.S. population, both adults and children, is becoming more overweight.[3] Thus there is need for concern.

For simplicity, the body can be broken down into two compartments: fat-free mass and fat mass. Fat-free mass is comprised of bone mass, muscle mass, and all the organs. Fat-free mass is sometimes referred to as lean body mass. However, technically speaking, lean body mass does contain some minor fat stores found in the nervous system, bone, and internal organs (<3%).[1] Fat-free mass is approximately 75 to 80% of the total body weight in a normal healthy adult.

Fat mass is composed of the adipose fat and fat found around and in the various organs. Body fat content can be broken down into two deposits: *Essential fat,* which is fat stored in the organs and is necessary for normal physiologic functioning. It also includes sex-specific fat, which is about four times as much in women as men (6 to 8% vs. 2 to 3%, respectively).[1] *Storage fat* is the fat that accumulates in the adipose tissue. This is the fat reserve that can be used for energy and is the majority of fat in the human body. The normal range of body fat percentage appears to be about 15 to 20% for adult men and 20 to 25% for adult women.[1,2] Obese individuals are typically over 30% body fat for men and 35% body fat for women. Newburgh has stated that between the ages of 45 to 50, life expectancy is reduced roughly 1% for every pound of excess fat.[4] Conversely, there is a minimum amount of fat that is necessary. Without this essential fat, the body will not function normally. Thus, estimating body fat is an important consideration for a total fitness assessment.

BASIC ASSESSMENT METHODS

The most basic way to assess weight status is to measure the person's height and weight, then consult the *standard height weight tables* (see Appendix B). These tables were designed by statisticians and represent the range of weights for a given height at which the lowest mortality rates (all cause death) occur. In general, a weight greater than 10% above the normal range is considered overweight, and 20% above the normal range is considered obese. The tables typically are divided into three weight categories based on frame size: small, medium, and large. Thus, frame size needs to be determined in addition to the height and weight. There are several methods to estimate frame size using the circumference of the calf muscle, the circumference of the wrist just above the bony protrusions (styloid processes), or the width of the elbow at the bony protrusions (epicondyles). The simplest is the height to wrist ratio in which the height in inches is divided by the wrist circumference in inches and Table 4.1 is used.

TABLE 4.1
Frame Size Estimates Based on Height (Inches)
Divided by Wrist Circumference (Inches)

Frame Size	Men	Women
Small	>10.4	>11.0
Medium	9.6–10.4	10.1–11.0
Large	<9.6	<10.1

The use of these height/weight tables has been challenged for several reasons. One reason is the tables have not taken into consideration the high death rate among low-weight smokers. Thus, removal of these low-weight smokers actually *reduces* the ideal weight ranges. Another reason is that the tables were not designed for use in non-Caucasians; they were underrepresented in the initial sampling. Also, the tables do not consider age nor do they consider body composition. It is assumed that all the weight above the "normal" range is fat mass. However, we know athletes can have an above average weight (for a given height) and yet have a low fat mass.

Another simple way to assess weight status is to compute *body mass index* (BMI). Height and weight are measured and converted to metric measures, height in meters (m) and weight in kilograms (kg). The weight is then divided by the height squared: wt_{kg}/ht_m^2. BMI does have a somewhat higher association with body fat than the height/weight tables. In addition, studies have shown a direct relationship between decreasing BMI and improved health status.[1,5] BMI is used by a number of researchers and clinicians. Thus, the ease of assessment and the existence of norms makes BMI a better alternative.

Individuals with BMI in the range of 20 to 25 appear to have the lowest health risk. However, desirable ranges are from 21.9 to 22.4 for men and 21.3 to 22.1 for women. That means that a 5'10" (1.78 m) man should have a weight of approximately 153 lb (69.5 kg), while a 5'6" (1.68 m) woman should weigh 133 lb (60.5 kg). BMIs ranging from 25 to 30 define the person as being overweight, and BMIs over 30 are considered obesity.[1,2]

As with the height/weight table there are problems with using BMI. Once again, racial status and age were not taken into consideration when the norms were devised. The major problem is the potential to misclassify someone with above average muscle mass as being fat when in fact they are not fat. One example is a weight lifter. This person may be only 70 in. (1.78 m) tall but weigh upwards of 200 lb (90.7 kg) and have a body fat content of 12%. However, the person's BMI would compute to be 28.6, or a classification of overweight. In addition, the height/weight table would classify this person as being 25% above ideal weight and therefore obese! That is why it is better to estimate body fat than to judge an individual strictly by weight norms. Thus, the use of BMI and weight tables should serve only as cursory guides. More precise measurement of proper weight should be used in an athletic or fit population.

MEASUREMENT OF BODY COMPOSITION

There are many methods of determining body composition, ranging from simple tables of age, height, and weight (see Appendix B, Table B-2 and Table B-3) to sophisticated and expensive computerized tomography (CT scan). The following is a synopsis of the more popular methods to assess body fat content.

DETERMINING PERCENTAGE OF BODY FAT

UNDERWATER WEIGHING

One of the most reliable methods of fat determination is based on the density of various body components and specific gravity of the body.[6,7] Specific gravity is the ratio of the mass of an object to the mass of an equal volume of water at the same temperature — the ratio of the weight of the body to its loss in weight when submerged in water. The concept of specific gravity was developed by Archimedes. The legend is that he was asked by the king to determine whether or not a certain crown was made of pure gold. He knew what the density of gold was because he could weigh a given amount, but he could not weigh the crown without melting it down. He hit on the idea of weighing it under water to determine its density. In like manner, we cannot cut up the human body into parts but must deal with the whole individual. However, we do know that the density of fat is 0.90 g/cc, lean tissue is 1.34 g/cc, and bone is 3.00 g/cc.[6,7] Thus, the greater the density, the lower the fat content.

Typically, a person will float due to air in the lungs. Thus, when using underwater weighing to measure density, the air in a subject's lungs must be totally expelled and then the residual volume of air in the lungs (the air remaining in the lungs after maximal expiration) must be accounted for. That means that in addition to a water tank and scales, pulmonary function equipment is necessary. Because the subject must blow out all his air and remain still for about five to six seconds, he needs to be very comfortable in the water. Although this method is considered the most accurate (the "gold standard"), it is relatively expensive, very time-consuming, and labor-intensive.

The accuracy of underwater weighing is affected by several factors. The accuracy declines when the subject tends to be claustrophobic or hydrophobic. The ability of the subject to relax in the water with no air in the lungs is important, because the longer the person remains calm underwater, the better the reading. Also, water weight gain or loss during menstruation may have a small impact on the results.[1] Finally, if the person does not naturally sink after full expiration, then weight must be added to the person to submerge him or the test is invalid. Despite those problems underwater weighing has good validity, reliability, and reproducibility.

Methodology

A. The subject is weighed on a metric scale while wearing swim attire. The reading (weight in air) is recorded.
B. The instructor directly measures the residual volume or vital capacity (VC) of the subject and then estimates the residual volume (Men: RV = 23.1% VC; Women: RV = 28% VC).
C. The subject climbs into a tank filled with warm water (90 to 95°F).
D. The subject then squeezes out any air bubbles that might have been trapped inside the bathing costume or body hair.
E. The subject then sits on a sling suspended from a balance while the water calms.
F. The subject then breathes out as hard as possible while slowly lowering himself underwater.
G. The instructor measures the underwater weight at the end of the forced expiration. The process requires the subject to sustain maximal expiration for at least six seconds before surfacing.
H. Subjects usually need a series of practice tests to become acquainted with the procedure.
I. Typically, three readings are taken. The largest number is assumed to correspond to the most complete expiration.
J. The information is then put into the following equations to get the percentage of body fat:

$$BD = \left(Wt\ in\ air\right) \Big/ \left(\frac{wt\ in\ air\ -\ underwater\ wt}{Density\ of\ water}\right) - residual\ volume$$

$$\%\ fat = ((4.57/BD) - 4.142) \times 100$$

SKINFOLD MEASUREMENTS

The specific gravity method is the best technique for determining body fat. But because it involves heavy and expensive apparatus, it is not always feasible. A relatively accurate and practical technique involves the measurement of skinfolds by the use of calipers. This method assumes that 50% of body fat is superficial (under the skin) and 50% is within and around the organs.[1,2,6] Skinfold measurements of body fat are generally within 5% of underwater weighing. However, practice with the technique can reduce error to less than 2%.

The measurement of skinfolds is a fairly simple technique to learn.[2] Pincer-type calipers, accurate to the millimeter and producing a constant pressure, are used to measure the thickness of skinfolds at specific sites on the torso and appendages. There are formulas that involve two to seven sites. The more sites involved, the greater the accuracy. The best methods use gender- and race-specific formulas and factor in the age of the subject. Skinfold calipers range in price from about $10 for plastic models to well over $200 for the most accurate models. There are also battery-operated electronic calipers with microchips that compute fat percentage automatically. They cost about $300. Care should be taken when purchasing these electronic calipers. Be sure to get the model that has the most appropriate skinfold sites and uses equations for the population(s) being tested. Generally speaking, the following method affords a good estimate of specific gravity from skinfold measurements in adult men and women regardless of race.

The major sources of error focus on the technique of obtaining the skinfold. The skinfold should contain all the subcutaneous fat but not the underlying muscle tissue. This may be difficult at sites such as the chest, thigh, and abdomen where the skin may be too tight or the fat mass to large to differentiate fat from muscle. With individuals with very tight skin, placing them in a supine position often helps to make the skinfold more accessible. Placing the calipers too high on the fold will cause the body fat to be underestimated, while placing the calipers too deep will result in an overestimation of body fat (see Figure 4.1). The other major problem is the specific site location. At some sites, such as the iliac crest, placing the caliper 1 cm forward or behind the proper site can make a 2% difference in the body fat content. Therefore, it becomes important to obtain the proper site and use the proper depth to place the calipers.

Methodology

A. The subjects should wear swimming attire; two-piece suits are best for women.
B. Obtain subjects' ages and present weights.
C. Measure three skinfolds at the gender-specific sights on the right side of the body. Make all measurements three times and average the two closest readings.

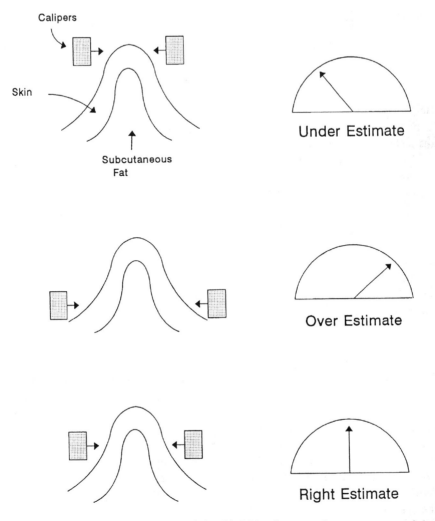

FIGURE 4.1 Effect of the placement of the skinfold calipers on the measurement of the skinfold thickness.

D. Sites[8,9]

    Men: 1. Chest: Diagonal fold half way between axilla (armpit) and nipple.

              2. Abdomen: Vertical fold about 1 in. from the umbilicus.

              3. Thigh: Vertical fold on the front of the thigh, halfway between knee and inguinal fold.

  Women: 1. Triceps: Vertical fold over tricep, halfway between the shoulder and elbow.

              2. Suprailiac: Horizontal fold on the crest of the ilium hip bone.

              3. Thigh: Vertical fold on the front of the thigh, halfway between knee and inguinal fold.

E. Add the three skinfold measurements and use the following equations to calculate body density (BD) then body fat. The sum can also be used to obtain body fat from Appendix B, Table B-4 and Table B-5.

Women: $BD = 1.0994921 - 0.0009929 \text{ (sum)} + 0.0000023 \text{ (sum}^2) - 0.0001392 \text{ (age)}$

Men: $BD = 1.10938 - 0.0008267 \text{ (sum)} + 0.0000016 \text{ (sum}^2) - 0.0002574 \text{ (age)}$

Percent Body Fat $= ((4.95/BD) - 4.500) \times 100$

Ultrasound can also be used to obtain the skinfolds rather than calipers. This allows for a more precise measure of subcutaneous fat. A sound wave passes through the fat and bounces back off the surface muscle and bone beneath. The time to bounce back is then converted to a distance score, and an image is presented on a screen. From the screen image the thickness of the subcutaneous fat can be directly measured. Ultrasound may be useful in obese subjects on which calipers cannot be used. The technique may also be useful for mapping regional fat deposition and assessing nutritional status of hospital patients.

CIRCUMFERENCE METHOD

An additional alternative, simple, and inexpensive procedure for measuring body fat is to measure body girths or circumferences. It is easy to take measurements with a cloth measuring tape, and accuracy can be achieved with a minimum of practice. Experiments involving a sample of normal adults found the predicted values for body fat were within 5 to 10% of values determined by underwater weighing. However, it should be emphasized that equations used to predict percent body fat from circumferences may not be valid when applied to athletic men and women, or to individuals who can be visually classified as thin or obese.

BIOELECTRICAL IMPEDANCE ANALYSIS (BIA)

There are three varieties of these machines on the market today; all work on the same principle. The theory is that electrical flow through hydrated fat-free tissue and body water is greater than through fat tissue.[2,6,10] Thus, electrical resistance increases as the body fat percentage increases. The machine typically attaches to the feet and hands, although there are also some models that the person simply stands on in bare feet. A small electrical signal from a battery is introduced, and the impedance (or resistance to flow) is measured. The machine, through a microchip, then converts the ohms of resistance to body density, which is converted to a body fat percentage using a standard equation. The exact methodology is dependent upon the machine.

The major problem with this method is its dependence upon the subject's state of hydration.[3] Dehydration can increase the body fat measure by more than 10%. Conversely, hyperhydration will underestimate body fat. Body fat estimates by BIA are also affected by skin temperature. Subjects with warm skin will have their body fat underpredicted, while subjects with cold skin will have their body fat overpredicted.

The home-version of the BIA that the person simply stands on seems to overestimate body fat compared with underwater weighing. However, newer versions of the machine will probably correct this problem. BIA machines are relatively expensive for their present precision (about $2,000, plus the cost of a printer), but newer home models have reduced the price tremendously to less than $500. At the present time, BIA is simply another way of providing an estimate of body fat, so long as environmental temperatures and state of hydration are controlled. BIA works best in a test/retest situation in which fat content is measured in the same person over time.

INFRARED INTERACTANCE

This method was originally developed for the U.S. Department of Agriculture.[2,6] An infrared light beam is emitted through a device held against the skin. The beam penetrates to the bone and is reflected back to a silicon detector on the device. The device contains a computer chip that measures the reflectance and then computes the body fat based on the individual's age, height, weight, and normal physical activity level. Studies have shown that the infrared measure significantly underestimates body fat compared with underwater weighing.[6] The method does show promise, but at this time it needs further improvement.

OTHER TECHNIQUES

Other techniques include obtaining body fat directly from dual-energy X-ray absorptometry (DEXA), computerized tomography (CT scan), and magnetic resonance imaging (MRI). Machines that make these scans are quite expensive, some costing upwards of $1 million, and are usually located at hospitals. Thus, due to cost of the scans and access to these machines, their use for a simple body fat analysis is limited. These machines and techniques have the potential to be quite accurate, but at the present time their use in the fitness community is questionable because of the expense and time needed to obtain the scans.

DESIRABLE BODY WEIGHT

There appears to be no single ideal weight that can be applied to all individuals. That is because genetics has endowed humans with a variety of body structures and frame sizes. In addition, some very athletic, competing adults strive for a body weight that makes them most competitive for their height. Since height/weight table and body mass index measures may not fit all individuals, the computation of a desirable weight could be beneficial. Ideal body weight can be estimated regardless of the method used to determine the fat free mass and the desired percentage of body fat. This method can serve only as an estimate because it assumes all the weight lost or gained is related to changes in body fat. In many situations, that is not entirely true. Dieting causes considerable loss of both muscle and fat mass as well as water, thus the use of this formula should serve only as a guide.

$$\text{Desirable Weight} = (\text{Fat Free Mass})/(1 - \text{Desired \% Fat})$$

Example: A 190-lb man who is 25% body fat and wishes to attain a body fat content in the normal range (20%).

	English Units	Metric Units
Fat Mass:	190 lb × .25 = 47.5 lb	86.2 kg × .25 = 21.5 kg
Fat Free Mass:	190 lb – 47.5 lb = 142.5 lb	86.2 kg – 21.5 kg = 64.7 kg
Desirable Weight:	142.5 lb/(1 – .20) = 178 lb	64.7 kg/(1 – .20) = 80.9 kg
Fat Mass Loss:	190 lb – 178 lb = 12 lb	86.2 kg – 80.9 kg = 5.3 kg

CONCLUSION

Presently, there is no one simple method of measuring body fat that is extremely precise. The best that can be expected is an estimate of fat content. Methodologies that rely on height/weight tables provide a rough estimate of ideal weight but do not account for individuals with above-average muscle mass. Underwater weighing presently provides the best estimate of body fat, with about a 3% error. Because this method is costly, time-consuming and expensive, fitness instructors have looked to other simpler methodologies. Presently, skinfolds provide a fairly good estimate of body fat. The procedures are easy to learn, and the monetary and time costs are low. The circumference method also provides an alternative to hydrostatic weighing. Cost is very low and techniques are simple. However, accuracy is questionable in lean and overweight populations. Newer methods such as the BIA and infrared interactance are being developed, but at the present time their accuracy is also questionable.

REFERENCES

1. McArdle, W.D., Katch, F.I., and Katch, V.L., *Exercise Physiology: Energy, Nutrition, & Human Performance*, Lea & Febiger, Philadelphia, 1996.
2. Nieman, D.C., *Fitness and Sports Medicine: An Introduction*, Bull Publishing Company, Palo Alto, CA, 1990.
3. Flegal, K.M., Trends in body weight and overweight in the U.S. population, *Nutr. Rev.*, 54, S97-S100, 1996.
4. Newburgh, L.H., Obesity. *Arch. Intern. Med.*, 70, 1033-1096, 1942.
5. NIH Consensus Development Panel on the Health Implications of Obesity: Health Implications of Obesity, *Ann. Intern. Med.*, 103, 1073-1077, 1985.
6. Berning, J.R. and Steen, S.N., *Sports Nutrition for the 90s*, Aspen Publications, Gaithersburg, 1991.
7. Brozek, J., Grande, F., Anderson, J.T., and Keys, A., Densiometric analysis of body composition: Revision of some quantitative assumptions, *Ann. N.Y. Acad. Sci.*, 110, 113-140, 1963.
8. Jackson, A.S. and Pollock, M.L., Generalized equation for predicting body density of men, *Brit. J. Nutr.*, 40, 497-504, 1978.
9. Jackson, A.S., Pollock, M.L., and Ward, A., Generalized equation for predicting body density of women, *Med. Sci. Sports Exer.*, 12, 175-182, 1980.
10. Dolgener, F.A., Hensley, L.D., Becker, T.E., and Marsh, J.J., A comparison of bioelectric impedance and hydrodensiometry in lean males, *J. Appl. Sport Sci. Res.*, 6, 147-151, 1992.

5 Flexibility, Warm-Up, and Cool Down Exercises

Purpose: To define and explain the principles and proper techniques of warm-up, flexibility training, and cool down.

Objectives:

1. To know the benefits of and proper techniques for warm-up.
2. To know the definition of flexibility.
3. To be able to name and define three types of stretching exercises and understand which type of stretches are the safest.
4. To know the benefits of incorporating flexibility exercises into a regular exercise routine.
5. To know the reasons for incorporating a cool down segment into each exercise session.

INTRODUCTION

Warm-up, cool-down and flexibility exercises are important parts of a well-rounded fitness program. Many times they are minimized or neglected entirely. When correctly incorporated into a fitness program, warm-up, cool-down, and flexibility exercises improve performance, improve safety, reduce the possibilities of exercise-induced injuries, and reduce the risk of lower back pain. Before focusing on the main topics, it is important to understand some key terms used when describing body movements and positions. Table 5.1 presents these terms and definitions.

DEFINITION AND IMPORTANCE OF FLEXIBILITY

Generally, flexibility is the ability of a joint to move freely through its full range of motion.[3] Flexibility is further defined by Anderson and Burke as "range of motion of a joint or series of joints that are influenced by muscles, tendons, ligaments, bones and bony structures."[3] Maintenance of full range of motion of the joints of the body protects the joints and muscles from injury during physical exertion. In everyday life, we are sometimes required to make rapid and/or strenuous movements that we are not accustomed to making. Tight muscles and connective tissues are easily overstretched or torn during such activities.[4] Low levels of flexibility are a major cause of low back pain. Low levels of flexibility also limit movement, resulting in decreased levels of exercise performance.[2] Stretching can also improve circulation and air exchange and is associated with a decreased muscle soreness after exercise.[5]

TABLE 5.1
Definitions of Terms that Refer to Bodily Movements and Directions[1,2]

Anatomical Position: The body standing erect with feet and hands facing forward

Anterior: The front of the body or body part

Posterior: The back of the body or body part

Prone: The body lying in a face-down position

Supine: The body lying in a face-up position

Planes of Motion: The direction that each part of the body can be moved within; there are three planes of motion

    A) the sagittal plane divides the body into left and right parts

    B) the frontal plane divides the body into front and back parts

    C) the transverse plane divides the body into upper and lower parts

Flexion: A movement that decreases the angle at a joint. Example: The angle of the knee joint is 180° when it is straight. When the knee bends (flexes) the angle is reduced to about 90° (a right angle).

Extension: A movement that increases the angle at a joint. Example: The angle of the hip joint is about 90° (a right angle) when a person is sitting in a chair. When the person stands up, the angle of the hip joint is 180° (a straight line).

Hyperextension: Extension beyond the anatomical position. Example: A back bend done in gymnastics. Joints commonly hyperextended are the cervical, thoracic and lumbar vertebrae, the shoulder, the elbow, the wrist, the hip, the knee, and the ankle.

Lateral: Refers to the outside of the body or body part and is also a directional term meaning to the side of the body. Example: Tilting the head to the right is right lateral flexion of the neck.

Medial: Refers to the inside of the body or body part and is also a directional term meaning toward the center of the body. Example: The medial side of the right knee is the left side of the knee.

Abduction: Movement of a part of the body away from the midline of the body. Example: See example in adduction.

Adduction: Movement of a part of the body toward the midline of the body. Example: A jumping jack is an example of abduction followed by adduction of the arms and legs.

Circumduction: Movement using flexion, lateral movements and extension in a series. The shoulder, hip, wrist, and vertebral joints allow this type of movement. Example: Full arm circles.

Inversion: Movement of the bottom of the foot to face the midline of the body. Another term used commonly with regard to the ankle is supination, which is a combination of plantar flexion (pointing the foot) and inversion of the ankle. Example: The ankle collapsing to the lateral side (outward).

Eversion: Movement of the bottom of the foot to face away from the midline of the body. Another term commonly used with regard to the ankle is pronation, which is a combination of dorsiflexion (flexing the toes up toward the front of the shin) and eversion of the ankle. Example: The ankle collapsing to the medial side (inward).

Pronation: Rotation of the forearm so that the palm faces backward or downward

Supination: Rotation of the forearm so that the palm faces forward or upward

Elevation: Raising of the shoulders and clavicle (collar bone)

Depression: Lowering of the shoulders and clavicle (collar bone)

Protraction: Action of moving the scapula (shoulder blades) away from the midline of the body (pulling the shoulders forward)

Retraction: Action of moving the scapula (shoulder blades) towards the midline of the body (pulling the shoulders back)

Note: Some of these terms are specific to certain joints. Others are more generally applied to the entire body.

TABLE 5.2

Persons with the Following Should Not Participate in Stretching/Flexibility Exercises Without the Permission of their Physician[5]

Pregnancy	Extreme joint laxity
Unhealed fracture	Infection of joint area
Any sharp pain when stretching	Inflammation of joint area
Contractures (functional shortening)	Any bone problem limiting joint motion

Different activities require different levels of flexibility. Running does not require a high level of flexibility, whereas sports such as basketball require moderate levels of flexibility, and gymnastics and martial arts require an exceptional level of flexibility.

Levels of flexibility differ widely among and within individuals. One person may have exceptional flexibility of the shoulder joint with low flexibility in his back and hamstrings, while another person may be the exact opposite. Individuals with naturally loose ligaments and tendons should not be allowed to stretch to extremes because the joints can become unstable, which can result in injuries.[5] In addition, pregnant women who normally have loose joints should not stretch because it can lead to low-back and permanent joint looseness after pregnancy.[5] Table 5.2 points out other situations in which stretching exercises may not be in a person's best interest. Each person should stretch to stay within his limits so as not to strain or tear tissue.[3]

PHYSIOLOGY OF STRETCHING: THE STRETCH REFLEXES

Muscles have reflexes that protect themselves from being damaged by overstretching.[1] Stretch receptors located in muscle fiber sense the degree of stretch that is being applied to the muscle. Those receptors send information to the parts of the brain that control muscle contraction. When the brain determines that the muscle is becoming overstretched, it sends signals back to the muscle to partially contract, thus antagonizing the stretch on the muscle. The greater the stretch applied to the muscle, the greater the antagonistic contraction. The speed at which the stretch is applied also affects the messages sent by the stretch receptors. The more rapidly the stretch is applied, the greater the opposite resulting muscle contraction will be to resist the stretch.[3]

Another important stretch reflex is called the inverse stretch reflex.[6] Receptors for this reflex are located in tendons that are attached to muscles. Those receptors sense tension in the tendons. When tension builds up in the tendons, the receptors send messages to the nerves to release muscle contraction.[1] That is the body's way of preventing the muscles from contracting so strongly that tendons are damaged. Because of the way these stretch reflexes work, stretches that are most effective are those that are created slowly and held for at least 10 seconds.[4]

TYPES OF STRETCHING

BALLISTIC OR DYNAMIC

This form of stretching involves quick, repetitive stretching and releasing of a particular muscle or muscle group — bouncing.[3,4] This type of stretching is effective but has a high potential for injury. The momentum of quick bouncing movements can overstretch joint tissues and lead to injury. Also, ballistic stretching activates the "stretch reflex" in the muscle. Repeated ballistic stretches activate this reflex, which makes the muscle contract to resist the sudden stretch. That undermines the purpose of stretching.[3,4]

STATIC

This form of stretching is considered safest and most effective for the general population.[1,3,4] In static stretching, a muscle is moved through the range of motion until slight tension is felt. The stretch is then held for at least 10 seconds, but it can be held for as long as desired. Holding the stretch means the movement is controlled and unlikely to cause injury. Holding a stretch allows for the stretch reflex to be overcome and the inverse stretch reflex to be activated. That leads to greater lengthening of the muscle being stretched. As the stretch is held, the feeling of tension should subside a little. This indicates that the muscle has lengthened. The stretch should not be painful. Pain indicates that the muscle is being strained, and that is counterproductive. Lasting improvement in flexibility comes from regular, mild stretching and not from straining.[2-4]

PROPRIOCEPTIVE NEUROMUSCULAR FACILITATION (PNF)

This third type of stretching is also known as the "contract and relax" method.[2-4] It is a specialized way of stretching muscles in which the joint being stretched is pushed to its limit of motion and held there. When the joint is extended to the point that tension is felt, the muscles being stretched are contracted isometrically against the direction of stretch. The contraction is held for a short time, released, and the joint is pushed (extended) a little further to a slightly greater range of motion. This series is repeated as many times as necessary. This technique is very effective in improving flexibility, but it is more painful and has a much higher potential for injury if done incorrectly than static stretching. This type of stretching is used by athletic trainers and physical therapists to improve range of motion in athletes and during rehabilitation of injuries.[2-4]

FLEXIBILITY TRAINING

Stretching can be incorporated into the warm-up or cool down or can be done anytime.[5] Stretching exercises can also be combined with relaxation techniques such as deep breathing and progressive relaxation. Incorporating flexibility exercises into the cool down ensures that the exerciser does not leave the session with an elevated heart rate. Research has found that the period immediately following exercise is the

---

TABLE 5.3
Guidelines for Flexibility Exercises[4,5]

1. Keep the body properly aligned at all times.
2. Always avoid locking the knees or elbows. They should be "soft" (have a very slight bend) rather than perfectly straight.
3. Avoid lateral or front and back flexion of the trunk. Too much flexion in any direction places a great deal of strain on the thoracic (upper back) and lumbar (lower back) vertebrae (spinal bones).
4. Feel the stretch. Take time to make the stretch correctly completed.
5. Go into stretches slowly and hold stretches for at least 10 to 15 seconds.
6. Avoid bouncing during the stretching exercise.
7. Avoid forcing a stretch while holding the breath.
8. Slowly reposition after the stretching exercise.
9. Repeat stretches at least two to three times during intensive flexibility training.
10. Avoid hyperextension of any joint.

---

time during which people are most likely to have heart complications. In general, to improve flexibility, muscles should be stretched slowly to a point where mild tension is felt.[1,3] Initially, the stretch should be held for about 10 to 15 seconds, but gradually over a period of weeks it can be held for longer (45 to 60 seconds) if desired.[5] The person should try to hold the stretch until the tension subsides. When the tension subsides, it means that the muscle has relaxed and lengthened. The stretch should be gradually released and then repeated two or more times. With each stretch repetition, the person should try to stretch a little further (within comfortable limits). To improve flexibility most efficiently, stretches should be performed three to four times per week. When the desired level of flexibility is obtained it can be maintained by stretching one to two times per week.

When stretching, it is important to pay attention to position and posture. Proper alignment of the trunk and pelvic area are important in preventing injury because it prevents hyperextension of the lumbar (lower back) vertebrae. The stretches listed here are appropriate for almost everyone. However, some commonly used stretching exercises may be unsafe.[4] Descriptions of these can be found in the chapter on Contraindicated Exercises (Chapter 9).

Table 5.4 lists recommended flexibility exercises for the entire body.[2-7,9] The following list gives definitions of terms generally used to describe bodily movements. Use these resources to create your own stretching program.

WARM-UP BEFORE EXERCISE

The purpose of warm-up is to prepare the body for physical activity.[10] Warm-up increases range of motion and puts the body in a state of readiness for vigorous activity, which can enhance athletic performance.[5] The warm-up also has the potential to reduce the risk of injury, especially during repetitive exercises, such as running.[5] Many people equate stretching with warm-up. Although stretching exercises should be included in the warm-up, the most important part of the warm-up is the circulatory warm-up. The purpose of the circulatory warm-up is to increase

TABLE 5.4
Recommended Flexibility Exercises for the Entire Body

Neck Area	Stretch
Side of neck and top of shoulder	Tilt head laterally to the right side until a slight stretch is felt, hold, and release. Repeat on left side.
Back of neck and upper back	Look down and press the chin toward the chest until a stretch is felt in the back of the neck and upper back, hold, and release.
Side and back of neck	Turn the head to the right (so you are looking over the right shoulder) until you feel a gentle stretch on the left side of the neck. Hold, release, and repeat looking to the left.

Chest, Shoulders, Sides, and Arms	
Chest and shoulder muscles	Keeping arms straight, reach behind the back and lace fingers together with palms facing each other, then lift upward slightly until tension is felt. Hold and release. Keep upper body (chest) upright.
Arms, shoulders, and upper back	Hold arms straight out in front of the body, lace fingers together with palms facing outward, bring hands over head keeping arms straight, push hands and shoulders slightly upward and back.
Sides	Standing with feet shoulder width apart and knees slightly bent, reach over the head as high as possible with the right hand and downward with the left hand, hold and release. Repeat exercise on other side. Do not laterally flex the trunk (bend over to the side).
Tricep (back of upper arm)	Bend arm at the elbow, bring arm up so that the hand of the bent arm is touching or almost touching the top of the shoulder blade on the back. If necessary, use the other hand to press the arm back to increase the stretch. Do not try to pull arm behind head.
Arms, shoulders, and upper back	Place hands, forearms, and elbows together. Lift arms up, keeping them together until a stretch is felt in the arms, shoulders, and upper back.
Deltoid and tricep (back of shoulder and arm)	Hold arm out straight at shoulder height, then bring the arm across the body until slight tension is felt in the back of the arm and shoulder.

Upper and Lower Back	
Upper and lower back	Bring the arms in front of the body, lace the fingers together, and push the arms and shoulders outward rounding the upper back. At the same time, contract the abdominal muscles and tuck the buttocks under, rounding the lower back, hold, and release.
Upper back	Hold arms out straight from the body, flex at the elbows to place hands on shoulders, bring elbows together, hold, and release.
Upper and lower back and hamstrings	Lie supine on the floor, bring both knees into the chest and hold, release. (Make sure to hold knees inside the bend of the knee to protect against over flexing the knee).
Lower back and hamstrings	Lie supine on the floor, bring one knee to the chest, keeping the other leg softly straight on the floor, hold, and release. Repeat with the other leg.
Lower back	Lie supine on the floor with legs bent. Press the lower back into the floor while tightening the abdominal muscles and squeezing the gluteus maximus muscles (butt muscles). This is called pelvic tilt.
Upper back	Get on hands and knees, press back upwards toward the ceiling or sky, hold, and release.

TABLE 5.4 (continued)
Recommended Flexibility Exercises for the Entire Body

Hips and Thighs

Hamstrings (hip extensors)	Sit on the floor with right leg straight out in front of body and the left leg bent with the bottom of the left foot touching the inside of the right leg. Push forward from the hip, keeping the back relaxed and straight until a stretch is felt in the hamstring (on back of upper leg) and hold. Repeat on other side. If necessary, put hands on floor beside hips to support back and facilitate tilting pelvis forward.
Hamstrings (hip extensors)	Stand with weight on bent right leg, bring the left leg forward and place the heel on the ground, keeping the left leg straight and foot flexed (dorsiflexed). Bend forward at the hips and down with right knee until a stretch is felt in the hamstrings of the left leg. If necessary, support upper body with hands on right leg. Repeat on other side.
Quadriceps (front of thigh)	Stand on right leg (knee slightly bent) using a wall or chair for balance, bend the left leg at the knee and bring the foot close to the buttocks. The hips should face straight ahead, and the back should be straight (no arching in the lower back). Hold the left foot with hand, and press the left foot into the hand while pushing the left knee downward until a stretch is felt in the quadriceps muscles (front of thigh). The knee will not move down, but pushing down improves the stretch without overbending the knee. Repeat on other side. This stretch can also be done while lying on side.
Iliopsoas muscles (hip flexors)	While standing in a lunge position with the feet pointing straight ahead, bend the back leg, slightly lifting the heel of the back foot off the floor, tilt the pelvis back (tucking the buttocks under) until you feel a stretch in the front of the thigh and inner hip area. Repeat on other side.
Hip adductors (inner thigh) and groin	Sit on the floor and put the soles of the feet together and knees apart in a butterfly position. Push the knees down slowly until a stretch is felt in the inner thighs. Make sure the back is straight, if necessary put hands beside the hips to support the back.
Hip adductors (inner thigh) and groin	Stand with feet farther than shoulder width apart. Bend the right knee (always keep the knee directly over the foot) and shift the body to the right until a slight stretch is felt in the left inner thigh. Repeat on other side.
Hip abductors, including sartorius, and iliotibial band (muscles on outer thigh)	Sitting on the floor with the right leg straight out in front of the body, bend the left leg at the knee and hip and cross it over the right leg. Pull the left leg towards the chest until a stretch is felt along the outer thigh. Keep upper body facing straight ahead. Do not rotate or twist the spine.

Calves and Ankles

Gastrocnemius (large muscle in calf)	Standing with feet in a lunge position (front knee bent, back leg straight) with toes pointing straight ahead, press the back heel into the ground or floor and lean forward with the body until a stretch is felt in the gastrocnemius (the large muscle of the calf). The back leg must be straight in order to stretch this muscle. The hands can be placed on the front leg for support, or a wall or fence can be used. Repeat on other side.

TABLE 5.4 (continued)
Recommended Flexibility Exercises for the Entire Body

Soleus (calf muscle underneath gastrocnemius)	Standing with feet in a modified lunge position (front knee bent, back leg bent but with heel still flat) with toes pointing straight ahead, press the back heel into the ground or floor and lean forward with the body until a stretch is felt in the soleus (a smaller muscle of the calf attached to the Achilles tendon in the heel). The back leg must be bent in order to stretch this muscle. The hands can be placed on the front leg for support, or a wall or fence can be used. Repeat on other side.
Gastrocnemius (Achilles tendon)	Lean against a fence or wall with both legs straight behind the body and heels pressed into the ground or floor until a slight stretch is felt in the gastrocnemius.
Soleus	Lean against a fence or wall with both legs slightly bent behind the body and heels pressed into the ground or floor until a slight stretch is felt in the soleus.
Anterior tibialis (muscle in front of calf)	Standing on right leg, bend left leg with left toe pointed. Place toe on ground slightly behind right foot and then press gently on the top of the foot until a stretch is felt in the ankle and front of the calf.

body and muscle temperature and increase blood flow to the working muscles.[1,2] Increased body temperature increases metabolic rate, which facilitates the production of energy for exercise. Increased temperature of the blood improves the release of oxygen into muscles. Increased blood flow increases oxygen delivery to the muscles. Fats and carbohydrates are utilized as energy more efficiently in direct proportion to increased availability of oxygen in themselves. Nerve impulses travel faster in a warm body. Muscle contractions occur more quickly and efficiently. A warm-up gradually increases the load on the heart, which helps prevent abnormal cardiac rhythms.

The warm-up will result in mild elevation of heart rate and ventilation and perhaps light perspiration, but it should not be fatiguing.[4] The circulatory warm-up should include moderately intense exercise lasting 5 to 10 minutes. In general, the colder the ambient temperature, the longer the warm-up should be. The intensity of the planned exercise session also should be taken into account. The more intense (harder) the planned workout, the longer the warm-up should be. Many people believe that warmed muscles, tendons, and connective tissue are more elastic and therefore less likely to be injured during physical activity, but there is very little scientific evidence to support that belief.

A warm-up can be general or specific.[10] A general warm-up includes exercises that might be different from the planned exercise session. For example, to warm-up for a weight-training session a person might run for 5 to 10 minutes. A specific warm-up includes the exercise that you will be doing in the exercise session. An example of that type of warm-up might be a very slow jog to prepare the body for running at the planned speed. Warm-up can incorporate both general and specific activities. A person warming up for a weight-training session may do light stationary cycling as a general warm-up, then at the beginning of each group of weight-training exercises, do a set with light weights to prepare that muscle group for more intense sets. Specific warm-ups are especially helpful in preventing injury and improving performance. They help the body get used to the activity gradually. That can be especially helpful in activities such as aerobic dance or competitive sports (for example, golfers hitting balls on the driving range before a round of golf). Also, a specific warm-up can help to focus the exerciser on performing his best.

Flexibility exercises should be performed after the circulatory warm-up.[4] Light stretching helps to prevent injury by relaxing contracted muscles and lengthening tendons, muscles and other connective tissue. That helps reduce stress on these tissues brought about by exercise. Flexibility exercises increase range of motion and decrease the chance of overstretching during vigorous activity. That can be especially important in competitive contact sports such as soccer, racquetball, and basketball. The focus of the flexibility warm-up should be the muscle groups that will be used during the planned exercise session, but it is best to include all of the major muscle groups. If the planned exercise is a run, then the muscles of the legs should be lightly stretched. Because the muscles of the upper body are not used, it is not as important to stretch them. The flexibility portion of the workout should take three to five minutes. In general, stretch at the beginning to reduce injury and stretch at the end of the workout to improve flexibility.[4] Table 5.5 gives examples of circulatory and flexibility warm-up activities for common exercises.[10]

TABLE 5.5
Circulatory and Flexibility Warm-Up for Common Exercise Activities

Activity	Circulatory Warm-Up (5–10 minutes)	Flexibility Warm-Up (3–5 minutes)
Brisk or race walking	Slow walking or marching in place	Stretch out gastrocnemius, soleus, quadriceps, hamstrings, thigh adductors (inner thigh muscles), thigh abductors (outer thigh muscles)
Jogging or running	Brisk walking, slow jogging, marching in place, jogging in place	Stretch out gastrocnemius, soleus, quadriceps, hamstrings, thigh adductors (inner thigh muscles), thigh abductors (outer thigh muscles)
Stationary or road cycling	Slow cycling, slow jogging, jogging or marching in place, brisk walking	Stretch out lower back, gastrocnemius, soleus, quadriceps, hamstrings, thigh adductors (inner thigh muscles), thigh abductors (outer thigh muscles)
Mountain biking	Slow cycling, jogging or marching in place	Stretch out lower back, gastrocnemius, soleus, quadriceps, and hamstrings, shoulders, upper back, thigh adductors (inner thigh muscles), thigh abductors (outer thigh muscles)

TABLE 5.5 (continued)
Circulatory and Flexibility Warm-Up for Common Exercise Activities

Activity	Circulatory Warm-Up (5–10 minutes)	Flexibility Warm-Up (3–5 minutes)
Aerobic dance, step aerobics	Low-intensity aerobic dance moves. Be sure to include lateral moving activity such as side lunges or grapevine walking. Make sure to include arm movements such as slow arm swings and circles.	Stretch out gastrocnemius, soleus, quadriceps and hamstrings, anterior tibialis, illiopsoas muscles (hip flexors), thigh adductors (inner thigh muscles), thigh abductors (outer thigh muscles), arms, shoulders, chest, sides, upper back
Cross-country skiing	Slow skiing, brisk walking with arm swing, slow jogging, marching in place with arm swings	Stretch upper back, chest, triceps, biceps, sides, gastrocnemius, soleus, quadriceps, hamstrings, thigh adductors (inner thigh muscles), thigh abductors (outer thigh muscles)
Stair climbing	Low-intensity stair climbing, marching in place, brisk walking	Stretch out gastrocnemius, soleus, quadriceps, hamstrings, thigh adductors (inner thigh muscles), thigh abductors (outer thigh muscles)
Rowing	Low-intensity rowing, brisk walking with arm swing, marching in place with arm swing, jogging	Stretch out upper and lower back, chest, sides, shoulders, hamstrings, quadriceps, thigh abductors (outer thigh muscles), gluteus maximus
Weight training	Low-intensity cycling, stair climbing, rowing, brisk walking, slow jogging. For each weight training exercise or muscle group being worked, do one set with light weight.	Stretch out each muscle group being worked in the routine
Swimming	Low-intensity swimming, swimming with the kickboard, walking in the shallow end with arm swing, marching in place with arm swing, brisk walking with arm swing, slow jumping jacks	Stretch out upper and lower back, shoulders, chest, triceps, biceps, sides, quadriceps, hamstrings, thigh adductors (inner thigh muscles), thigh abductors (outer thigh muscles)

COOL DOWN AFTER EXERCISE

Cool down is an important part of a workout, particularly for untrained exercisers or individuals that have one or more cardiovascular disease risk factor.[11] Research has shown that the highest number of cardiovascular complications occur during the cool down portion of exercise.[9] Cool down is basically warm-up in reverse. It is important to bring the heart rate down gradually. Abruptly halting intense exercise (intense exercise can be defined here as exercise in the training heart rate range) places a large load on the heart.[2,11] When a person is exercising, the working muscles in the arms and/or legs help to push the blood through the body and back to the heart. That mechanism is referred to as the muscle pump. When a person stops exercising abruptly, the muscle-pumping action stops and gravity causes a portion of the blood to pool in the lower extremities, reducing the amount of blood returning to the heart. When "venous pooling" happens, the heart must beat faster and harder to circulate the blood. Even though exercise has stopped, the body still has an increased need for blood. The body must clear waste products and get rid of the excess heat produced by exercise. By reducing the intensity of exercise gradually, the heart can keep adequate blood flow to the skin for thermoregulation and to the muscles for waste removal. That way the heart has the continued help of muscle pump to do its job without undue strain. Another problem with abruptly stopping exercise is that venous pooling of blood in the extremities may cause dizziness and fainting in some people.

Similar to the warm-up, the cool down has two parts: a circulatory cool down and a flexibility cool down. The circulatory cool down consists of rhythmic exercises gradually decreasing in intensity and can also include calisthenics such as sit-ups and push-ups. It is advisable that the heart rate be below 120 bt/min. before the person stops moving continuously and begins to do calisthenics or flexibility exercises. The flexibility cool down can include comprehensive flexibility training and sometimes relaxation exercises. Proper cool down helps muscles to recover more efficiently. The more intense the exercise session, the longer the cool down should be. Also, in warm weather it will take longer to bring the heart rate down than in cooler weather. The activities recommended for circulatory warm-up can be found in Table 5.5.

CONCLUSION

Flexibility is an important part of fitness and lower back pain prevention. Care should be taken to perform flexibility exercises safely. Each person has the ability to maintain and improve his personal level of flexibility. An effective warm-up prepares the body for exercise and makes the transition to higher-intensity exercise safer. Properly done, the cool down helps the body begin its recovery process more efficiently. These components of an exercise program are important and should not be omitted or minimized.

REFERENCES

1. McArdle, W.D., Katch, F.I., and Katch, V.L., *Exercise Physiology: Energy, Nutrition, and Human Performance.* Lea & Febiger, Philadelphia, 1986.
2. Van Gelder, N. and Marks, S., *Aerobic Dance-Exercise Instructor Manual,* IDEA Foundation, San Diego, 1987.
3. Anderson, B. and Burke, E.R., Scientific, medical, and practical aspects of stretching, *Clin. Sports Med.,* 10, 63-86, 1991.
4. Branner, T.T., *The Safe Exercise Handbook.* Kendall/Hunt Publishing Co., Dubuque, 1989.

5. American College of Sports Medicine, *ACSM's Resource Manual for Guidelines for Exercise Testing and Prescription*, 3rd ed., Williams & Wilkins, Baltimore, 1998.

6. Noakes, T., *Lore of Running: Discover the Science and Spirit of Running*, Leisure Press, Champaign, 1991.

7. Hoeger, W.W.K., *Lifetime Physical Fitness and Wellness: A Personalized Program*, 2nd ed., Morton Publishing Company, Englewood, CO, 1989.

8. Katch, F.I. and McArdle, W.P., *Introduction to Nutrition, Exercise, and Health*, Lea & Febiger, Philadelphia,1993.

9. Kosich, D., Stretching the "Hot Spots," *IDEA Today*, March, 37-39, 1991.

10. Kravitz, L. and Cisar, C., Warm-up techniques, *IDEA Today*, May, 46-49, 1991.

11. Pollock, M. L. and Wilmore, J. H., *Exercise in Health and Disease: Evaluation and Prescription for Prevention and Rehabilitation*, W. B. Saunders Company, Philadelphia, 1990.

6 Principles of Aerobic Fitness Training

Purpose: To gain an understanding of the principles of aerobic fitness training, which will enable the exerciser to prudently develop an effective training program.

Objectives: At the end of this chapter the participant will be able to do the following:

1. List the benefits of aerobic fitness training.
2. Understand the relationship among the components that affect aerobic fitness training.
3. Know the advantages and disadvantages associated with specific aerobic activities.
4. Review calculation of the target heart rate range using the heart rate reserve method.
5. Be able to help an individual select a suitable training activity.
6. Understanding the principles of progression and program flexibility as they apply to exercise prescription.

INTRODUCTION

What comes to mind when you think of aerobic fitness? The marathon runner, the triathlete, a cyclist in the Tour de France? Certainly those athletes possess qualities that enable them to perform those grueling feats. But do you necessarily need to be a competitive athlete to become aerobically fit? Consider the couple who walks a mile each evening after dinner, the person who bikes three miles to work each day, or the people at the gym who participate in an aerobic dance exercise program. Although those people may not be preparing for athletic competition, they can be aerobically fit.

The aerobic revolution began in the early 1970s following the research of Dr. Kenneth Cooper and his development of aerobic training programs for use by the general population. Those training programs, which were based on a system of points or credits assigned to popular aerobic activities, provided the public with an easy introduction to the benefits of aerobic training. Subsequently, more and more people have begun exercise programs, including walking, jogging, cycling, in-line skating, swimming, and other aerobic activities to improve and maintain their physical fitness.

WHAT ARE AEROBIC ACTIVITIES?

Aerobic activities are those activities that are completed for sufficient time to evoke the aerobic energy system (longer than five minutes) but are not completed at an intensity of greater than 85% of maximal capacity. Examples of those activities include walking, jogging/running, aerobic dance, cycling, swimming, cross-country skiing, stair stepping, and rowing.

Physical activities activate the body's three energy production systems (ATP-CP system, glycolytic system, and aerobic system) to varying degrees depending on the duration and intensity of the activity.[1] In many cases, all three energy systems operate at different times during an exercise. Brief high-power outputs lasting up to 10 seconds rely almost exclusively on the immediate energy generated from the ATP-CP system.[1] All-out exercise lasting up to four minutes, with power output diminishing, relies mostly on anaerobic glycolysis, which provides a high rate of energy production but causes one to fatigue quickly.[1] Prolonged exercise at a lower intensity relies predominantly on the aerobic energy system and depends less on the ATP-CP system and anaerobic glycolysis.[1] Although the stores of energy from ATP-CP and anaerobic glycolysis are limited, the body has sufficient energy stores to exercise aerobically for hours.

The human body, being a dynamic system, is capable of changing in response to a stimulus such as exercise. When "optimal" exercise is presented to the body, "optimal" training effects occur.[2] Exercise, when repeated at regular intervals of sufficient duration, frequency and intensity, produces beneficial training effects that enable the trained person to function at a higher or more efficient level.

An important principle of exercise training is *specificity*: The body responds specifically to stressors presented to it.[1,3] Responses and adaptations are specific to organs, tissues, and systems used during training. Thus, aerobic training necessitates choosing activities that sufficiently stress the aerobic system — moderate-intensity activities lasting longer than 5 to 10 minutes. Aerobic activities focus on the involvement of the cardiorespiratory system, because they are performed in a continuous and rhythmical manner and require the use of large muscle groups. Thus, this form of exercise training increases the transportation and uptake of oxygen by skeletal muscles. Along with the improvement in oxygen transport and utilization, this form of training also causes several health benefits (Table 6.1).

TRAINING FOR AEROBIC FITNESS

Aerobic fitness is usually defined in terms of aerobic power, or maximal oxygen uptake (VO_2max). VO_2max is the maximal amount of oxygen that an individual can utilize.[1] It is usually measured in terms of milliliters of oxygen per kilogram of body weight per minute (ml/kg/min). As an individual becomes more aerobically trained, his VO_2max increases. For example, a typical unconditioned middle-age woman may have a VO_2max of 35 ml/kg/min. As she trains using aerobic exercises, it is highly likely that the VO_2max will increase to over 40 ml/kg/min. Highly trained endurance athletes can have VO_2max greater than 70 to 80 ml/kg/min. However, 35 to 45 ml/kg/min appears to be the normal range for most adults.

TABLE 6.1
Benefits of Aerobic Training[2-4]

1. Increased capacity to generate ATP aerobically, including increased size and number of mitochondria and increased levels of aerobic system enzymes.
2. Increased capacity of muscle to mobilize and oxidize fat. At any submaximal work rate, a trained person uses more free fatty acids for energy than an untrained person.
3. Increased capability of trained muscle to oxidize carbohydrates.
4. Decreased resting and submaximal exercise heart rate.
5. Increased stroke volume during rest and exercise.
6. Increased maximum cardiac output.
7. Increased heart weight and volume.
8. Increased plasma volume and total hemoglobin.
9. Reduced systolic and diastolic blood pressures during submaximal exercise and decreased resting blood pressures of individuals with hypertension.
10. Increased ability of muscle to extract oxygen from the circulating blood.
11. Increased lung function and maximal ventilation capacity.
12. Decreased body fat in obese and borderline obese individuals.
13. Improved heat dissipation and ability to tolerate heat and cold.
14. Decreased rate of the age-related physiological decline.
15. Reduced risk of cardiovascular disease.
16. Improvement in immune system functioning.
17. Decreased fatigue during daily activities.
18. Improved glucose tolerance and insulin sensitivity.
19. Enhanced sense of well-being.

Another means of measuring aerobic energy besides oxygen uptake is the metabolic equivalent (MET) system. One MET is considered the equivalent to resting energy expenditure. In oxygen uptake terms, 1 MET equals 3.5 ml/kg/min. Thus, an activity that requires 3 MET of energy expenditure elevates metabolic rate three times resting or 10.5 ml/kg/min. Maximal MET capacities of 10 MET or above are considered normal; over 15 MET is considered highly aerobically trained, while less than 10 MET is poorly trained.

There are four basic principles that apply to all aerobic training that results in increases in VO_2max: overload, intensity, duration, and frequency.

OVERLOAD

To elicit a training response, the body must be stressed above a normal level of exertion.[1,2,4] That level is sometimes called the training threshold.[2] The threshold is dependent upon the training status of the individual. For example, a sedentary person may be able to improve aerobic fitness by simply walking (a 3–4 MET activity) for 30 minutes, because the walking is above the normal level of exertion for this person. Conversely, a person that can run for 30 minutes at 8 mph (an 11 MET activity) would actually lose fitness if he changes to a walking program. Therefore, the overload principle must be individually applied to the exercise prescription, taking into consideration the present state of fitness.

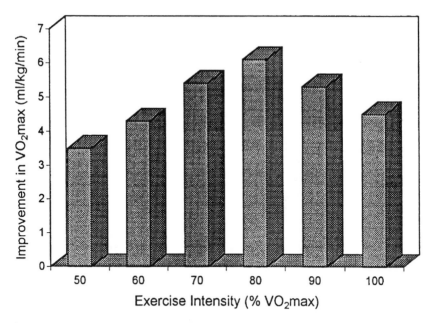

FIGURE 6.1   The effect of exercise training intensity on improvement in VO$_2$max when training three to four days a week.

INTENSITY

There appears to be an optimal level of intensity for improving and maintaining aerobic fitness. Figure 6.1 illustrates the effects of intensity on VO$_2$max. The magnitude of change in VO$_2$max increases as exercise intensity increases from 50 to 85% VO$_2$max and begins to fall as intensity exceeds VO$_2$max.[5] At exercise intensities above 85%, the duration of exercise is usually reduced because the exerciser quickly fatigues. That is why there is a reduction in fitness gains. Another point illustrated in Figure 6.2 is that higher intensities of exercise training are associated with increased injury.[3]

The American College of Sports Medicine (ACSM) recommends physical activity that corresponds to 40 to 85% VO$_2$max or 50 to 85% maximal heart rate reserve (HR$_{reserve}$).[2,4,6] The use of HR as an estimate of intensity of training is the common standard because there is a relatively linear relationship between HR and exercise intensity as long as environmental conditions, psychological stimuli, or disease do not interfere and the exercise is aerobic. Heat, anger, fever, isometric contractions, and weight lifting all will cause an increase in heart rate that does not reflect an increase in VO$_2$. Situations in which any of these factors are involved should not use heart rate to estimate metabolic rate. The key to improving aerobic fitness is to increase the metabolic rate. Increases in heart rate independent of changes in metabolic rate may cause limited or no training improvements. For example, heart rates during weight lifting can be maximal, but there will be little change in VO$_2$max as a result of weight lifting.

It is customary for the instructor to provide a training intensity range because individuals can easily vary the intensity 10% above or below the average intensity for the entire workout. Two commonly used methods for determining training intensity are stipulating a fixed percentage of maximal HR ($\%HR_{max}$) and determining the percent difference between maximal and resting heart rate ($HR_{reserve}$) and adding it to the resting heart rate. HR_{max} can be estimated simply by subtracting the current age in years from 220. Although easy to calculate, the $\%HR_{max}$ method for determining target heart rate range is not valid, as demonstrated by the following examples.

TABLE 6.2
Example Calculations of 50–85% Target Heart Rate Range for a 35-Year-Old

1. Percent HR_{max} Method:

```
 220
-35 years old
 185 (HRmax)                   185
×.50                           ×.85
  93 bt/min        —           157 bt/min (target heart rate range)
```

This heart rate range would result in the person exercising between 20 and 65% VO_2max.

2. Heart Rate Reserve Method: Assume a resting HR of 80 bt/min.

```
 220
-35 years old
 185 (HRmax)
-80 (resting HR)
 105 (HR reserve)             105
×.50                          ×.85
  53                           89
+80 (resting HR)              +80
 133 bt/min       —           169 bt/min (target heart rate range)
```

This heart rate range would result in the person exercising at 40 to 80% VO_2max. This is considerably higher than in the percent HR_{max} method.

Table 6.2 shows a comparison of target heart rates calculated using the two methods. It shows that the HR_{max} method calculates target heart rate range much lower than the $HR_{reserve}$ method. Calculation of 50% HR_{max} (Example 1) is 93 bt/min. for this individual, which corresponds to about 20% VO_2max (2–3 MET), an intensity that is probably not sufficient to produce a training effect. Therefore, the $HR_{reserve}$ method (Example 2) should be used for calculating target heart rate range.

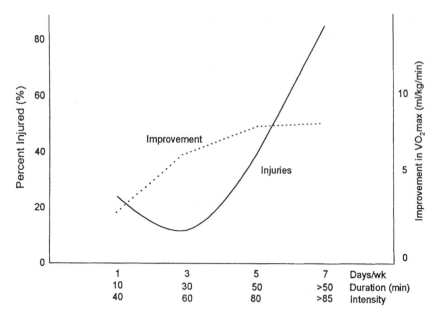

FIGURE 6.2   Percentage of injuries that occur based on workout parameters with respect to gain in VO$_2$max.

In Example 2, using the HR reserve method, if the individual lowers resting HR from 80 to 60 bt/min, then the target heart range is also lowered — 50 to 85% is now calculated to 123 to 166 bt/min.

Activities undertaken in the horizontal position (swimming, recumbent cycling) favor maximal venous return to the heart, which reduces the heart rate achieved during maximal exertion compared with activities undertaken in the upright position. A reduction of 6 to 12 bt/min must be made in the prescribed target heart rate whenever supine exercise is used during aerobic training.

Because resting heart rate is lowered by training, it is important to re-evaluate it periodically and adjust the target heart rate range. One thing to keep in mind is that persons with a lower initial level of fitness will begin to make gains at a lower intensity than persons who are more fit.[1,3] Because high intensity is associated with injury, it is particularly important that individuals begin their aerobic training program at a low intensity to allow them to adjust to new stresses. That will help prevent the unnecessary soreness that can occur if a "breaking-in" phase is not incorporated into the design of the exercise program. Injury or soreness will dishearten even the most highly motivated person who is just getting started. So the neophyte should go slowly the first week or two and then begin to gradually increase the intensity of the workout until the training produces the prescribed target heart rate.

DURATION

The American College of Sports Medicine recommends 20 to 30 minutes of aerobic exercise of moderate intensity for individuals beginning an exercise program.[2,4,6]

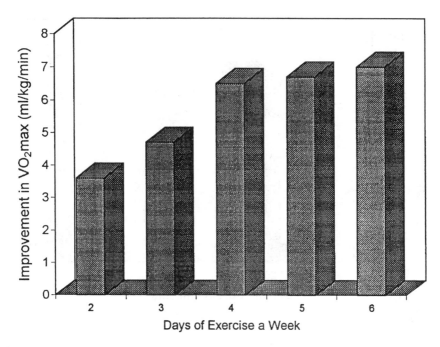

FIGURE 6.3 Influence of the number of days a week of training at ~60% VO_2max on improvement in VO_2max.

Sessions of 5 to 10 minutes performed at a high intensity can produce significant improvements in VO_2max, but they are not desirable for most participants because they carry a *high* risk of injury and burn fewer calories compared to longer, moderate-intensity exercise sessions. Figure 6.4 shows the effect of exercise duration on VO_2max. Improvements in VO_2max are the same for 15- to 25-minute sessions and 25- to 30-minute sessions at the same exercise intensity, but improvements increase when duration exceeds 35 minutes.[1,4-6] If weight loss is the primary consideration, one should keep in mind that exercising longer will result in more calories being burned. However, as Figure 6.2 points out, training for longer sessions may increase the risk of injury unless intensity is somewhat reduced.

FREQUENCY

Most studies indicate that improvement in VO_2max occurs if exercise is performed three to four times per week for at least three weeks.[1,3-7] There are reports of significant improvement in individuals who train only one day per week. However, the subjects in those studies were sedentary individuals with their VO_2max so low that almost any training provided a sufficient overload to produce improvement. Studies also show that improvements from training four to five times per week are only slightly greater than training three times per week. For the average individual, that means that those added workout sessions are not going to be all that beneficial. However, if weight control is a consideration, it is necessary to keep in mind the

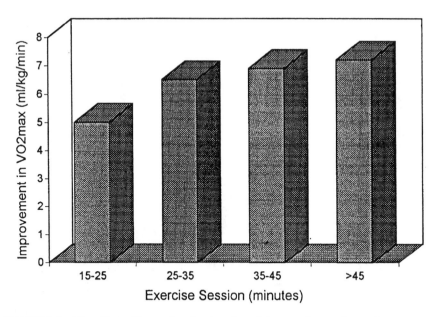

FIGURE 6.4 The effect of increasing the duration of the exercise session on improvement in VO_2max when training at ~60% VO_2max four days a week.

total number of calories that need to be burned. In that case, more frequent exercise provides a more optimal environment to lose weight (i.e., burn more calories). As Figure 6.3 illustrates, when intensity and duration of exercise is held constant, VO_2max greatly improves as frequency increases up to six times per week with minimal difference between the amount of change produced by five and six sessions per week. In addition, training more than five days a week is associated with a significant increase in injury rate (Figure 6.2).[3]

ACTIVITY MODE

If intensity, duration, and frequency of training are similar (total caloric expenditure is equal), then training adaptations are not dependent on the type of aerobic activity that is used. For example, comparing running, walking and cycling for 30 minutes, 60% $HR_{reserve}$, three days a week results are nearly equal training improvements.[7] That is an important point to keep in mind because it permits the individual to mix different activities from workout to workout (or within a workout session for that matter) without sacrificing the training effect. Incorporating different activities into the workout program may help prevent boredom. In addition, the staleness and injuries caused by repeated or overuse of the same muscle groups doing the same exercises may be avoided.

INITIAL LEVEL OF CARDIOVASCULAR FITNESS

An individual's fitness level affects the relative contributions of each of the three energy systems.[2] As a person becomes more aerobically fit, an exercise previously

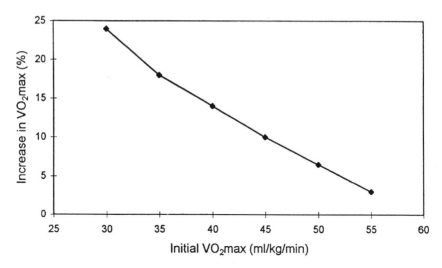

FIGURE 6.5   Expected increases in aerobic power (VO_2max) based on initial VO_2max.

relying predominantly on the ATP-CP and glycolytic systems for energy (an anaerobic activity) will become aerobic because the increased fitness now permits the individual to meet the energy requirements through aerobic metabolism.[1] Running an 8-minute mile may have been an all-out activity for an untrained individual that required anaerobic metabolism to meet the energy demands. The predominant use of the anaerobic metabolism would cause the exerciser to fatigue quickly. However, as this exerciser becomes more aerobically trained, the capacity to transport and utilize oxygen increases such that the energy demands of the 8-minute mile can be met by the aerobic system. Thus, the person does not fatigue as quickly and can exercise at a faster pace (than in his untrained state) for a longer time.

Improvement in aerobic power (VO_2max) depends on the individual's initial aerobic capacity. Increases in VO_2max are inversely related to the initial fitness level. Those who are unfit at the start of a training program have considerable room for improvement and can expect to have greater gains within a given amount of time than those who are highly fit.[1,5,7] That implies that as the fitness level increases, the amount of improvement in VO_2max with subsequent training will decrease even though intensity, duration, or frequency may be increased. As a guideline, those who are classified "average" for VO_2max can expect to improve 5 to 25% following a 12-week program of aerobic training. Conversely, individuals with very high VO_2max can train for 12 weeks and only improve VO_2max by 1 to 2%. That is illustrated in Figure 6.5. It is important for exercisers to understand the significance of initial fitness levels so that they can set proper goals for their fitness programs.

HOW MUCH EXERCISE IS NECESSARY?

The amount of exercise that is necessary is dependent upon the goals of the exerciser. Research has shown that exercise that causes only small improvements in VO_2max can cause considerable health benefits.[2] That research has led to statements by the

U.S. Centers for Disease Control and Prevention (CDC), the American College of Sports Medicine (ACSM), and the U.S. National Institute of Health (NIH) to issue guidelines indicating that moderate-intensity physical activity for 30 minutes for most days of the week is all that is necessary for health benefits to accrue. That would amount to walking at 3 to 4 mph (3–4 MET activity) for 30 minutes, five to seven days a week.

The same reports continue by saying that exercise at intensities and durations above this minimum will cause further benefits to accrue, including an increase in aerobic power. Based on that evidence, the following recommendations are made regarding the quantity and quality of training for developing and maintaining aerobic power:[2,6]

- Frequency of training: three to five days per week
- Intensity of training: 50 to 85% of $HR_{reserve}$
- Duration of training: 20 to 60 minutes of continuous aerobic activity
- Mode of activity: any activity that uses large muscle groups, can be maintained for a prolonged period, and is rhythmic and aerobic in nature

Studies indicate that when aerobic exercise is performed above the minimum intensity threshold (50% $HR_{reserve}$), the total amount of work accomplished is an important factor in fitness development and improvement.[1,3,5] The duration of exercise and intensity of exercise needed to improve VO_2max are related. Thus, improvement in VO_2max may be similar for various aerobic activities performed at lower intensities for longer durations, compared with higher-intensity activities of shorter duration, as long as total energy expenditure is equal.

Training for maintenance of aerobic power differs from training for improvement. Once the desired level of VO_2max is attained, then exercising at that training intensity should produce sufficient stress to cause the aerobic power to be maintained. Some research suggests that if training intensity is maintained, then frequency and duration can be reduced without affecting fitness, e.g., cutting back to two to three days a week instead of five days a week. However, if intensity is reduced while the frequency and duration are maintained, then a significant decline in aerobic power occurs.

CHOOSING THE APPROPRIATE AEROBIC ACTIVITY

As mentioned earlier, training adaptations are nearly equal for various types of aerobic activities as long as intensity, duration, and frequency are similar (resulting in equal energy expenditure). In choosing an activity, there are numerous considerations.[8] Can the activity easily fit into the individual's schedule? Does the activity require being outdoors? Will it be affected by bad weather? Is this an activity that can be performed with other individuals? What equipment or accessories are needed? Will the individual be motivated enough to continue with this activity long enough and at a sufficient intensity to achieve training benefits? Is the activity safe? What are the risks and injuries associated with the activity? Perhaps the most important question to answer is whether or not it is an activity that the individual will enjoy. Those are only a few of the apparent considerations (see Table 6.3).

TABLE 6.3
Advantages, Disadvantages, and Concerns of Typical Aerobic Exercises

Exercise Mode	Advantages	Disadvantages & Concerns
Aerobic Dance	Routines can be easily adapted to one's fitness capacity. All muscle groups can be effectively used during a properly choreographed routine. Low-impact can be low-stress on the joints.	Need music source, adequate space, resilient floor surface (for high intensity). Energy expenditure for various form can vary greatly. Easy to get high heart rate with low metabolic rates.
Step Aerobics	High intensity workout can be achieved quickly and maintained. Good for back, buttocks, and legs. Can vary step height for individual.	May aggravate knee or ankle conditions. Limited upper body involvement. Equipment cost: $20–$100.
Bicycling	Good aerobic workout. Great for lower body. Opportunity to vary environment.	Limited upper body involvement. Is difficult for a novice to get a good workout. Sessions usually last long. Traffic can be a problem. Need helmet. Cost of bicycle.
Stationary Cycling	Done in a safe and controlled environment. Easy to control intensity. Relatively few injuries.	Limited upper body involvement. Can be boring if session is prolonged. Does not appear good for weight loss. Cost $200–$2,000.
Rope Skipping	Excellent activity for aerobic fitness, agility, and coordination. Low cost. Can take equipment everywhere.	May aggravate knee and ankle problems. Need good shoes with cushioning. Exercise may be too intense causing DOMS. Most people cannot skip for long enough to get a good workout. Limited upper body involvement.
Rowing & Rowing Machines	Easy to adjust intensity to provide a good aerobic workout. Uses upper and lower body musculature. Good for strengthening muscles.	Potential low-back injury, so start easy with proper technique. Cost of equipment high: $150–$1,000.
Running/Jogging	Good aerobic training. Good for weight loss. Easy to adjust training intensity (pace). Opportunity to change environments. Only equipment needed is shoes.	Limited upper body involvement. May aggravate back, hip, knee, or foot problems. Not recommended for very overweight individuals. Shoes cost $40–$200.
Skating or In-line Skating	Can get a good aerobic workout. Good for strengthening lower body musculature. Fun. Opportunity to change environments.	Requires balance and coordination, requires safety (pads and helmet) equipment and safe, flat surface. Limited upper body involvement.
Ski Machines & Cross-country Skiing	Good aerobic workout. Machines allow for tension and resistance settings to control intensity. Can strengthen legs and arms.	Requires balance and coordination. May take some time to master the techniques. Machines cost $250–$800. Skiing requires snow and a large area. Cost: $100–$600.

TABLE 6.3 (continued)
Advantages, Disadvantages, and Concerns of Typical Aerobic Exercises

Exercise Mode	Advantages	Disadvantages & Concerns
Stair Climbing & Stair Stepping	High-intensity workout can be achieved quickly and maintained. Good for back, buttocks, and legs. Can vary step height for individual.	May aggravate knee or ankle conditions. Limited upper body involvement. Equipment cost: $100–$500.
Swimming	Good overall workout: aerobic and some strength. Good for lower back. Can adjust intensity of workout by time for a given distance.	Need a pool at least 20 yards long. Does not appear good for weight loss. Requires skill.
Water aerobics	Good overall workout: aerobic and some strength. Low-impact can be low stress on the joints. Can adjust intensity fairly easily.	Requires a pool. May be hard for very fit persons to get a good workout.
Walking	Good aerobic workout for sedentary or moderately trained persons. Low-impact — easy on joints. Easy to adjust intensity (pace). Requires only comfortable walking shoes.	Not very good for weight loss. May be hard for very fit persons to get a good workout.

PRESCRIBING AN AEROBIC TRAINING PROGRAM

There is a tendency by many fitness instructors to oversimplify the art of exercise prescription. It is easy to simply plug numbers into a formula: *aerobic activity at a heart rate of "X" bt/min for "X" minutes "X" times per week = exercise prescription.* However, development of a successful exercise prescription needs to be more individualized based on the desires, needs, goals, and capacity of the person.

People begin aerobic training programs for a variety of reasons: to lose or maintain weight, to gain health benefits, to enhance self-esteem, or to improve athletic performance. Although the training goals of the exerciser need to be realistic, the exerciser should make increased habitual physical activity an overall goal. Often the training principle of *progression* is overlooked by the participant and sometimes by the fitness instructor. Instead, progression is replaced by the rules of "no pain, no gain" and "more is better," which lead the new participant to alter an originally well-designed program with increased intensity, duration and/or frequency in hopes of speeding up the training process. Negative consequences may follow, such as delayed onset muscle soreness (DOMS), overuse injuries, or chronic fatigue. If progression is stressed from the start of the program, those problems can be avoided.

Well-designed training programs for unconditioned individuals start out with a "breaking-in" or conditioning period of at least one to two weeks. During that period, the exerciser may perform the workout at an intensity that is lower than required to produce a training effect. This break-in or starter program allows the exerciser to start to adapt to the stress of exercise, increasing the strength of tendons, ligaments, and muscles without DOMS. At the same time, it gives the exerciser a feeling of success. As the individual begins to adapt to the stress of exercise, then the intensity and duration of the session can gradually be increased until the participant is comfortable following the program prescription. By periodically reassessing the participant's fitness level and evaluating progress toward goals, problems can be identified early and reinforcing feedback that may be much needed by some exercisers can be provided.

A too rigid exercise program can cause exercisers to lose interest quickly. Because different individuals respond differently to the same amount of training, exercisers should not compare their responses to others and should maintain a certain degree of program flexibility. Changing the exercise prescription or participating in alternative exercises can sometimes be an easy means for keeping involved.

Getchell and Anderson provide useful examples of progressive exercise programs in their book *Being Fit*.[8] They include programs for walking, running, bicycling, stationary cycling, and swimming. The appropriate starting point depends on the individual's fitness level.

TYPICAL EXERCISE SESSION

A typical exercise session should include 5 to 10 minutes of warm-up exercises at the beginning to gradually prepare the muscles for the upcoming demands. That is followed by the aerobic activity portion or the strength training portion of the workout. The order of those two parts of the workout can occur interchangeably. In some cases, either the aerobic or strength portion can be omitted, depending on the needs and goals of the exerciser. A 5 to 10 minute cool-down phase should follow the completion of the aerobic workout. During the cool down, or tapering period, the activity is continued for several minutes at a lowered intensity level. That allows the working muscles to continue to assist in pumping blood from the extremities to the heart. Warm-up exercises can be repeated during this period. It is also an opportune time to stretch because the muscles are warmed up.

CONTINUOUS VS. INTERMITTENT TRAINING FOR AEROBIC FITNESS

Continuous training is submaximal exercise performed at moderate to high intensity for a considerable period of time (20 minutes, three times a week, ~60% intensity). This form of training is recommended for people who have attained a moderate level of fitness or for those exercising for weight control.[5,9]

Intermittent training is exercise completed for shorter periods of time but performing multiple short periods, e.g., three, 10-minute periods per day. Recent evidence suggests that improvement in fitness and health benefits can be obtained by intermittent periods of exercise.[2,5]

Interval training is high-intensity training with alternating periods of exercise and rest to allow a person to accomplish a large, intense amount of exercise with minimal fatigue,[1] e.g., 10, 400-m sprints with one minute of rest between sprints.

The training prescription is based on the intensity and duration of the exercise interval, length of recovery time, and number of repetitions. Quick recovery from brief, intense work intervals allows repetition of the exercise. This method eventually places considerable demand on the aerobic system. Due to the intensity of the exercise intervals, this form of training is not recommended for people starting a program.

CONCLUSION

Understanding the principles of aerobic fitness training is a prerequisite for prescribing an exercise program. Once a program has been designed, the instructor should help the individual set realistic goals, monitor progress toward those goals while offering feedback and support, and, if necessary, make changes in the exercise prescription.

REFERENCES

1. McArdle, W. D., Katch, F. I., and Katch, V. L., *Exercise Physiology: Energy, Nutrition, and Human Performance*, 4th ed., Williams & Wilkins, Baltimore, 1996.
2. Holly, R. G. and Shaffarth, J.D., Cardiorespiratory endurance, in *Resour. Man. Guid. Exer. Test. Exer. Prescr.*, American College of Sports Medicine, Eds., Williams & Wilkins, Baltimore, 1998, 437-447.
3. Pollock, M. L. and Wilmore, J. H., *Exercise in Health and Disease*, 2nd ed., W.B. Saunders, Philadelphia, 1990.
4. American College of Sports Medicine, The recommended quantity and quality of exercise for developing and maintaining cardiorespiratory and muscular fitness in healthy adults, *Med. Sci. Sports Exer.*, 22, 265-274, 1990.
5. Wenger, H.A. and Bell, G.J., The interactions of intensity, frequency and duration of exercise training in altering cardiorespiratory fitness, *Sports Med.*, 3, 346-356, 1986.
6. American College of Sports Medicine, *Guidelines for Exercise Testing and Prescription*, 5th ed., Williams & Wilkins, Baltimore, 1995.
7. Pollock, M. L., Dimmick, J., Miller, H. S., Kendrick, Z., and Linnerud, A. C., Effects of mode of training cardiovascular function and body composition of middle-aged men, *Med. Sci. Sports Exer.*, 2, 139-145, 1975.
8. Getchell, B. and Anderson, W., *Being Fit: A Personal Guide*, John Wiley & Sons, New York, 1982.
9. Katch, F. I. and McArdle, W. D., *Introduction to Nutrition, Exercise, and Health*, 4th ed., Lea & Febiger, Philadelphia, 1993.

7 Strength-Training Techniques

Purpose: To gain an understanding of the principles of strength training, which will enable the reader to prudently prescribe and complete an effective strength-training program.

Objectives:

1. Explain the principles of strength training.
2. Compare the various strength-training methods.
3. Demonstrate correct techniques for exercising all major muscle groups.
4. Design a strength-training program.

INTRODUCTION

Many leisure and occupational tasks require muscular strength (e.g., moving, lifting, or holding heavy objects). Maintaining or increasing strength enables an individual to perform those tasks with minimal physiological stress and reduces the risk of injury. Strength training also reduces the risk of lower-back injury that commonly occurs due to lifting or moving objects. In addition, maintaining strength is important to reduce the age-associated loss of muscle tissue. Thus, strength training is a necessary component of any well-rounded fitness program.

TERMINOLOGY

Strength can be simply defined as the maximal force or tension generated by the muscle.[1] It refers to the ability to generate a peak force during a maximal voluntary contraction. Strength is often measured by a one-repetition-maximum lift (1-RM).

Power is defined as the maximum strength-producing capability of the individual relative to time.[1,2] It is often equated with "explosive" strength.

Muscular endurance is the ability of a muscle to sustain contractions of a given force over time.[1] It is measured by determining the number of repetitions of a given exercise (e.g., bench press, sit-ups, pull-ups) that can be performed in a specific period of time or the number of continuous repetitions that can be done before the muscle fails.

Strength curve refers to the variation in peak force that can be developed by a muscle through the range of movement. Each muscle has its own unique strength curve. There is a position during the muscle contraction at which the muscle is "strongest" and at which the muscle is "weakest" (sticking point).

Overload refers to the muscle contracting against a resistance that is normally not encountered.[1,3] The overload principle must be applied to gain strength.

Volume refers to the total number of repetitions performed during a specified time.[4] It is a function of frequency and duration of training.

Periodization refers to a type of training that involves cycles of variation in volume and intensity of training.[4,5] Periodization brings about the greatest strength gains of all training methods.

Progressive resistance exercise refers to an increase of stress placed on the muscle as it becomes stronger.[1] That is achieved by increasing the resistance or volume over time.

Specificity refers to the concept that the changes in muscular strength are dependent upon the way in which the muscle is trained.[1,2] Specificity involves changes in the nervous system as well as within the muscle.

BASIC PRINCIPLES OF STRENGTH TRAINING

The concepts of overload and specificity are the basis of any strength-training program.[1,2] They are related to the ability of muscle to adapt to imposed stress. Both concepts cause structural and functional changes in the muscle to increase strength. The overload principle refers to placing greater than normal physical demands on the muscle. To produce strength gains, muscles are progressively overloaded by increasing the number of repetition, resistance, or the overall intensity of the exercise as the training program progresses. The specificity principle is related to the nature of changes that occur in an individual as a result of training. The Specific Adaptation to Imposed Demands (SAID) principle is the basis for program design.[1,2] Applying that principle to strength training involves consideration of the specific movement patterns and the particular muscles to be strengthened. Programs used for the development of muscular strength are different than those used to develop muscular endurance. Strength is best achieved with high resistance and a low number of repetitions, whereas muscular endurance is best achieved with low resistance and a high number of repetitions (DeLorme's Principles).

TYPES OF STRENGTH TRAINING

Isometric exercise involves static contraction of a muscle group when the joint angle and the muscle length remain constant.[2,5] That type of training is normally performed against an immovable object such as a wall or on a weight machine loaded beyond the individual's maximal strength. Isometrics can also be performed by contracting a weak muscle group against a strong muscle group (e.g., bending the left elbow while resisting the movement by pushing down on the left hand with the right hand).

Isotonic exercise involves dynamic contractions that occur through a range of motion against resistance.[1,2,4] The speed of movement is not fixed. The movement is divided into two phases: the concentric or positive phase, which involves the shortening contraction of the muscle (the lifting phase of a biceps curl), and the eccentric or negative phase, which involves a "lengthening contraction" of the muscle (the lowering phase of a biceps curl). Lengthening contraction is somewhat misleading because the muscle does not actually lengthen but instead returns to its resting or original length. Isotonic exercise is also subdivided into constant resistance exercise and variable resistance exercise. During constant resistance exercise, resistance remains the same throughout the muscle's range of movement. The amount of weight that can be lifted is limited by the weakest points in the range of motion of the exercising muscle. Variable resistance exercise, which requires equipment that utilizes cams, levers, pulleys, etc., attempts to vary the resistance experienced by the working muscle through its range of motion so that will match the strength curve. (Nautilus,® Eagle,® Icarian,® and Soloflex® machines provide variable resistance).

Isokinetic exercise involves contraction at a constant speed against an accommodating resistance.[4] The equipment controls the speed of movement and ensures that resistance is proportional to the force exerted by the muscle at each point through the full range of motion. That method permits maximal muscle tension through the full range of motion. Those principles serve as the basis for Cybex® machines. The machines are very sophisticated and are quite expensive. They are generally found in rehabilitation clinics.

TABLE 7.1
A Summary of the Types of Strength Training

	Isometric	Isotonic	Isokinetic
Maximal contraction?	Only at angle of pull.	Maximal at weakest point in range of motion.	Throughout the entire range of motion.
Strength increased throughout the range of motion?	Only if performed at several points throughout the range of motion.	Yes	Yes
Advantages	Good to use with patients who have limited range of motion due to pain or injury; does not require equipment or assistance.	Lifting stacks of weight can be motivational for some people; variety of exercises makes it possible to work all muscle groups.	Muscle soreness is minimal or nonexistent; lower risk of injury; spotters are not required; fast nature of muscular contraction permits a decrease in the workout time.
Disadvantages	Motivation may become a problem because there is no visible movement of weights.	Spotters are required if free weights are used.	Motivation may become a problem because there is no visible movement of weights.
Cost	None	Minimal to moderate	Expensive

METHODS OF STRENGTH TRAINING

A person will gain strength by performing any type of resistance training as long as maximal muscle contractions are accomplished. Table 7.1 lists the advantages and disadvantages of the various types of strength training. When comparing the three types of training, studies have found isotonic training produces the best overall strength gains but has the highest potential for injury.[1,2] In a rehabilitative setting, isokinetic training produces the greatest gains with the least potential for injury.[4]

The DeLorme light-to-heavy system is the foundation for all strength-training programs. This progressive resistance program produces significant gains in strength over short training periods.[1] The program uses three sets of 10 repetitions with the resistance progressing from 50% to 66% to 100% of a 10-RM (maximum weight that can be lifted 10 times).

Periodization is a training model that produces superior results compared to other strength-power programs.[5] This method reduces overtraining and brings performance to optimum levels by varying training volume and intensity. This variation occurs over the entire training period which can last one to four years (macrocycle), within smaller periods such as several months (mesocycle), and weekly (microcycle). Within each cycle, the participant goes through a hypertrophy phase in which he lifts a large total volume of weight (many repetitions/low resistance, e.g., three sets of 20 repetitions), a strength phase involving fewer repetitions of increased resistance (e.g., three sets of six repetitions), a power phase that includes only a few repetitions and maximal resistance one to three sets of three maximal repetitions), and a maintenance phase that involves one to three maximal lifts only one to two times per week. Individuals who are interested in that type of strength training should obtain more information about those training regimens.

TABLE 7.2
Suggested Order for Strength-Training Exercises for a Beginning Lifter

1. Leg press	6. Leg extensions
2. Bench press	7. Sit-ups
3. Leg curls	8. Biceps curls
4. Lower legs	9. Triceps curls
5. Latissimus pull-down	

BEGINNING A STRENGTH-TRAINING PROGRAM

Prior to performing any strength-training exercise, a proper warm-up is needed. This increases blood flow to the muscles and increases body heat, which improves muscle function. The warm-up can be accomplished by easy jogging, running in place, or cycling. Warm-up exercises should be followed by gradual, progressive stretching of all muscles. Finally, the warm-up should include lifting light weights in the manner they will be used during the training session. That practice reduces the risk of injury.

Strength-training exercises for all major muscle groups of the upper body, lower body, and torso should be included. Table 7.2 presents a basic program for a beginning weight lifter. The program was designed to use the larger muscle groups before the smaller groups and so that no two consecutive exercises involve the same muscle groups. Each muscle group should be worked through its full range of motion. Lifts should be performed slowly using good form. The overhead press or military press exercise has been omitted from the beginning program. This exercise has been omitted due to the increased risk of back injury if the exercise is not done incorrectly. Once the back becomes stronger and the individual feels more comfortable with weight training, then the overhead press can be added to the program, probably between exercises six and seven. For some individuals who have been strength-training for some time, this program may be too basic. Those individuals may organize their programs so that an entire session is devoted to upper- or lower-body exercises. But within the sessions, the lifter should still adhere to the large before small muscle groups and alternating push-pull exercises.[6] Tables 7.3 and 7.4 found at the end of this chapter list the techniques for performing various exercises. Table 7.3 lists free-weight exercises. Table 7.4 lists exercises performed with typical weight machines.

Determining the correct starting weight for the beginner is dependent on the size and strength of the exerciser. There is no magic number of sets and repetitions. Some people can sufficiently overload a muscle group in one set of exercises whereas others require multiple sets to accomplish the same degree of stimulation. The American College of Sports Medicine recommends a minimum of 8 to 10 exercises involving the major muscle groups performed a minimum of two times a week for the average healthy adult. A minimum of one of those sets should be completed to fatigue.[3,6] The person should first determine the maximum amount of weight he can lift 8 to 10 times (8–10 RM). The beginner should start with two to three sets of 8 to 10 repetitions for each muscle group. The first set should involve lighter weights (less resistance) than the second set. The third set should involve heavier weights (more resistance) than the second set. The number of sets and repetitions do not have to be the same for all the exercises. Once the chosen number of sets and repetitions can be performed using good form, the weight can be increased by 5 to 10%. The first four to six workout sessions should be performed with light weights. That will permit the muscles to adjust to the movements and help prevent injury and reduce muscle soreness. This preconditioning period enables the individual to learn and practice correct form. Recording the weight, number of repetitions, and number of sets is particularly useful to provide motivation and to monitor the progression. The rate of progression should be about 2 to 5 lb increases when two or more repetitions above the standard number of repetitions can be completed, e.g., the standard set is 10, the lifter can complete 12, then weight can be increased.

Rest is a component that must not be overlooked in the strength-training program.[1,2] At least one day of recovery between training sessions is needed for any given muscle group. Two days recovery is recommended for beginners. Some programs alternate upper body and lower body workouts. That type of program allows for successive weight training days without working the same muscle groups on consecutive days. Relatively long rest periods (several minutes) should be used between sets when heavy resistance is used to increase strength.

TABLE 7.3
Typical Free Weight Exercises

Exercise	Muscle Groups	Starting Position	Movement
Dead Lift	Lower back, thighs, buttocks	Stand with the feet apart about shoulder width while gripping a barbell or a pair of dumbbells, arms extended downward.	Slowly bend at the knees and waist to the lowest possible depth, then return to standing position.
Half Squats	Thighs, buttocks	Position bar on shoulders behind the neck. Stand with legs straight.	Sink downward until thighs are parallel to floor. Keep back as straight as possible and heels flat. Rise up until knees are straight.
Toe Raisers	Calves	Place barbell on the shoulders or dumbbells in each hand. Put balls of feet and toes on a 2-in. rise.	Rise on toes as high as possible and then drop down until heels touch floor. Rise back up.
Bench Press	Chest, shoulders, triceps	Lay prone on a bench with knees bent and feet flat on floor, back flat on bench. Bar gripped about shoulder width apart or a little wider, palms upward. Dumbbells can be used.	Lower bar toward chest in a straight line. Press the bar upwards in a straight line until arms are fully extended. Use a spotter.
Incline Press	Chest, shoulders, triceps	Lay face up on an inclined bench, feet on floor. Extend arms up to bar. Dumbbells can be used.	Lower the weight to the top of the chest, then extend arms forward and upward to full extension. Use a spotter.
Flying Exercises	Chest	Lay face up on a bench. Hold dumbbells in each hand, palms inward, arms extended over chest.	Slowly lower the dumbbells outward while keeping arms fairly straight, dumbbells parallel. Squeeze chest muscles together as the weights are returned to starting position.
Overhead Press	Shoulders	Stand while holding the barbell in front of thighs using overhand grip, hands are slightly greater than shoulder width apart.	Pull bar upward, with a quick snap bring elbows under bar so that bar rests on chest. Align hips under bar. Thrust the hips forward slightly while the bar is pushed overhead. Keep the bar close to the body while thrusting it upward. Try to fully extend arms overhead, body directly under bar.

Exercise	Muscles	Starting Position	Action
Behind the Neck Press	Back, chest, biceps	While seated, raise the barbell or dumbbells overhead using a forward grip.	Slowly lower the bar until it touches the shoulders behind the neck. Press the bar upward overhead.
Shoulder Shrugs	Shoulders, upper back	Standing upright, hold the dumbbells in front of the thighs using an overhead grip.	Shrug the shoulder, like trying to touch shoulders to ears.
Upright Rowing	Shoulders	Standing upright, hold the dumbbells in front of the thighs using an overhead grip.	Pull bar to chin while trying to keep elbows raised as high as possible. Lower slowly. Repeat.
Bent Lateral Raisers	Shoulders	Lean forward (~75°). Dumbbells extended downward.	Keeping the arms nearly straight, raise dumbbells to sides as high as possible and return to original position slowly.
Side Lateral Raisers	Shoulders	Standing upright with arms by side, dumbbells in hand, overhand grip.	Raise dumbbells sideward until they are almost parallel to the head. Pause a moment, then lower to original position.
Frontal Raisers	Shoulders	Arms hanging at sides, grip dumbbells using overhead grip.	Raise one arm forward at a time, elbows extended. Raise to chin level and return to original position.
Curls	Biceps, forearms	Stand erect, arms extended with bar resting on thighs using an underhand grip.	Flex arms to bring bar to chest and return to original position.
Reverse Curls (Triceps extension)	Triceps, forearms	Lift bar or dumbbells over head keeping elbows close to the head.	Slowly lower the weights behind the head until touching the back. Straighten the arms to the overhead position.
Wrist Curls	Forearms	While seated, grip bar or dumbbells with underhand grip. Forearms resting on thighs, arms extended past knees.	Raise and lower weights by moving hands, wrist, and fingers only.
Reverse Wrist Curls	Forearms	While seated, grip bar or dumbbells with overhand grip. Forearms resting on thighs, arms extended past knees.	Raise and lower weights by moving hands, wrist, and fingers only.

TABLE 7.4
Typical Weight Machine Exercises

Exercise	Muscle Groups	Starting Position	Movement
		Universal Machine	
Leg Press	Legs, buttocks	Sit with seat positioned so knees bent about 90°, both feet on foot pads.	Straighten both legs and return to original position.
Leg Extensions	Quadriceps (front of thigh)	Sit upright with bar (pads) across ankles and knees snug against seat (or table). Grip sides with arms.	Straighten legs smoothly, then lower back to original position.
Leg Curls	Hamstrings (back of thigh)	Lie face down on bench. Place ankles under bar (pads) with knees just over the edge of the bench.	Curl legs by trying to touch feet to buttocks. Lower back to original position. Avoid arching back.
Bench Press	Chest, shoulders, arms	Lie flat on back with head close to machine, feet on floor or flexed on bench. Grip bar slightly wider than shoulders.	Press weight upward while exhaling. Return to original position. Keep back flat on bench.
Seated Press (overhead press)	Chest, shoulders, arms	Sit close and facing the machine, arms on bar about shoulder width apart.	Press weight upward while exhaling. Return to original position. Keep back flat.
Lat Pull-Downs (Lat machine)	Back, shoulders, arms	Sit (or kneel) on floor facing bar. Fully extend arms overhead to grip bar, using a wide grip.	Tilt the head forward and pull the bar to the base of the neck. Return to starting position. Avoid arching the back.
Triceps Extension (Lat machine)	Triceps, forearms	Stand erect and grasp bar palms downward, elbows close to body. Bar shoulder height.	Press downward, keeping elbows next to body, and return to original position.
Curls	Biceps, forearms	With arms extended toward knees, grasp bar using underhand grip.	Bring bar to chest and return to original position.
Upright Rowing (curl machine)	Chest, shoulders, arms	Adjust bar so it rests across thighs with arms extended.	Pull bar toward chin and return to starting position.
Wrist Roller	Forearms	Grip wrist roller palms downward or upward.	Flex or extend wrists in a rotation-type motion.

Nautilus Machine

Exercise	Body Areas	Position	Movement
Hip and Back	Hips, back, thighs	Lie on back with legs over roller pads, hip joint aligned with cams. Fasten seat belt and lightly grip handles.	Extend both or one leg(s) fully. Return to starting position.
Hip Abduction	Hips	Use lever on side of machine to adjust until both movement arms are together. Move thigh pads to outer position. Sit on machine with knees and ankles on movement arms, thighs and knees against resistance pads, shoulders against seat back.	Spread knees to widest position possible, then bring knees together.
Hip Adduction	Hips and thighs	Use lever to adjust range of movement. Move thigh pads into position so that inner thighs are against pads. Sit back and fasten seat belt.	Pull thighs together with feet pointed inward. Return to original position.
Calf Raisers	Calves	Adjust belt around waist. Place balls of feet on first step and hand on front of carriage.	With knees locked, elevate the heels as high as possible (point toes), then lower slowly. (Can also stretch at the bottom by lowering heels.)
Decline Press (double chest machine)	Chest, shoulders, arms	Use the foot pedal to raise handles to the starting position. Keep body erect.	Press bar forward, keeping the elbows wide, and lower bar to original position.
Arm Cross (double chest machine)	Chest, shoulders	Adjust seat so shoulders are directly under axis of cams. Place forearms behind and firmly against the pads. Grasp handles.	Push with forearms, trying to touch elbows together in front of chest. Return to original position.
Lateral Raisers (double shoulder machine)	Shoulders	Adjust seat so shoulder joints align with cams. Sit with thighs on seat and ankles crossed. Fasten seat belt.	Pull handles back until knuckles touch pads. Raise both arms leading with elbows until parallel with floor. Return to original position.
Overhead Press	Shoulders, triceps	Raise seat to obtain full range of motion and grasp handles above shoulders.	Press handles overhead and return to original position. Do not arch back.
Pullovers	Back, abdominals	Adjust seat so shoulder joint is aligned with cams. Assume erect position and fasten seat belt. Place elbows on pad, adjusting seat as needed. Hands open, resting on curved bar.	Rotate elbows back as far as possible and stretch. Rotate elbows downward until bar touches midsection. Return to original position.
Rowing Machine	Shoulders, back	Sit with back toward weight stack. Place arms between pads and cross arms.	Bend arms in a rowing fashion as far as possible. Return to starting position.

TABLE 7.4 (continued)
Typical Weight Machine Exercises

Exercise	Muscle Groups	Starting Position	Movement
Behind the Neck (neck/torso/arm machine)	Back	Adjust seat so shoulders are in line with cams. Place back of upper arms between movement arm pads. Cross forearms behind neck.	Move arms downward until perpendicular to floor. Return slowly to crossed arm position behind the neck.
Behind the Neck Pull-downs (neck/torso/arm machine)	Back, biceps	Lean forward and grasp the bar with both hands.	Pull the bar behind the neck, keeping the elbows back. Return to original position.
Neck and Shoulder Machine	Shoulders, neck	While seated, place forearms behind pads with palms open and back of hands pressed against bottom of pads.	Straighten up until weight stack lifted. Shrug shoulders as high as possible (shoulders toward ears) and return.
Biceps Curls (biceps machine)	Biceps	Place elbows on pad and in line with axis of cams. Adjust seat so shoulders are slightly lower than elbows.	Curl both arms toward chest. Return to original position.
Triceps Curls (triceps machine)	Triceps	Place hands on the movement arm and elbows on pads, in line with axes of the cams. Adjust seat so that shoulders are slightly lower than elbows.	Extend arms fully. Return to original position.
Triceps Extension (multiexercise machine)	Triceps	Loop a towel through the weight belt. Grasp one end of the towel in each hand. Face away from machine. Arms overhead with elbows to ears. Adjust grip until weight stack separates.	Extend arms. Return to original position.
Wrist Curls (multiexercise machine)	Forearms	Attach a small bar to the movement arm. Grasp handles with palms upward or downward, forearms against thighs.	Using hands and wrists curl bar upward or downward. Return to original position.

Precautions

Holding one's breath during weight lifting can be dangerous. It is called Valsalva and can cause dizziness or even blackout. The lifter should always attempt to exhale during the movement or contraction. Inhaling during the contraction or movement can lead to the Valsalva.

When performing an isotonic program using barbells or even dumbbells, always have a spotter for the heavy lifts.

Maximal or near maximal efforts in isometric and slow dynamic muscle contractions produce relatively high blood pressures and heart rates, particularly if a large muscle mass is involved. That can be hazardous for individuals with cardiovascular disease. High-risk individuals should avoid high-resistance exercises and concentrate on developing muscular endurance rather than high levels of muscular strength. To avoid the exaggerated blood pressure responses, the individual could do single-limb exercises rather than double-limb exercises.[6] For example, instead of doing arm curls with a bar and using both arms, the person could use dumbbells and do one arm at a time. As with any exercise, the person should stop exercising if signs or symptoms such as dizziness, localized pain, unusual shortness of breath, or abnormal heart rate occur.

Muscle Soreness

Delayed-onset muscle soreness (DOMS) is a type of soreness that typically occurs 48 to 72 hours after exercise. It can last several days or more. Eccentric contractions result in a higher incidence of DOMS than do concentric or isometric contractions. DOMS usually occurs after doing a new activity or exercise too intensely. The incidence of DOMS can be reduced or eliminated by slowly increasing the training regimen (weights, repetitions, sets) over a period of weeks. In general, if correct form cannot be maintained during a lift, the amount of weight should be reduced.

CONCLUSION

Muscular strength is an important component of fitness. All successful strength-training programs adhere to the principles of overload and specificity. An understanding of the advantages and disadvantages of various types and methods of strength training is helpful in designing a proper strength-training program. A variety of equipment is available that allows exercise of most muscle groups. Knowledge of the various pieces of equipment will also aid in developing a good training program. Correct exercise technique is important for both safety and a program's success.

REFERENCES

1. DiNubile, N.A., Strength training, *Clin. Sports Med.*, 10, 33-62, 1991.
2. Tuten, R., Moore, C., and Knight, V., *Weight Training Everyone*, Hunter Textbooks, Inc., Winston-Salem, 1986.

3. American College of Sports Medicine, The recommended quantity and quality of exercise for developing and maintaining cardiorespiratory and muscular fitness in healthy adults, *Med. Sci. Sports Exer.*, 22, 265-274, 1990.
4. Fleck, S.J. and Schutt, R. C., Types of strength training, *Clin. Sports Med.*, 4, 159-168, 1985.
5. Stone, M.H., O'Bryant, H., Garhammer, J., McMillan, J., and Rozenek, R., A theoretical model of strength training, *Nat. Str. Cond. Assoc. J.*, 4(4), 36-39, 1982.
6. Bryant, C.X., Peterson, J.A., and Graves, J.E., Muscular strength and endurance, *ACSM's Resour. Man. Guid. Exer. Test. Pres.*, Williams & Wilkins, Baltimore, 1998, 448-455.

8 Low Back Pain and the Effects of an Exercise Program

Purpose: To familiarize the reader with the causes of low back pain and prevention methods that can be used to correct muscular-elasticity causes of low back pain.

Objectives: At the end of this chapter, the reader should know the following:

1. The basic anatomy of the lower back.
2. Causes of low back pain.
3. Ways to prevent low back pain.
4. Exercises that can be used to reduce the occurrence of low back pain.

INTRODUCTION

Low back pain is one of the most common complaints of adults. Between 10 and 17% of the general population have low back pain each year, and 60 to 80% of all adults at some point will experience low back pain.[1] The rate of incidence is second only to heart problems. In adults, low back pain is the second leading cause of visits to primary care physicians.[1] Furthermore, low back pain is the number one cause of worker's compensation claims, representing more than 20% of all claims and over $100 billion per year in direct and indirect costs.[2] Low back pain can be acute or chronic. Chronic low back pain is usually related to an abnormality of vertebrae or disks between vertebrae.[2] Acute low back pain is related to muscle weakness or loss of flexibility.[2] Although congenital or disease etiologies account for about only 2 to 5% of all cases, about 90 to 95% can be attributed to mechanical problems, such as muscular weakness or inelasticity.[2]

The spine sits on the pelvis and is kept in equilibrium by four sets of muscles (Figure 8.1): the abdominal muscles, the quadriceps in front of the leg, the hamstrings in the back of the upper leg, and a number of small back muscles. The lack of strength in the abdominal muscles is the major contributor to low back pain. Lack of strength in those muscles allows the abdomen to "slide" forward, which tends to pull the spine with it. The major muscle group related to a loss of elasticity is the hamstrings. As these muscles shorten they pull on the pelvis, which changes the angle between the spine and pelvis and causes pain. Knowing the causes and how to prevent muscle pain is the key. This chapter will focus on those issues.

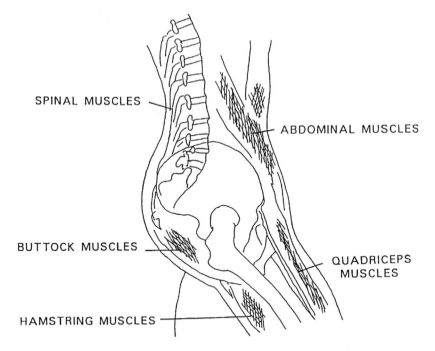

SPINAL MUSCLES

ABDOMINAL MUSCLES

BUTTOCK MUSCLES

QUADRICEPS MUSCLES

HAMSTRING MUSCLES

FIGURE 8.1   Anatomy of the musculature controlling the back.

CAUSES OF CHRONIC BACK PAIN

SLIPPED OR RUPTURED DISCS

Although uncommon, these are notorious for causing severe pain and disability.[2] The disk between the vertebrae may slip, shift, or bulge and stimulate nerve endings in its tough capsule. In some advanced cases, it may actually rupture (herniate), like a tire blow-out, and pinch the spinal nerves. This type of pain usually radiates down the back of the thigh and leg and is referred to as sciatica. If pressure or pinching of the spinal nerves continues, nerve damage can occur and cause either numbness or muscle weakness in the leg. Most patients with slipped discs improve with nonsurgical treatment, but a small percentage may require surgery.

WEAR AND TEAR ARTHRITIS (OSTEOARTHRITIS)

This seems to be part of the aging process. Osteoarthritis affects the disks and bones of your back in varying degrees.[2] It narrows the discs and can cause irritating spurs to appear on the vertebral bodies, producing pain. However, osteoarthritis often causes no discomfort at all. Age-related spinal degeneration and facet syndrome, where some of the bone wears off at the facets of the vertebrae, can also result in low back pain.

CONGENITAL ABNORMALITIES

These types of abnormalities occur in the development of the spine.[2] They include spina bifida, in which there is incomplete closure of the neural tube and abnormally developed vertebrae, sponylolysis or displaced vertebrae due to abnormal vertebral growth, segmentation abnormalities where the shape and number of vertebrae are not normal, and curvature of the spine (scoliosis).

MISCELLANEOUS CAUSES

These include any condition that may affect the various back structures or nearby areas.[2] Most notable are spinal trauma (fractures and dislocates), spinal bacterial infections, inflammatory causes of noninfectious origin, and tumors. Metabolic disorders, particularly osteoporosis is becoming a more common cause. Other indirect causes, like male prostate trouble or female menstrual problems, are more common. For whatever reason, any severe, persistent or chronic backache should be brought to your doctor's attention.

CAUSES OF ACUTE BACK PAIN

POOR POSTURE, LACK OF EXERCISE AND OVEREATING

This triad is the back's worst enemy and probably the cause of most back pain. Poor posture strains the lower back and makes it more vulnerable to injury.[1-4] Weak abdominal muscles and protruding pot bellies deprive your back of its greatest support. Overweight also adds to the strain — the back muscles have to work harder.

BACK SPRAINS

These can occur when back muscles or ligaments are stretched or torn.[2,4] Back sprains usually result from common activities done improperly, such as bending, lifting, standing, or sitting. Back sprains may also occur as a result of wrenching, or whiplash, caused by an automobile accident or athletic mishap.

TENSION AND EMOTIONAL PROBLEMS

The stresses of everyday life are important factors in causing back pain.[4] Economic worries, family pressures, and fatigue can cause back spasms and pain.

EXERCISE

Certain exercises have the potential to cause back pain.[1,5] Those exercises are discussed in the chapter on contraindicated exercises. Generally they focus on exercises that put extreme hyperextension of hyperflexion on the spine, such as straight leg toe touching, windmills and cobras. In those positions, the vertebrae tend to pinch on one side, which tends to force the disk between to be displaced or can even pinch the disk (see Figure 8.2). Sit-ups with the hand placed behind the head encourage

Normal Alignment   Hyperextension

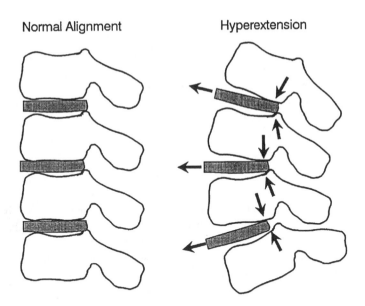

FIGURE 8.2 Relationship of vertebrae to disks during hyperextension and hyperflexion.

neck problems. In addition, many aerobic exercises such as step aerobics, aerobic dance, jogging, and rowing have the potential to cause back pain either because the person overexercises or the back is not sufficiently strong to handle the stress. Finally, weight lifting can cause back pain if the back does not have the strength to handle the stress or if the exercises are not done correctly. The dead lift, upright rowing, bench press, and overhead press present the biggest risk. However, most of these potential problems with exercise can be eliminated by using proper progression of intensity and duration and/or proper techniques.

PREVENTION

The following suggestions focus on the prevention of *acute* low back pain. These suggestions may not have any effect on chronic low back pain due to disk, osteoar-thritis, or any congenital defect. Therefore, before a person attempts any low back program a consultation with a physician is needed to determine what therapies could help and which could make the situation worse.[1-4] However, there are some basic habits that should be developed to reduce the risk of low back pain.[4,5]

Lifting

Lifts should not be attempted with the body bent over and legs straight. The knees should be bent, not your back — "Be an elevator not a crane." The lift should be accomplished with the leg muscles while object is held close to the body. The further away from the body an object is held, the greater the stress on the spine. When possible, lifts above shoulder level should be avoided; objects should be lifted only chest-high. When the load is heavy, the person ought to use help, plan ahead to avoid sudden load shifts, and be sure the footing is adequate.

STANDING/WALKING

When a person stands for long periods of time, he should change positions often. It also helps to stand for short periods of time with one foot up or bend the knees and keep the back straight. Also, it is not a good idea to bend forward while holding legs straight. Good posture can help avoid low back pain. The head should be held high, chin tucked in, pelvis forward and toes straight ahead. Comfortable shoes are also a benefit. High-heeled or platform shoes need to be avoided when standing or walking for long periods. For some individuals, standing with one foot forward and the other slightly backward and rocking weight from one leg to the other can relieve minor low back pain due to standing. In addition, tilting the pelvis upward and downward during standing can relieve minor pain. Placing a 4 to 6 in. step under one foot while standing and switching the support leg can also reduce the potential for pain during prolonged standing.

DRIVING

The driver should not sit far back from the steering wheel while driving. Stretching for the pedals and wheel increases low back curve and strain. The driver is better off with the car seat moved forward to keep the knees bent higher than the hips. Sitting straight and driving with both hands on the wheel are also healthful. Vibrations from the vehicle can contribute to low back pain, so keep the engine tuned and the wheels balanced and aligned.

SITTING

Sitting actually puts about 50% more stress on the lower back than standing.[6] Sitting in a chair that is too high or too far from the work surface should be avoided. Also, leaning forward and arching the back, or sitting back and slumping can cause back or neck pain. A person should sit in chairs that are low enough to enable him to place both feet on the floor and keep the knees higher than the hips. Legs can be crossed and feet can be raised on a stool. The back should be upright and firmly placed against back of the chair.

VIDEO DISPLAY MONITORING

Working at a display monitor is becoming one of the most common worksite duties and is fast becoming a major cause of back pain. Monitoring a video display or working at a computer compounds the effect of sitting on the low back with potential neck problems.[5] The display and chair should be situated such that the person can sit comfortably and not have to adjust the head position to look upward or downward to see the monitor. If those adjustments to the head become a chronic work condition, neck pain can result. To reduce or eliminate the pain, the terminal workers should stretch the neck from side to side, holding the stretch for 4 to 6 seconds on each side. In addition, stretching the top of the neck for 4 to 6 seconds at a time by gently pulling forward on the top of the head can also help, as can tucking the chin in and pushing it out. Finally, stretching the trunk can reduce potential back pain. There are two stretching exercises that may help. One is completed by placing one arm over the head (like a ballet dancer) and leaning away from the side of that arm. Hold the stretch for about six seconds and switch arms. The other exercise is completed by stretching the arms backward over the edges of back rest of the chair. Hold the stretch for about six seconds and repeat a few times.

SLEEPING

A good night's sleep on a firm mattress is good for the back. When possible, avoid sleeping or lounging on soft, sagging, no-support mattresses or cushions. Swayback and back strain can result, especially when sleeping on the stomach. To reduce the possibility of sleep-induced low back pain, sleep on one or the other side of the body with knees bent or on the back with a pillow under your knees. Avoid sleeping on the stomach and sleeping with both arms over the head.

EXERCISE PROGRAM

Participation in an exercise program significantly reduces the risk of acute low back pain. Exercise increases the strength and endurance capacity of the back muscles. It also improves pain tolerance and reduces anxiety and depression, conditions known to exacerbate pain. In addition, exercise can contribute to weight loss, and being overweight is an independent risk factor for low back pain.[1] Research has shown that a carefully planned exercise program is better than bed rest when back pain is due to an uncomplicated mechanical problem.[1] The program typically consists of aerobic exercise (walking, jogging, swimming, cycling), strengthening exercises (especially the abdominal muscles), and stretching exercises (hamstrings and hip flexors).[1] The person should keep in mind that when recovering from a back problem, avoid possible further injury by doing *only* the exercises the doctor has recommended. At the same time, exercise should be stopped if there is pain. Consult a doctor if pain is experienced while exercising. Avoid overdoing it. This is typically a case where of repetitions can be helpful, but too many may be hazardous. Daily exercise is best.[2,4] Occasional exercising may actually be harmful to the back.

The typical program consists of about 30 minutes a day, three to five days a week.[1] Like any therapeutic programs, the exercise should be graduated. At first, the 30 minutes each day appears to work best when split into two parts, preferably 15 minutes in the morning and 15 minutes at night. As the individual becomes stronger and gains endurance, the program should evolve to 30 to 45 minutes of continuous activity a day. Begin the exercise session with a warm-up period lasting two to three minutes. Use the proper starting positions for all strengthening and stretching exercises. Limber up arms and legs by alternately tightening and relaxing muscles.[2,4] Any change in the program should occur only in consultation with the physician.

If the individual is recovering from low back pain, an exercise program should not be initiated until it is cleared by a physician. Some physicians will use the ability to sit upright for 15 to 20 minutes as a guide because it actually causes more tension in the back than walking.[6] Once cleared, walking becomes the first exercise attempted. Some experts suggest that a walking program should be started three to four days after reduction of pain.[1] However, that rule should be applied on a case-by-case basis.

SPECIFIC EXERCISES

1. Knee-to-Chest Raise: To help limber up a stiff back.
   * Starting either by lying on the back or standing.
   * Raise right knee to chest.
   * Hold, count to five, release.
   * Repeat five times.
   * Repeat steps 1 to 4 with left leg.
   * Repeat steps 1 to 4 with both legs.
     Note: Do not lift legs with arms or hands.
2. Pelvic Tilt: To strengthen front and back muscles and reduce swayback.
   * Starting either by lying on the back or standing upright.
   * Firmly tighten buttock muscles.
   * Hold, count to five.
   * Relax buttocks.
   * Repeat five times.
     Note: Keep lower spine flat against floor.
3. Single Leg Raise: To help limber up and stretch hamstring.
   * Lie on the stomach.
   * Slowly raise right leg as high as you comfortably can.
   * Hold, count to five.
   * Return leg to floor.
   * Repeat five times.
   * Repeat steps 1 to 5 with left leg.
     Note: Do not swing legs up fast or use hands to help.
4. Nose-to-Knee Touch: To stretch hip muscles and strengthen abdominal muscles.
   * Starting by lying on the back.
   * Raise left knee slowly to chest.
   * Pull left knee to chest with both hands.
   * In a separate motion, raise head, touch nose to knee.
   * Hold, count to five, release.
   * Repeat five times.
   * Repeat steps 1 to 6 with right knee.
     Note: Keep lower back flat on the floor.
5. Half Sit-Ups: To strengthen abdominal and back muscles.
   * Assume starting position on the back, knees bent upward.
   * Slowly raise head and neck to top of chest.

- Reach both hands forward, place on knees.
- Hold, count to five.
- Slowly return to starting position.
- Repeat five times.
  Note: Keep mid and lower back flat on the floor.

6. Abdominal Bracing: To strengthen abdominal muscles and relieve stress on lower spine.
   - Lie on the back on a firm surface with knees bent upward.
   - Brace the stomach muscles so that the back is flattened against the surface.
   - Hold for about 10 seconds.

7. Hamstring Stretch: To stretch hamstring muscles.
   - Assume sitting position, legs together and straight.
   - Lean forward from the pelvis.
   - Do not try to touch toe with hands.
   - Repeat five times, holding for about six seconds each.
     Note: Feel stretching of hamstrings.

8. Hip Stretch: To stretch back muscles and hamstrings.
   - Put foot on a chair with leg extended and hands on that knee.
   - Lean forward from the hip, keeping the back straight.
   - Feel the stretch in the weight-bearing leg.
   - Hold for about 10 seconds and switch legs.

9. Aerobic Exercise: Aerobic exercise is the cornerstone of a low back program. There is gathering data that shows that participation in 20 to 30 minutes of aerobic exercise reduces the risk of low back pain.[1] The aerobic exercise should start easy, for example, 20 to 30 minutes of walking, gradually becoming more strenuous up to about 70% of maximal intensity for 30 to 45 minutes.[1] There appears to be little benefit for low back pain above this intensity and duration of exercise. The exercises that appear most beneficial are swimming, recumbent cycling, aerobics, aerobic dance, step aerobics, rowing, jogging, upright cycling, or in-line (roller) skating. Some experts suggest that swimming, front or back crawl, is the optimal aerobic exercise. That is because the water gives support, and the swimming motions tend to simulate some of the stretching exercises mentioned above.[5] Participation in those forms of aerobic exercise makes the assumption that there is no back pain to begin with. Some of those aerobic exercises, such as step aerobics, upright cycling, rowing, or jogging may actually exacerbate back pain if the pain exists before the exercise program starts.[1,5] That is why it is best to check with your physician.

ADVANCED EXERCISES

These exercises should be used by someone who can easily complete the above exercises.

1. Scissors: To limber and stretch abdominal, hip, back, and hamstring muscles.
   - Assume starting position on the back.
   - Raise both legs until balanced.
   - Slowly scissor legs up and down 10 times.
   - Slowly scissor back and forth (crosswise) 10 times, alternating right leg over left, left over right.
   - Return knees to chest, then feet to floor.
   - Repeat once.
   Note: Keep good balance and lower back flat on floor.
2. Hip Hyperextension: To stretch, strengthen hip, buttock, and back muscles.
   - Lie on stomach.
   - Stiffen left leg straight.
   - Slowly raise leg from hip.
   - Return leg to floor.
   - Repeat five times.
   - Repeat steps 1 to 5 with right leg.
   Note: Do not lift pelvis to raise leg. Keep leg straight.
3. Alternate Arm and Leg Lift: To strengthen lower back and hamstring muscles.
   - Lie face down with arms and legs extended.
   - Raise the right arm and left leg simultaneously and keep them extended a few seconds.
   - Return to starting position.
   - Now raise the left arm and right leg simultaneously.
   - Alternate.
   - Repeat 5 to 10 times on each side.
   Note: Do this exercise slowly. Do not jerk the legs up and down.

CONCLUSION

Low back pain can be described as an "adult's nemesis." Overexertion, weak musculature, and loss of flexibility account for most of the cases. However, the incidence of this debilitation can be reduced by using proper sitting, lifting, and driving techniques. *Chronic* back pain related to a congenital, degenerative, inflammatory, metabolic, or neoplasm condition may not respond to standard programs. Individuals with those problems should work one-on-one with a physician. For those individuals with *acute* back pain, the incidence can also be dramatically reduced by an aerobic exercise program, along with increasing the strength of the abdominal and back muscles and increasing the flexibility of the hamstring muscles. A carefully chosen exercise program may be better than bed rest when back pain is related to uncomplicated mechanical problems. Keep in mind that proper treatment includes a partnership between the injured individual and his physician. Learning proper techniques and appropriate exercises and adhering to the recommendations of the physician are important to minimizing low back problems.

REFERENCES

1. Deyo, A., Exercise in the prevention and treatment of low back pain, in *Exercise for the Prevention and Treatment of Illness,* Goldberg, L. and Elliot, D.L., eds., FA Davis Company, Philadelphia, 1994, pp. 158-170.
2. Pope, M.H., Andersson, G.B.J., Frymoyer, J.W., and Chaffin, D.B., *Occupational Low Back Pain: Assessment, Treatment and Prevention,* Mosby Year Book, St. Louis, 1991.
3. Getchell, B., *Physical Fitness: A Way of Life*, Macmillan Publishing Company, New York, 1992.
4. Patient Information Library, *Back Owner's Manual*. PAS Publishing, Dale City, 1981.
5. Oliver, J., *Back Care: An Illustrated Guide*, Butterworth-Heinemann Ltd., Oxford, 1994.
6. Nachemson, A., The lumbar spine: An orthopedic challenge, *Spine*,1, 59-71, 1976.

9 Contraindicated Exercise

Purpose: To define and identify contraindicated exercises.

Objectives: At the end of this instructional session, the reader will be able to do the following:

1. Be aware of what constitutes a contraindicated exercise.
2. Be familiar with commonly used contraindicated exercises and understand why they are contraindicated.
3. Know and understand guidelines for identifying contraindicated exercises.

INTRODUCTION

Exercise has physical and emotional benefits, but exercise also has some inherent risks. Generally, the benefits of exercise outweigh the risks. However, not all exercises have a similar risk/benefit ratio. Exercises that present a high risk of injury are contraindicated because the risks outweigh the benefits derived from regularly performing them. Many exercises now considered risky were incorporated into exercise programs for many years. As knowledge of kinesiology and the musculoskeletal system has improved, so has the ability to evaluate exercises to determine their usefulness in improving fitness and reducing the risks of injury. The best exercise programs combine fitness and low risk of injury. Therefore, the purpose of this chapter is to point out the most commonly used contraindicated exercises and explain why they are undesirable. Guidelines given will also help identify unsafe exercises.

WHAT IS A CONTRAINDICATED EXERCISE?

Contraindicated exercises are those that have a high potential for causing injury. According to Lindsay and Corbin, exercise can cause acute or chronic injury.[1] Acute injuries include sprains or strains that produce immediate pain. Chronic injuries usually occur from microtrauma due to repetitive movements performed several days per week as part of an ongoing fitness program. Microtrauma is a small injury to tissue. An example of microtrauma is the wear and tear that occurs in the intervertebral disks as a result of repeated side flexion (side bends).[1] The intervertebral disks are the soft cushioning structures between the bones of the spine. When the spine is flexed sideways, those cushioning structures are squeezed. Over time, that repetitive squeezing causes degeneration of the intervetebral disks, which leads to back pain and/or later injury. Contraindicated exercises are associated with either one or both types of injury.

Individuals differ widely in genetic makeup and ability to perform different exercises. Certain individuals may be able to perform contraindicated exercises and never suffer any lasting injury, but for others that will not be the case. It is virtually impossible to predict who will or will not be injured.[2] However, even though it is impossible to avoid all injuries or microtraumas, it is possible to reduce their potential by avoiding exercises that ignore normal joint movements.

GUIDELINES FOR SPOTTING CONTRAINDICATED EXERCISES

As we learn more about the human body, we are better able to identify exercises that have more costs (injuries) than benefits. The field of exercise is always changing. Fitness instructors have a responsibility to update their knowledge periodically. The following guidelines should help identify contraindicated exercises.[2]

The exercise is probably contraindicated if it involves the following:

1. Hyperextension of the back, neck or knee.
2. Forward flexion or more than 20° of side flexion of the spine.
3. Twisting the spine or knee.
4. Ballistic movements.
5. Hyperflexion of the neck or knee.

COMMONLY USED CONTRAINDICATED EXERCISES

The following exercise descriptions were based on the writings of Lindsay and Corbin[1] and T. Branner.[3]

BACK ARCHING ABDOMINAL STRETCH/COBRA

This exercise stretches the abdominal muscles by hyperextending the back (and sometimes the neck as well) while the person is lying prone or doing a back bend (Figure 9.1). Hyperextension of the spine may cause injury due to compression of the vertebrae, possible pressure on a nerve, and/or possible herniation of the intervertebral disk and other spinal structures. The abdominal muscles are typically too long and weak in most people to warrant stretching.

DONKEY KICK

The purpose of this exercise is to strengthen the muscles in the buttocks. It involves kneeling on all fours and bringing the knee to the nose then kicking the leg backwards as high into the air as it will go (Figure 9.2). This causes hyperextension of the back and sometimes the neck. Also, injuries are more likely to occur when the movement is done quickly with great momentum. This exercise can be safely performed by not allowing the leg to kick up higher than the back and keep the head down.

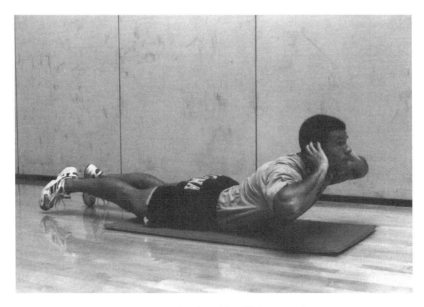

FIGURE 9.1   Back arching/Cobra exercise.

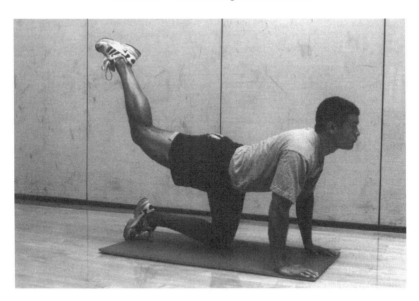

FIGURE 9.2   Donkey kick.

STRAIGHT-LEG SIT-UPS OR DOUBLE LEG LIFTS

Although usually done with the objective of improving abdominal strength and endurance, these two exercises actually work the iliopsoas, or hip flexor, muscles. Keeping the lower back from hyperextending during these exercises is very difficult

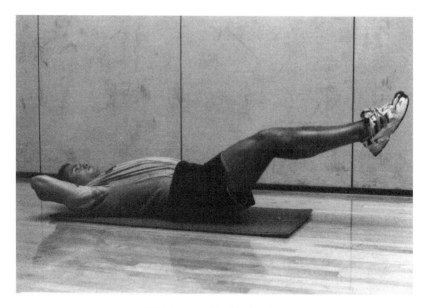

FIGURE 9.3   Double leg lift.

if not impossible for most people (Figure 9.3). Even if there is adequate abdominal strength to keep the lower back flat, these exercises still create a great deal of pressure on the discs of the lumbar (lower) spine. Most people do not need to strengthen hip flexors because those muscles tend to be strong; over-development of the hip flexors is undesirable and can lead to lower back problems. Single-leg scissors exercise mentioned in the last chapter may not put the pressure on the back because only one leg is elevated at a time.

ELBOW TO KNEE SIT-UPS/HANDS BEHIND THE HEAD SIT-UPS (FULL OR CRUNCHES)

Elbow to knee sit-ups work mainly the hip flexors and are not very efficient abdominal exercises. Both of these types of sit-ups usually involve placing the hands behind the neck. That is not recommended because participants may start to use their hands to pull up their upper body. This pulls the head and neck into hyperflexion and can excessively stretch ligaments in the back of the neck. The hands should be placed across the chest or on the ears to prevent this problem.

YOGA PLOUGH/VERTICAL BICYCLING/SHOULDER STAND

These exercises require lying supine on the floor with the legs up in the air over the lower body (Figure 9.4). In the *Yoga Plough,* the feet are lowered over the head causing hyperflexion of the back and neck. In *Vertical Bicycling,* the lower body weight is supported on the upper back, shoulders, and neck. Both of those positions place a great deal of stress on the lower back, compress the cervical vertebrae, and can cause overstretching of muscles and ligaments. These exercises should be avoided.

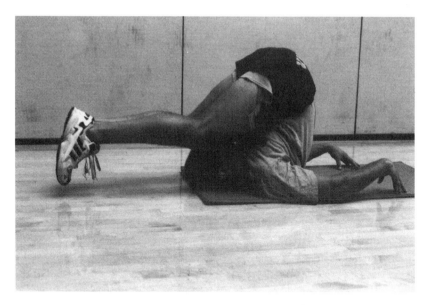

FIGURE 9.4 Yoga Plough.

STANDING TOE TOUCHES/WINDMILLS/FORWARD FLEXION OF THE SPINE

These exercises involve forward flexion of the spine (bending forward at the waist) and are generally done to stretch the hamstrings (Figure 9.5). This motion places a great deal of stress on the intervertebral discs and can, over time, lead to disc deterioration. Adding twisting motion to forward flexion such as during windmills increases stress on the spine. Standing toe touches require the hamstrings to stretch and contract at the same time. If forward flexion is done with the knees straight, the knees can be pulled into hyperextension, which creates abnormal amounts of stress on the knee. Also, forward flex flat-back positions with straight knees create similar problems for the knees. Keeping the head below the heart for prolonged periods can elicit an abnormal blood pressure response in certain people. These positions should be avoided.

SIDE STRETCHES/SIDE FLEXION OF THE SPINE

The problems with these exercises are similar to those associated with forward flexion. A traditional side stretch is done by bending to the side as far as possible. Like forward flexion, side flexion places stress on the intervertebral discs. Side stretches can be done safely by reaching upward with one arm and limiting side flexion to 20°.

FULL NECK CIRCLES

Tilting the head back (hyperextension of the neck) places considerable strain on the cervical (neck) vertebrae and can result in acute and/or chronic injury. This movement does not contribute to flexibility or strength and is best left out of an exercise program.

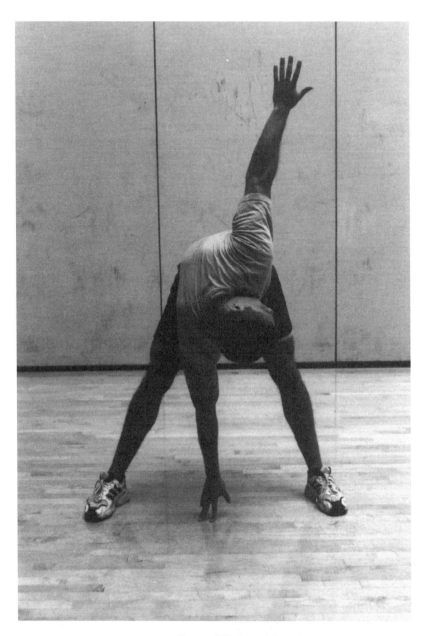

FIGURE 9.5   Forward flexion of the spine.

Leg Stretches at the Ballet Bar

These stretches are done with one leg raised more than 90° with the knee straight and the foot or ankle resting on a ballet bar. They are intended to stretch the hamstrings and back. This exercise is problematic because the leg is held in a position

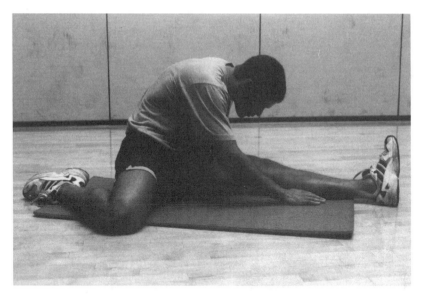

FIGURE 9.6 Hurdler's stretch.

that exceeds the natural range of motion. Problems such as sciatica have been associated with this exercise, especially in those who have below-average flexibility. A safer version of this stretch can be performed by putting the foot on the seat of a chair, keeping the knee straight, and bending forward from the hips until a stretch is felt.

HURDLER'S STRETCH/THE HERO

In these exercises the leg is bent so that the foot and knee are turned outward (Figure 9.6). This places torque on the flexed knee, which can overstretch the ligaments and tendons. These exercises are done to stretch the quadriceps and hamstrings. To reduce the overstretch, simply maneuver the bent leg so that the bottom of the foot is next to the straight leg and the knee is pointed outward. (See Chpater 5 for safe stretches for these muscles.)

DEEP KNEE BENDS/HYPERFLEXION OF THE KNEE

When the knee is flexed so that the calf touches the back of the thigh, the ligaments and joint capsule of the knee can be overstretched. Flexion beyond 120° is not recommended. A deep knee bend that puts the person in a squat past 90° of flexion, like that of a catcher on a baseball team, can cause injury especially if it is done with weights. The foot needs to be kept directly aligned with the knee (as much as possible) to reduce stress on the joint. Certain quadriceps stretches also hyperflex the knee. It is not necessary to hyperflex the knee to stretch the quadriceps. Simply bring the heel of the foot toward the buttocks with the opposite hand. Extend that leg at the hip and press the foot into the hand to feel a stretch.

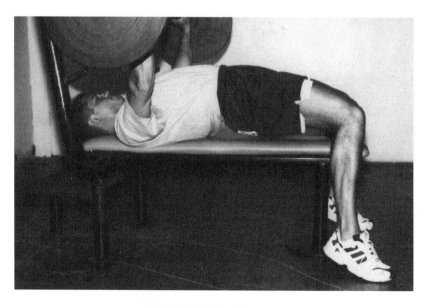

FIGURE 9.7 Bench press.

BENCH PRESS/PUSH-UPS

These exercises are done to strengthen the chest and upper body. Those who are beginning an exercise program should be taught the correct way of doing these exercises in order to avoid lumbar (lower back) hyperextension (Figure 9.7). The bench press should be done with the feet on the bench. This helps keep the lower back from hyperextending. Many weight lifters, in order to lift more weight, will push their feet against the floor. That leads to hyperextension of the lumbar spine. Injuries are very likely because the large amounts of weight used will place a great deal of pressure on the spine. If a person cannot lift the weight with proper form, then he should decrease the weight. Traditional push-ups done on the toes with legs straight may be a problem for those with weak trunk muscles and low upper body strength. The spine should be kept in proper alignment throughout the push-up. A modified push-up done with the knees on the floor is easier and safer for those unable to do traditional push-ups properly. Wall push-ups are suggested for people with very low upper body strength.

CONCLUSION

Regular exercise involves risks as well as benefits. Exercises that may be appropriate for one person may be dangerous for another.[1] Therefore, contraindicated exercises should be avoided when leading groups in which there may be some concern that individuals are performing the exercises correctly. In many cases, it is best to learn proper form first, in a one-on-one situation, then work individually or in groups without supervision. In addition, it is important that fitness instructors be aware of movements and exercises that are associated with more "costs" than "benefits." The goal of exercise to improve health is to maximize benefits and minimize injury.

REFERENCES

1. Lindsay, R. and Corbin, C., Questionable Exercises — Some Safer Alternatives, *J. Phys. Educ., Rec., Dance*, 60 (10), 26-31, 1989.
2. Van Gelder, N. and Marks, S., *Aerobic Dance-Exercise Instructor Manual.* IDEA Foundation, San Diego, 1987.
3. Branner, T. T., *The Safe Exercise Handbook*, Kendall/Hunt Publishing Co., Dubuque, 1989.

10 Fitness Equipment

Purpose: To familiarize the reader with the fitness equipment presently on the market.

Objectives: At the end of this chapter, the reader should have an idea of the characteristics of fitness equipment, what each machine does, and what to look for when making a purchase. The specific equipment covered will include the following:

1. Exercise treadmills
2. Exercise cycles
3. Stair climbers
4. Rowing machines
5. Cross-country ski machines
6. Weight training equipment

INTRODUCTION

There is a wide variety of fitness equipment on the market. Furthermore, the fitness equipment industry is ever-evolving and expanding, as indicated by the fact that sales of equipment rose $233.5 million between 1995 and 1996.[1] Machines have become an important mainstay in the fitness industry because people believe they can just use any piece of equipment for 20 to 30 minutes and get a complete workout, and because people find machines provide added motivation to exercise. Some machines are valuable because their use can result in a good workout and cause calorie expenditures of 500 to 700 kcal/hr. However, some machines are simply gimmicks and may even cause harm to the user. In addition, none of the equipment presently on the market will provide a *total* workout.[1-3] Therefore, the consumer must make some decisions and obtain some knowledge before purchasing. Fitness instructors are the most often asked persons regarding the purchase of equipment for home or institutional use. Therefore, it is in the best interest of the instructor to have basic knowledge about equipment, to be able to advise others and at the same time make smart purchases for their clients and their own facilities. Because equipment designs are continuously being changed, there is some need on the instructor's part to keep acquainted with what is available and to know how to seek the opinions of other professionals.

Generally speaking, aerobic equipment can be divided into six categories: treadmills, stationary cycle ergometers (bikes), steppers and climbers, cross-country ski machines, aerobic riders, and rowing machines. The basic assumption of these aerobic machines is that the calorie burn is about the same for all when an individual exercises at the same heart rate intensity. That is not true because some machines involve more muscle mass than others and therefore result in a greater caloric use. In addition, some of these machines cause a greater isometric (static) component during the exercise, which causes a greater heart rate at a given metabolic rate. Therefore, if the user is basing metabolic rate on heart rate response, a greater isometric component will result in less calorie utilization than expected.

Strength or resistance training equipment falls into three general categories: isometric, isotonic, and isokinetic equipment. Isometric equipment generally produces very slow movements and has a very high static component. Exercising a joint through a range of motion may take 10 to 30 seconds. Also, those pieces of equipment cause very high blood pressures that are usually sustained throughout the movement. Isometrics can cause a Valsalva maneuver — attempting a forced expiration but keeping mouth and nose closed. The valsalva, combined with the prolonged muscle tension, results in a reduction in blood flow back to the heart and eventually the brain, which can lead to syncope (fainting). Thus, isometric equipment is not generally recommended for the general public. Isotonic machines move the joint through a range of motion using a constant resistance. Isotonics include free weights, dumbbells, and some resistance machines. Isotonic equipment allows the exerciser to lift as much weight as the weakest point of the range of motion, a biceps curl, for example. The arm can exert only 60 to 80% of its maximal force with the elbow straight. But when the elbow is at 90°, maximal force can be exerted. In addition, once the weight is in motion, it is easier to keep it in motion, which actually reduces the effort on the part of the lifter. The third type of machines are isokinetic machines. Those machines increase or decrease resistance through the range of motion so that maximal force can be exerted throughout the range of motion. The machines also control speed. These are expensive pieces of equipment and are usually found in a rehabilitative setting. As with aerobic equipment, not all resistance training equipment are created equal. This chapter will focus on the major types of fitness equipment, discussing the intended purpose, pros and cons, and approximate price for purchasing these machines.

AEROBIC EQUIPMENT

EXERCISE TREADMILLS

Exercise treadmills are good for anyone who can walk or jog. They are popular because walking and running are natural movements familiar to all normal people. Because the movements are natural, learning to exercise on a treadmill takes little time. A treadmill can provide a high caloric use, provide good aerobic fitness improvements, and increase the tone of the legs. However, the use of treadmills provides limited fitness benefits for the upper body.

Treadmills can be purchased in motorized and nonmotorized models. The non-motorized versions are those in which the exerciser's walking or running causes the belt to move. These treadmills cause the exerciser to change their stride in order to move the belt, thus they take considerable practice to keep a steady pace. Nonmotorized treadmills are usually the least expensive treadmills, but they do not seem to work well for most individuals. The motorized treadmills are better because they set the pace/speed for the exerciser. Some motorized models have adjustable elevation, which gives a more strenuous workout. Those types are preferable to level, "speed only" treadmills. Many models come with side and front rails to help balance the exerciser. Those rails can increase the comfort and safety of the beginning exerciser, but they may get in the way as the exerciser becomes more acquainted and comfortable, especially when the treadmill is narrow. The more sophisticated treadmills can be programmed for a variety of intensities to give a "complete workout": warm-up, easy work, hard work, interval exercise, and cool down. Some display speed, grade, miles covered, and caloric usage. Although the speed, grade and mileage readout are usually correct, the caloric use indicators may be unreliable and should not be taken at face value.

Some treadmills provide "kill" switches that will automatically shut the treadmill down if the exerciser loses balance, falls, or cannot keep up with the speed or grade. Many also have interfaces with heart rate monitors, so the exerciser can monitor how hard he is exercising. Although the calorie use readout may not be accurate, there is fairly good agreement between heart rate and metabolic rate during treadmill exercise, e.g., 60% of maximal heart rate is approximately 50 to 55% of maximal metabolic rate. Conversely, treadmills are not appropriate for persons who have debilitating illness or orthopedic or balance problems.[2] Another problem is that the measurements of blood pressure and heart rate can be difficult during high speeds.

Treadmills are expensive. The consumer will be expected to pay at least $1,000 for a reliable walking model.[4] If the exerciser is an experienced runner or the treadmill is expected to sustain hard use, the cost will increase dramatically from $1,500 to $10,000. Cheaper models are available, but they usually do not last. The more costly models are usually for institutional, heavy use and are quite large. Models are usually signified by belt size. A model 18 by 54, means that the width of the belt is 18 in. and the length of the walking surface is 54 in. The largest treadmill presently available is an 18 by 65 model. A minimum of 16 in. width is recommended, and a length of 48 in. is the smallest anyone should consider buying. Even that size may feel small.

Treadmills also take up considerable space. Even the smallest will require a 4-ft by 8-ft space, so storage may be a problem. In addition, treadmills are noisy. The sound of the motor and the pounding of the feet may make it difficult to hear a radio or TV without turning up the volume, which then may disturb others.

The purchaser should look for the following features in a good treadmill: 1. A surface that is of adequate length for the person's stride, wide enough to feel comfortable, and with some cushioning. 2. Speed and incline controls that are located so they can be easily adjusted during exercise. 3. An emergency stop switch that is easily accessible. 4. A strong motor (1.5 horsepower or greater) that can handle higher speeds (5 to 10 mph) or heavy loads (over 175 lb). 5. Be careful of gadgets. Some electronic peripherals can be cheaply made gadgets that tend to malfunction quickly and may be on the machine solely to inflate price. Make sure these extra functions are really needed, and check their warranty. The purchaser should also run or walk on the treadmill before making an acquisition. If planting the foot firmly on the belt causes the belt to slip or hesitate, or the motor to groan or grind, then this is not the treadmill to purchase.

Care needs to be taken when mounting or dismounting the treadmill to prevent injuries. The exerciser should begin by straddling the belt on the machine when starting it. He should try to get a feel for the speed by "pawing" the belt before stepping onto it, then step onto the belt with a slightly longer forward stride to compensate for the movement of the belt. Typically, the treadmill is started at a slow speed and increased when the exerciser feels comfortable.

EXERCISE CYCLES

Exercise cycles are usually less costly than treadmills. They also take up less space. Some are even portable. The cycle can be used for persons who have difficulty walking, problems with balance, some forms of back problems, some orthopedic problems, or weight problems.[1,3,4] Cycling is also low-impact and puts less strain on the joints and back than running or jogging. However, cycles focus on the muscles of the thighs and at high work loads may aggravate knee problems. The ergometers are easy to use because the cycling motion is familiar to most individuals. However, some individuals find it uncomfortable to sit on the seats for prolonged periods of time. Cycles exercise only the lower body, therefore people generally have a hard time losing weight using cycling programs. If the cycle is being used for exercise testing, the technician will find that it is fairly easy to set a precise resistance and measure heart rate or blood pressure even at high work rates. There are six types of cycles available: stationary leg cycle ergometer, stationary arm cycle ergometer, arm and leg wind trainers, recumbent (reclining) ergometers, bicycle trainers, and standard bicycles.

Stationary leg cycle ergometers range in price from $150 to over $2,000, but a good model can be purchased for about $300 to 400. The wide range is related to the features. The inexpensive cycles use friction to increase the work loads. They may be wobbly, noisy, and hard to pedal. The more expensive cycles are electronically braked, have controls that can be programmed for specific workouts, and have readouts of distance, time, work load, and calorie burn. Some models come with heart rate monitors that clip to the finger or earlobe. Like treadmills, the accuracy of the calorie count is questionable. The top-of-the-line units have a computerized video display that will allow the cyclist to simulate training in the mountains or racing against other cyclists. Some models are *recumbent*, allowing the person to sit with the back supported and pedal. The large seat and back rests give the body support not found in the typical cycle ergometer. Those models are good for individuals with neck, shoulder, and back problems. They may be useful for persons with borderline or true hypertension because blood pressure may not rise as much as during conventional cycling. A recumbent cycle works the muscles of the buttocks and hamstrings more than the conventional cycle. The major drawbacks of the recumbent ergometers are that they take up considerable space, and they tend to be costly, ranging from $500 to more than $1,000.

Arm and leg ergometers are usually air-braked. They contain no friction or electronic devices to produce the resistance, thus fewer parts to break down. These "wind trainers" are very useful because they can exercise both upper and lower body or each part individually. They usually have fewer parts to maintain, which reduces the long-range cost.[4] They also provide a breeze when they are being used, which cools the exerciser. Prices range from about $250 to $1,000, depending upon features. Like other stationary ergometers, monitors can give readouts of the amount of work, time, rpm, and calorie use. Once again, the calorie burn is just an estimate.

Arm crank ergometers are the least favorite because they use only the muscle of the upper extremities. They produce relatively high heart rates and blood pressures for a given metabolic rate. Arm ergometers should be avoided by those with a high risk of cardiovascular disease because high blood pressures and heart rates do occur at comparatively low work loads.[2] These ergometers are also comparatively expensive.

Regardless of the type of cycle ergometer, there are some common features a purchaser should consider.[1,4] The cycle should not feel unstable or frail; look for solid construction. The seat should be comfortable and adjustable to the user's height. (The knee should be only slightly bent when the leg is extended on the pedal.) The handlebars should also adjust to the person's reach. The pedals should have toe clips, or the capacity to accept toe clips, to keep the feet from slipping and to allow the legs to work on the upstroke. The cycle should have a means of indicating and setting the work load in watts or kpms. That is especially true if the ergometer is used for fitness testing. The work load or resistance should be able to be set using a friction belt or by electronics (unless the machine is air-braked). If the cycle is a friction-type, the friction device should be at least large pads and not simply a screw-down wheel. The better ergometers use friction belts around the entire wheel. As with treadmills, use of the cycle before making a purchase will help to make an informed decision.

Bicycles and *bicycle trainers* are a different issue. Bicycles need to be sized to the individual when purchased. There are many methods to figure the right frame size. The simplest involves straddling the bike and standing flat-footed. The top tube on the bike should be about an inch below the crotch of the rider. With mountain or all-terrain bikes (those with fat tires and straight handlebars), there should be as much as 5 inches clearance between the crotch and the top tube.

Handlebars on bicycles come in several varieties. The drop, or curved, underbars should be about shoulder width apart. If they are too wide, they can strain the shoulders and neck. They should be at the level of the seat or slightly lower. This type of bar gives the rider several different hand positions, which can reduce fatigue. There is also a proper distance from the seat to the handlebars. If it is too long, the rider can get back pain. To test, stand along the side of the bike, put an elbow at the tip of the saddle and reach for the bars. The fingertips should be within a half-inch of the bars. If not, the handlebar stem will need to be changed. Alternatively, on some bikes the seat can be moved forward or back an inch or two. Straight bars are commonly found on mountain bikes. These may or may not be slightly wider than conventional bars and should be at or just above seat height. Straight bars have only one position for the hands and arms, so, on long trips the arms of the rider can easily fatigue or cramp. To avoid the fatigue, modified mountain bike handlebars or "bar ends" can be purchased (cost: $40 to 125). Their fit can be tested like that of conventional handlebars.

Seat height is important to reduce stress on the back and knees of the rider. The rider's leg should be only slightly bent at the bottom of the downstroke, while at the top of the stroke the thigh should be parallel with the top tube.

Bicycles range in price from $150 to $4,000, depending on the type (touring, mountain, racing, or hybrid) and features. The purchaser should be prepared to spend about $300 to $500 to get a reliable bicycle. The purchaser should also tell the cycle technician (salesperson) the type of riding he intends to do (short-distance commuting, road racing, trail riding, long-distance touring) and other accessories or features he wants. Hybrids look like mountain bikes with skinny tires, but they usually cost less. In general, bikes with top tubes are sturdier and usually have better braking ability. Multispeed bikes may appear intimidating for the first-time rider; however, the availability of new "index shifting" on most bikes makes shifting almost worry-free. Because multispeed bikes permit inexperienced and marginally conditioned riders to tackle hills and go over rough terrain without excessive straining, learning to shift gears is well worth the effort.

The beauty of a bicycle is that it allows the exerciser to see the countryside and get out in the fresh air, making it less boring than stationary bikes. Of course bicycling in areas of high traffic congestion may not be advisable. But for the exerciser who wants to have the freedom of riding but cannot always get out into the countryside, the bicycle can be used as a stationary bike by mounting the frame on a *bicycle trainer* apparatus.

A *bicycle trainer* is a stand that fits on the rear wheel of a bike and typically has a roller that rests against the wheel. The exerciser simply attaches the trainer and pedals normally. A magnet or small turbine supplies the resistance/work load to the rear wheel. The amount of work is adjusted by using the gears and varying the pedal frequency. The simpler trainers do not require the removal of the front wheel to mount the bike on the apparatus. The trainers that are magnetically controlled are quieter but cost more than wind-resistance turbine designs. Many trainers fold up for easy storage. Bicycle trainers are priced from $95 to well over $200. Because the rear wheel is a few inches off ground level, the rider is forced to lean forward more than normal. That forward lean makes it difficult to balance without using the handlebars, thereby making it difficult to read or watch television during rides. However, a small block of wood can be put under the front wheel to level out the bike and make riding easier.

Another style of bicycle trainer is the "rollers." The cyclist pedals the bike while balancing on two sets of rollers (one for the front wheel and one for the rear). The rollers are the best at simulating actual road cycling. Resistance is changed by shifting gears. An exerciser will need some practice and a good sense of balance to effectively pedal on the rollers. Prices start at around $125 for a good set. Keep in mind that they will occupy considerable space.

STAIR STEPPERS/CLIMBERS

Stair steppers or climbers are two of the most recent and popular additions to the line of fitness equipment. Stair climbing is known to be one of the most stressful forms of exercise.[1,4] Training programs that include running up stairs usually result in formidable gains in aerobic capacity and strength of the legs and buttocks. Thus, simulating these motions should result in a good workout. Although the terms stepper and climber are used synonymously, they are actually somewhat different. *Stair steppers* provide only a lower body workout because the arms are not involved. However, *stair climbers* have grips at or above head level and require the person to push/pull with the arms while stepping, providing both lower and upper body workouts.

Workouts using these machines can be hard and can cause both aerobic and strength gains. Participants can reach very high heart rates and blood pressures very quickly, so beginners need to be careful not to overexert. These circulatory responses also suggest that heart and stroke patients should consult their physicians before attempting a stair climber program. Stair climbing is tough on the knees and could aggravate some knee problems such as chondromalacia. To reduce the possibilities of these injuries, the exerciser should be sure that his knees are aligned over the toes during stepping. Most machines tend to work the calf muscles more and the buttock muscles less than actual stair climbing. Also, many have rails or a monitor mounted in front that can be used to lean on. Leaning on the controls or rails reduces the intensity of the workout.

Stair steppers are available in two main varieties: escalator type and the pedal type. The larger (and more expensive) models operate like escalators and simulate real stair climbing. To modify the intensity of the exercise, the participant simply speeds up the rate at which the stairs are presented to or passed by the exerciser. These models can be equipped with a computer that will give the exerciser a complete workout profile (warm-up, exercise, cool down), time, and calorie burn. They may also include a heart rate monitor. Some of the large electronic versions have pedals so that the step height can be modified. The typical "home" variety has pedals for the exerciser to stand on and a front rail that can be used for balance. The exerciser simply pumps the pedals. The pedals can work independently or may be synchronized such that a downstroke with one causes the other to automatically upstroke. Pedal resistance is induced by either a piston (pneumatic, hydraulic, or air-filled), spring mechanism, or flywheel. The pedal-type stepper actually puts less stress on the knees than the escalator-type stair climbers. The major drawbacks of the pedal steppers are that the exerciser can use the hand rails to support the weight or can set the resistance so high that the person ends up taking small steps and does not use the lower body muscles through the complete range of motion. Either case provides a reduced workout.

A good stair stepper should keep the body in good alignment, with the back upright and the knees behind the toes.[1,2,4] The stepping action should be smooth, and the apparatus should be stable and not wobble at rapid step rates. The pedals should be large and self-leveling. The unit should have rails or handlebars. The resistance setting should be accomplished easily. Models with independent pedals provide more natural stepping actions and a better workout. For larger individuals, the piston (or shock absorber) type may not be the best choice because they tend to break down. Steppers range in price from $200 to $1,500.

The star climber should come with moving hand grips that will allow the exerciser to work the upper body as well as the legs. As with the stair stepper, the action should be smooth and the apparatus should be stable and not wobble at rapid step rates. When in position to use the climber the person should be fairly upright, like a vertical ladder. The climber tends to simulate rock climbing more than stepping. Stair climbers range in price from $600 to $2,200.

CROSS-COUNTRY SKI MACHINES

These machines can provide the most complete workout by simulating outdoor cross-country skiing.[1,4] The feet slide back and forth on rails while the arms complete a poling motion using either cords or poles. Some models allow the exerciser to increase or decrease the resistance and elevate the slope of the skis to increase the intensity of the exercise. They provide excellent aerobic conditioning and some muscle strength. Because these machines use most of the muscles of the body, they cause a high calorie use. They are good for almost all individuals. Ski machines are low-impact, placing little strain on specific joints, and normally do not aggravate knee problems. Some models allow the arms and legs to move independently. Those models may seem awkward at first and may take the exerciser some time to learn the coordination. Other models allow the exerciser to move the arms and legs synchronously and are easier to learn. The units with attached poles are easier to learn to use, but they do not seem to give as good an upper body workout because the poles can be used to lean on and reduce the effort.

Good cross-country ski machines have a long enough base to accommodate the stride of the exerciser. The resistance for both the arms and legs can be adjusted and do not have pistons or shock absorbers. Those pistons tend to malfunction sooner and do not take the beating of long strenuous workouts or large strong individuals. The "ropes and pulley" models tend to work more smoothly and are more easily repaired. As with other exercise machines, cross-country ski machines should have a sturdy base of support and be comfortable to use. These machines are expensive, ranging from $200 to $1,000. A purchaser should be prepared to spend about $400 to $500 to get a decent machine.

ROWING MACHINES

Rowing machines have the potential to cause both aerobic and strength gains — they condition the entire body, particularly the abdomen and back.[1,4] They are among the safest to use and burn a high number of calories. If the exerciser uses proper technique, there is little strain on the joints. However, if the person has back problems, a physician should be consulted before starting a rowing program. Rowers are probably the most popular items of fitness equipment.[4] But in the long run they also tend to be one of the least used and hence a great "dust catcher."

There are generally two types of rowing machines, and the price can vary dramatically — $100 to $3,000. The typical home machine has pistons or shock absorbers that provide the resistance. Those can be awkward to use; the piston can heat up and actually give out. The seat should not be fixed. A movable seat, sliding up and down a rail, insures that the whole body is used for each stroke. The second type is designed with a flywheel attached to a chain and handlebar. Many of those flywheels use wind resistance (such as the "wind trainers" cycle ergometers). Some even have the flywheel in a water tank. Those models all have movable seats on fixed rails. The exerciser sits on the seat and rows in the natural position, increasing the speed of rowing or adding more water to the tank increases the intensity of the exercise. Those ergometers feature digital readouts that give work rate in watts or kgms, strokes per minute, and calorie use rate. The deluxe units have a computerized video display that provides a complete workout profile or allows the exerciser to simulate racing other rowers.

The better rowing ergometers have sturdy, large comfortable seats that roll on rollers or ball bearings during the stroke action. The rowing action is smooth. Piston-type machines may "catch" during the power stroke, while the flywheel varieties are very smooth. The better units have footrests that pivot as the leg extends during the stroking action.

Proper rowing technique is important. The technique emphasizes the legs and not the back. To begin the stroke, the arms come forward before the knees are bent. The exerciser should not lean forward to begin the stroke. The legs (not the back) extend to begin the power stroke. As the legs are extending, the arms should come into play. Be careful not to finish the stroke with an exaggerated back pull.

AEROBIC RIDERS

Aerobic riders, or gravity riders, are one of the newest and most popular items in the fitness equipment market. Exercise is completed with the person in the seated position. The seat rises as the exerciser pushes with the feet and pulls with the arms. These machines are easy to learn to use and provide a low-impact workout. Although some of these machines apply the resistance via electronics, many use the exerciser's weight as the sole mechanism for applying resistance. Therefore, as the exerciser trains and loses weight, they actually get less resistance. The machines usually come with a computerized readout, including some indicator of effort, frequency, time, and caloric use. As with the other aerobic equipment, the calorie readout is not accurate.[3]

Some exercisers that use this type of machine have complained of low back pain. Therefore, this piece of equipment may not be appropriate for those exercisers with any type of chronic low back pain or weak back muscles. Beginners should probably use them with some caution, starting slowly.

The consumer should expect to pay between $200 and $500 for this form of machine. Good aerobic riders have adjustable seats and handlebars, a mechanism for adjusting resistance, and some form of electronic readout.

WEIGHT TRAINING EQUIPMENT

ISOTONIC EQUIPMENT

There is a considerable variety of weight training equipment on the market, ranging from simple free weights to complex computerized isokinetic resistance equipment costing thousands of dollars. There are $1,000 machines that will simply strengthen the neck and $200 machines that have numerous stations that strengthen the entire body. The variety of equipment and the misleading advertising make decisions difficult.

Free weights are dumbbells and barbells. They are the least expensive of all types of weight training equipment and can be used for a wide variety of exercises. Free weights may be better than any weight machine for general strength because they require more muscle mass to move the weight and stabilize the body against gravity. Also, motivation is easier because the exerciser knows how much weight he is lifting.

There are some disadvantages to free weights. Because the person is lifting the weight against gravity, he will need to develop the mastery of the lifting technique to avoid losing control and dropping the weight, which could lead to injury. Even during submaximal lifts, proper technique does not insure against losing control of the weight. For this reason and because of fatigue, a spotter, or assistant, is required. As mentioned earlier, the body can lift only the amount of weight that can be moved at the weakest point of the range of motion of the lift. For example, the weakest part of the range of motion of a curl occurs at the beginning when the arms are straight, while the strongest occurs when the elbow is bent about 90°. At the beginning, the person may be able to lift 30 lbs, but at 90° the person may be able to lift 50 lbs. Also, inertia can be used to reduce the amount of strength necessary to complete the lift. Inertia states that a body in motion will remain in motion unless acted on by an outside force. For example, an arm curl can be started by resting the weights against the legs and then using the legs to "snap" the bar in motion, making it easier to move more weight than when the lifter starts without the leg snap. Of course, it will also be harder to stop the motion of the bar at the end of the lift, which could cause injuries.

Free weights should have high-quality steel bars that are gnarled for better grip. They need not be chrome-plated or stainless steel, but that will reduce rusting. Olympic-style bars are best if the lifter is expected to lift very heavy weights. That type of bar can hold plates (weights) on one side without falling off its stand. The plates should be purchased in a variety of weight, ranging from 1/2 lb to 50 lb. Instructors should keep in mind that free weights make excellent door stops and tend to disappear. Thus, a way to keep them in the weight room is needed. An Olympic-style bar costs about $100. Each plate (weight) costs anywhere from $5 to $40 and is usually sold by the pound. A complete set can be purchased from a local sporting goods dealer for a few hundred dollars.

Along with weights, a solid, sturdy bench and a rack or weight stand are needed to complete the setup. They are relatively inexpensive for the increase in safety they provide. A variety of styles are available (e.g., curling bench, inclined bench press, and a standard bench). The most familiar and a very useful style is the bench designed for the standard bench press. The bench should be wide enough and long enough to accommodate the lifter. The upholstery should be heavy-duty with adequate padding underneath. The bench should be sturdily constructed and should not wobble when supporting the weight of the lifter. Some models permit bar height adjustments. Home benches start at $60. Gym quality benches start at $200.

Weight machines have been developed to reduce the potential for injuries related to problems controlling the weight. The weights cannot be dropped on the lifter! Many of these machines, such as the Eagle,® Nautilus,® Universal Gym,® Soloflex,® or Hydrafitness® have specific machines, or stations, for each exercise. Each machine was designed to cause the lifter to work through a specific range of motion. These machines allow for isolation of specific muscle groups, thus the gains in these specific muscle groups should be theoretically better.

Some machines are built for a "reference man," which is to say that the seats and pads used to position the parts of the body are designed for a specific sized person and are unadjustable. Small individuals, and especially women, may have problems using the equipment because they cannot get into the starting position or work through the range of motion. That could lead to injury. Larger individuals may find the machine is easier to use or harder to fit into. Many of these machines advertise that they are "isokinetic," which means they adjust to differences in strength throughout the range of motion of the exercise. In general, most of these machines are not truly isokinetic because they accommodate only for strength differences throughout the range of motion and do not control speed.

Weight machines come in a variety of forms. Some machines include stations for all major lifts. Those types are preferential because a whole upper and lower body workout can be obtained by working around the machine. They are also the most expensive, costing thousands of dollars. Many companies also sell specific stations, such as a bench press, arm curl, or back machine. In fact, one company has a station that exercises only the neck muscle and costs over $1,000! Separate stations are nice add-ons when there is a great deal of space available and a large number of lifters. All machines operate with cables, pulleys, chains, or levers and will need maintenance.

ISOKINETIC MACHINES

Isokinetic machines are the most expensive. For example, a simple knee extension machine costs thousands of dollars. These machines have accommodating resistance, which allows the person to lift maximally through the range of motion. The machines also allow the lifter to set the speed of motion. Isokinetic machines usually cause the least muscle soreness of all weight lifting methods. Their use results in fewer injuries. Besides expense, there are other shortcomings. Motivation is difficult with isokinetic machines because in many cases the person has no idea how hard they are working or how much weight they are lifting. It is also easy to "cheat" on the lifts. All the exerciser has to do is apply less resistance and he can still work through the range of motion. In summary, isokinetic machines have a more appropriate place in rehabilitation than in a standard fitness setting.

CONCLUSION

Exercise machines can be used to motivate individuals to exercise. These machines will cause the exerciser to increase aerobic capacity and strength, some better than

---

TABLE 10.1
Checklist for Purchasing Equipment[5]

Determine needs and budget

Evaluate present facilities for space, electrical, safety

Obtain product information (see list at end of chapter)

Evaluate product for ease of use, safety, design, electrical needs

Find out service history, availability of service contracts

Check warranties

Compare costs, including maintenance costs

Use the product, try it out

Find out the most effective payment plan

Purchase equipment

---

others. Conversely, use of the machines can result in injury and cause loss of motivation if the equipment is of poor quality or not appropriate for the person. However, there seems to be more pieces of fitness equipment in attics than in use. Therefore, several decisions need to be made before any equipment is purchased.[3] What is the goal of the exerciser: to lose weight, to gain strength, to increase aerobic power, or to train for a specific sport? What amount of money does the exerciser want to spend? How much floor and storage space is available for the equipment? Will the machine be used by one individual or a number of people? Finally, does the exerciser actually need this equipment? Because of the expense and the space many of these consume, it is important to be sure that the machine is suitable for the person and that the person will use it. It is also important for the exerciser to have a basic understanding of fitness equipment to make educated purchases. Thus, the exerciser should try a number of different types of machines and models to determine which is going to meet his needs and be within budgetary and spatial constraints. The best way to learn about fitness equipment is from trade shows, professional publications that examine equipment, or professional fitness organizations.

REFERENCES

1. Kuntzleman, C.T. and Wilkerson, R., A primer to recommend home aerobic equipment, *Heal. Fit. J.*, 1(6), 24, 1997.
2. Comparing aerobic-exercise machines, *University of California, Berkeley Wellness Letter,* 9 (12), 5, 1992.
3. Stamford, B., Choosing and using exercise equipment, *Phys. Sportsmed.,* January, 1977.
4. Burke, E.R., *Complete Home Fitness Handbook*, Human Kinetics, Champaign, 1966.
5. American College of Sports Medicine, *ACSM's Resource Manual for Guidelines for Exercise Testing and Prescription*, 3rd ed., Williams & Wilkins, Baltimore, 1998.

Appendix

Possible suppliers of fitness equipment, including addresses, phone numbers and equipment they supply.

Bally Fitness Corp., 9601 Jeronimo Rd., Irvine, CA 92718, 800-543-2925: Lifecycle, Liferower, weight equipment

Concept II Inc., 105 Industrial Park Drive, Morrisville, VT 05661, 800-245-5676: Rowing ergometers

Country Technology Inc., PO Box 87, Gays Mill, WI 54631, 608-735-4718: Cycle ergometers, stair climbers, rowing ergometers, treadmills, Olympic-style free weights

Cybex, 10 Trotter Drive, Medway, MA 02053, 800-677-6544: Eagle weight machines, isokinetic machines, treadmills, stair steppers

Heart Rate Inc., 3188-E Airway Ave., Costa Mesa, CA 92626, 800-237-2271: Stair climbers, VersaClimber

Icon Health & Fitness, 800-999-3757: Aerobic riders

Iso-Flex, 800-735-6518: Weight training machines

Lifecycle, 10601 West Belmont Ave., Franklin Park, IL 60131, 800-634-8637: Stationary cycles

Nautilus International, 709 Powerhouse Rd., Independence, VA 24348, 800-874-8941: Weight training equipment

Nordictrack, 105 Peavey Road, Chaska, MN 55318, 800-328-5888: Ski simulators and resistance exercise equipment

Pacemaker (Aerobics), 3310 Keller Springs Rd., Carrollton, TX 75006, 201-256-9700: Treadmills

Paramount Consumer Sales, 645 E. Bandini Blvd., Los Angeles, CA 90040, 800-854-0183: Weight equipment

Precor Co., PO Box 3004, Bothell, WA 98041, 800-786-8404: All kinds of fitness equipment, mainly treadmills and stationary cycles

Quinton Fitness Equipment, 3303 Monte Villa Parkway, Bothell, WA 98021-2791, 800-426-0337: Treadmills, stationary cycle ergometers, arm ergometers

Schwinn: 615 Landwehr Road, Northbrook, IL 60062, 800-SCHWINN: Stationary cycles, arm and leg ergometers, bicycles

Sportime, One Sportime Way, Atlanta, GA 30340, 800-283-5700: Step aerobic steps, cycle ergometers, free weights

Stairmaster, 12421 Willows NE, Suite 100, Kirkland, WA 98034, 800-635-2936: Stair steppers, cycle ergometers, treadmills, strength equipment

Tunturi Inc., 1776 136th Pl. NE, Bellevue, WA 98005, 800-827-8717: Cross-country skiers, cycle ergometers, rowing machines, treadmills

Universal Fitness Products, PO Box 1270, Cedar Rapids, IA 52406, 800-553-7901: Treadmill, wind-trainer cycle ergometers, weight training equipment

Water Rowers, 30 Cutler St., Warren, RI 02885, 800-852-2210: Rowing machines

11 Exercise Leadership and Motivation

Purpose: To familiarize exercise leaders with administrative problems and student concerns in conducting physical fitness programs.

Objectives: At the end of this chapter, the reader will be able to do the following:

1. Define leadership and list the identifiable traits of an effective leader in an exercise setting.
2. Design an organizational plan for facilities, equipment, and supplies for a fitness program.
3. Know how to schedule events and staff.
4. Design a fitness notebook that will adequately store fitness assessments, profiles, and exercise prescriptions and that will aid other instructors and help with liability concerns.
5. List the eight reasons for engaging in physical activity and the relationship between knowledge, attitude, and behavior.
6. Discuss the physiological responses that occur when a person exercises.
7. Identify the seven barriers to modifying fitness behavior.
8. List and explain the various ways of motivating individuals to continue in their exercise programs.

INTRODUCTION

There are numerous administrative matters that an instructor has to be aware of in order to organize and conduct a physical fitness program. The day-to-day challenge of ensuring that facilities, staff, and equipment are readily available is a major one. An instructor must also be concerned with the medical and physical capabilities of the participant and the types of exercise the participant can accomplish. How can the instructor motivate students to work hard at improving their fitness levels? Those are major problems that all exercise instructors must face and resolve.

LEADERSHIP

Leaders actively seek not only to define and interpret the aims, goals, and roles but also to build cohesive, value-infused social structure that drives the individual toward achieving the purposes. The qualities of leadership go beyond the means and process, the routine organizational maintenance, and includes the skills needed to build interpersonal leadership. Most importantly, a leader must have a firm grip on significant goals to be achieved.[1]

TABLE 11.1
Identifiable Leadership Traits[1,2]

Knowledge. The instructor has at least one of the following:
   Degree in physical education
   Certification by a respected institution
   Length of experience and activity
Class Control. The instructor:
   Gives confident instruction
   Warns and questions any orthopedic limitations
   Provides positive feedback
   Shows different levels of intensity and difficulty with exercises
Motivation. The instructor:
   Is enthusiastic
   Shows concern for students' well being
   Makes each student feel safe
   Offers encouragement
Appearance. The instructor:
   Appears clean, fresh, dressed appropriately
   Has good posture and bearing
   Is energetic
   Is a positive role model for participants

The physical fitness instructor will be the most important ingredient in the success or failure of a fitness program. Your professionalism and dedication will make the difference between a mediocre or well-run program. Being a good leader is the one trait that will determine how much impact you will have on the students and their motivation to adopt new fitness strategies. It has been said that good leadership accounts for approximately 50% of the success in a physical fitness program. You as the fitness leader will function as an agent for behavior change and as a role model for the students.

The instructor has three primary responsibilities as the exercise leader.[2] For a program to be a success, all three of these responsibilities must be met.

Recognize the individual: Design exercise programs based on individual fitness assessments; counsel individual students on nutrition, diet, and exercise programs; and motivate students to improve performance.

Organize group activities: Organize and plan specific group functions, i.e., plan time in the weight room, group runs, or group games (basketball, volleyball, aerobics).

Develop program management: Design a total fitness program that involves facilities, equipment, staff, and participant safety.

ORGANIZATIONAL PLAN

Facility: What type of facility will be used in the course? Is it a gym? Is there access to a weight room? Where can the participants run and do calisthenics workouts? Is there an area for aerobics, softball, swimming, or other activities? Is there access to

TABLE 11.2
Optimal Facility Features

a. Gymnasium	f. Administrative area to store records and equipment
b. Weight room	g. Obstacle course
c. Playing field	h. Locker and rest rooms
d. Classroom	i. Swimming pool
e. Track or running course	j. Parking

TABLE 11.3
Safety Considerations for Exercise Programming[3]

Clearly marked location for emergency supplies

Clear plan for emergencies, with phone numbers and scripts to report a problem

Regular staff emergency practices

All electrical equipment should be properly secured and grounded

Treadmills should have emergency cut-off switches

Specific weekly and monthly maintenance checklist

Mounted safety instruction in clear sight near the equipment

Be sure equipment

- Accommodates the size of all users (or is restricted)
- Does not force joint movement beyond normal range
- Does not force the body into an abnormal position (back hyperextension)
- Has wide benches that support whole body and weight of the body

Adequate racks for free weights, width to accommodate Olympic-style bars

No physical obstructions in exercise area (posts, steps, uneven floors)

a nearby telephone in case of an emergency? How safe are the facilities? Are there obstacles in the workout areas that could cause accidents (stairs, columns, railings, trees)? Can the instructor keep the participants in sight during the workouts? Is any indoor facility air-conditioned or heated? The instructor needs to determine the answers to those questions before the class starts because they will determine what your students will be able to do. The instructor may need to arrange for an off-site facility such as a school gym, recreation center, or even public areas such as parks and fields. Long-distance running may have to be completed on nearby city streets. Be sure that you have access to (and have reserved) the specific facility that you choose. It is your responsibility to make sure that you have the facility or training area reserved.

Equipment/Supplies: Many fitness courses can be initiated with minimal equipment and supplies. However, successful programs require the purchase of some equipment. It is the responsibility of the fitness instructor to advise the person in charge of financial decisions of program needs. In the interim, the instructor may have to be creative and either borrow the needed items, improvise, or make them. The following (Table 11.4) is a list of items needed to successfully conduct a complete fitness assessment.

TABLE 11.4
Equipment and Supplies Needed for Exercise Testing

a. Blood pressure cuff	h. Steel tape measure
b. Stethoscope	i. Scales
c. Stopwatch	j. Leg press machine
d. Step bench	k. Bench press machine
e. Metronome	l. Floor mats
f. Yardstick or Sit & Reach Box	m. Basic first aid kit
g. Skinfold calipers	

Staff: It is recommended that one instructor be responsible for the program.[4] That person is in charge of maintaining the records, assessing the participants, and designing exercise prescriptions. However, having a varied and challenging program will require several instructors. If it is not possible to have additional help with the fitness program, there should be at least one other person who is certified to teach and supervise the course in the instructor's absence. That person should understand the exercise prescriptions and how to monitor each participant's progress. The liability is too great to have an untrained instructor in charge if a serious injury should occur.

The staff could also include individuals the principle instructor has personally trained to assist with the weight program, fitness testing, etc. An advisory staff should also be a consideration. Those advisors should come from the medical, pharmaceutical, and legal professions.

Fitness notebook and records: Maintaining accurate records of participant performance is a good way to track improvement and assist in the event of a liability suit. Those records should be kept in a notebook or filing cabinet. Complete and up-to-date records are important in cases of liability. The records should include the following (Table 11.5):

TABLE 11.5
Fitness Notebook Items

a. Medical forms
b. Fitness assessments
c. Fitness profiles
d. Exercise prescriptions
e. Daily activity logs
f. Injury reports

Documents of medical condition: Each instructor should have a copy of the medical physical exam performed on each participant. The instructor should know the medical condition of each participant before conducting an assessment or deciding on an exercise prescription. The medical form is important because it will help the instructor decide the kind of exercise and the proper intensity of exercise for the participant.

TABLE 11.6
Elements of Designing a Successful Exercise Program[3]

Description of the benefits of exercise

Reasonable or realistic expectations of the exercise program

Teaching proper skills and techniques to enhance confidence

Experimenting to find best, most enjoyable program and locations

Monitoring progress: Daily or weekly log

                              Three- and six-month follow-up physical testing

Reinforcement: Social group interactions

                              Note accomplishments

                              Money, symbolic (awards), physical testing

Relapse prevention, coping strategies

Documents of participant performance: The fitness assessment forms clearly indicate the participant's strengths and weaknesses and document improvement.

Outlines of exercise program: The exercise prescription form will tell what type of program each student currently is participating in.

Documents of daily activities: It is a good idea to have the participants record their fitness activities and their intensity levels (heart rate). That helps the instructor know if the person is exercising safely (in their target heart rate range). That record may also help identify problems such as overtraining or failure to improve fitness.

Documents for accidents or injuries that occur during the program. For more details, see Chapter 15 on liability.

MOTIVATION

The physical fitness instructor has a limited amount of time in which to teach good fitness habits and practices. The end result should be that the participants appreciate the benefits of working out and continue to work out on their own. Many studies have shown that 50% of individuals who start exercise programs quit within the first six months.

Many people have positive attitudes about fitness but still do not exercise. A theoretical model has been identified that outlines how people adopt new fitness habits.[1]

Knowledge: Before many adults will engage or adopt a healthier lifestyle, they must first be educated. Imparting health, nutrition, and fitness information to them is the first step in modifying behavior. Many adults will not change their habits unless they are educated about why it is important to change and how the change can be made most easily.

Attitude: When individuals gain knowledge they can begin to adjust their beliefs and attitudes. If the instructor can convince the participant that he can benefit from the program, then the participant will be motivated to perform.

Behavior: Adjusting behavior will be difficult for participants and may be the hardest obstacle faced by instructors, even in their own fitness program.

REASONS FOR PHYSICAL ACTIVITY

Why do individuals pursue fitness and sports activities? There is not a single or simple answer to that question, but there are several factors that influence people to exercise:[1-6]

a. To improve health and fitness
b. For social experiences
c. To relieve tension — catharsis
d. To express artistic style — aesthetic
e. For ascetic — willingness to forego immediate pleasure now for the ultimate goal
f. To improve cosmetic appearance
g. To fulfill the need for competition
h. To experience the partial loss of body control, providing a sense of thrill — vertigo

To motivate the student, instructors need to understand the physiological responses to exercise and how exercise helps the body.[7-10]

1. Exercise reduces the risk of heart disease and some cancers by reducing blood clotting and improving the immune system.
2. Regular exercise changes the way the body metabolizes fats. Total serum cholesterol and triglycerides may decrease with regular aerobic exercise while HDL-C (the good cholesterol) increases; thus, the ratio of HDL to total cholesterol improves.
3. Exercise brings needed calcium to the bones. As a result of normal aging and weight loss, bones lose calcium and become brittle. It takes adequate calcium intake plus exercise to bring calcium to the bones.
4. Exercise burns calories both during the activity and for a while after exercise ceases (after burn).
5. Exercise maximizes fat loss and minimizes the loss of lean tissue. There is a difference between weight loss in terms of pounds and fatty tissue loss (weight loss vs. fat loss). A diet without exercise can result in about 60% fat tissue loss and 40% lean muscle loss. Combining exercise and diet will increase fat tissue loss, while maintaining muscle mass.
6. Regular exercise can reduce an individual's adverse response to stress.

BARRIERS TO MODIFYING FITNESS BEHAVIOR

Many individuals have started and stopped various exercise and weight loss programs throughout their lives. The excuses listed below seem to be the main reasons.[1,2,8]

"It can't happen to me." Denial is the first psychological barrier; it is a way of shutting out new input. Denial prevents us from seeing things the way they really are, even though reality is often obvious to everyone else around us. Unfortunately,

---

TABLE 11.7
Factors That Can Influence Participation[3]

Family influences, supportive or unsupportive
Access to proper facilities
Flexibility of scheduling
Weather conditions
Convenience for activity
Cues and prompts that promote physical activity
Visible short-term benefit

---

for some people, it takes a catastrophic health event (such as a heart attack or stroke) to make them confront and put aside their barriers.

"It's someone else's fault that I am the way I am." Wellness and lifestyle change begins with responsibility and taking ownership of your problems. Blaming others is a trap, a way of avoiding responsibility.

"It's too late to change." Nonsense! It is never too late. What is your definition of old? Push back your concept of aging because it is becoming more and more common to see healthy, vibrant, magnificent people in their eighties and nineties. If the quality of your day-to-day life is poor, you can be "old" at age 30. If it is good, you can be "young" at 80 years of age!

"I'll do it later." Remember that change is achieved in small steps, and the time to start taking those tiny steps is now. The rest of your life starts today, not after the holidays or when the weather gets warmer.

"I've got to give up or lose the things I love." Instead of focusing on the benefits of change, most people tend to focus on what they are losing. Instead of mourning the loss of your cigarettes, second piece of chocolate cake, or the comfort of the couch, focus instead on the gains: money saved, a better figure, a new wardrobe, more self-respect, etc.

"What if I fail? I'll look silly!" There is really no such thing as failure; there are only learning experiences. All of us have setbacks from time to time. Be secure with yourself. Know internally that what you are attempting is inherently good for you. The "silly" people are doing absolutely nothing to make themselves healthier.

"I don't deserve to succeed." The participant may feel that he does not deserve to be skinnier or in better physical condition. Some people even feel they do not deserve the luxury of the workout time. Well, they do deserve it! They owe it to themselves. They are worthy persons and have the right and the need to care more about their physical condition and methods to improve it.

SPECIFIC REASONS FOR QUITTING [1,2]

Insufficient time: This is the most common excuse for not exercising. People will say there is not enough time to work out after working an 8- or 12-hour day. Some say they live too far from the spa/workout facility. How far do they live from their running shoes and street? How much time do they spend doing passive things such as watching television, reading the newspaper, etc.?

Lack of self-discipline: Some people do not have the drive and discipline to stay with a workout routine. They get easily sidetracked by the issue of insufficient time. It is important for these people to have spouse or peer support to help them stay with the program. Group activities also work well for these individuals.

Lack of interest/boredom: Boredom can ensue if an exerciser completes the same workout every day. However, there is such a wide variety of activities to choose from that there should not be a reason to keep doing the same routine over and over again.

Instructors should realize that the best way to keep barriers from defeating the participant is by expecting some of them to occur. Instructors need to understand the origin of the barrier and have an alternate plan for breaking down the barrier/habit. Old habits, even though unproductive, are at least familiar and comfortable. They are what make behavior change so difficult. The instructor should look back at the barriers listed above and add others he can think of and then ask, "What can I do to help the exerciser overcome those obstacles?"

MOTIVATING TIPS

Provide individual attention: Take an interest in the participant's progress and encourage him on a regular basis. Be quick to point out all progress and offer suggestions for future improvements.

Set realistic goals: Do not set goals that are too hard for the individual to accomplish. Start with simple workout goals that can be accomplished within a short time. Example: A person with a goal of running three miles who cannot run a mile should be encouraged to set an initial goal of a one-mile walk/jog.

Group participation: Encourage group workouts. Also, having a workout buddy helps to keep each person motivated.

Involve the spouse: Try to get the spouse and other family members involved in the exercise program. Studies have shown that individuals stay in programs longer when they have family support.

Design programs that minimize risk of injury: The workout should not cause pain or injury. It should not be so strenuous that the participant tires quickly or has considerable delayed-onset muscle soreness. Pain diminishes motivation.

Positive role model: The instructor should work out and take care of himself on a regular basis. The instructor should "practice what he preaches" so that the participants take the program seriously.

Periodic assessment: The participant's progress should be assessed at least yearly. The assessment keeps the participant informed of his physical conditions and motivates the person to either continue to workout or to start their programs again.

CONCLUSION

The physical fitness instructor has a major responsibility. The person who takes this position needs to be truly motivated physically as well as professionally to teach participants about lifelong fitness and nutritional habits. A great deal of time and effort is required on the part of the instructor to ensure that each participant enjoys a positive fitness experience. It takes a dedicated leader to run a successful fitness program, one who can work with the individuals in the program and conquer the administrative problems that will undoubtedly arise.

REFERENCES

1. Stone, W.J., *Adult Fitness Programs: Planning, Designing, Managing, and Improving Fitness Programs,* Scott Foresman and Company, Glenview, 1987.
2. Institute for Aerobic Research, *Physical Fitness Specialist Course Notebook,* Institute for Aerobic Research, Dallas, 1979.
3. American College of Sports Medicine, *ACSM's Resource Manual for Guidelines for Exercise Testing and Prescription,* 3rd ed., Williams & Wilkins, Baltimore, 1998.
4. Tubesing, N.L. and Tubesing, D., *Structured Exercises in Wellness Promotion,* Vol. 3, Whole Person Press, Duluth, 1986.
5. Cooper, P.G., *Aerobics: Theory and Practice,* Aerobics and Fitness Association of America, Sherman Oaks, 1985.
6. Tubesing, N.L. and Tubesing, D., *Structured Exercises in Wellness Promotion,* Vol. 2, Whole Person Press, Duluth, 1984.
7. American College of Sports Medicine, *Guidelines for Exercise Testing and Prescription,* Lea & Febiger, Philadelphia, 1991.
8. Corbin, C. and Lindsey, R., *The Ultimate Fitness Book,* Leisure Press, Champaign, 1984.
9. Dintiman, G.B., Davis, R. et al., *Discovering Lifetime Fitness,* West Publishing Company, St. Paul, 1989.
10. *Wellness: Skills for Lifestyle Change,* Great Performance Inc., Beaverton, 1988.

Section III

Medical & Legal Implications

12 Exercise in Special Populations

Purpose: To provide the reader with sufficient background to determine whether or not individuals should exercise in a medically supervised or normal unsupervised programs.

Objectives: To provide adequate knowledge to determine which type of fitness program is best for the following special cases:

1. Persons with arthritis
2. Persons with asthma
3. Persons with cardiovascular disease
4. Persons with cancer
5. Persons with diabetes mellitus
6. Persons with chronic obstructive pulmonary disease
7. Persons with hypertension
8. Persons with obesity

INTRODUCTION

The training of fitness instructors involves a considerable amount of time practicing the "tools of the trade." Most of that practice involves a normal healthy person. However, once in the real world setting, the instructor finds that not all participants are young, healthy, and completely normal. Sometimes individuals need special programs. For many exercisers, participation in a medically supervised program may be temporary. But for other more chronically ill individuals, a medically supervised program will be their regular routine. There is a need to know when to send those special cases to other exercise programs. Such knowledge will improve the safety for the participant and at the same time reduce the liability of the fitness instructor. This section does not tell the fitness instructor how to prescribe exercise for an individual with a specific disease. It was designed to give the instructor sufficient background to make an educated decision concerning the most appropriate exercise program for the individual.

ARTHRITIS

There are two types of arthritis: *osteo* and *rheumatoid*. Both are characterized by pain, morning stiffness, and swelling in the joints, possibly accompanied by some restricted range of motion. *Osteoarthritis* is the most common form of arthritis.[1] It has a slow, noninflammatory degenerative effect on joint cartilage. The disease primarily affects those over 40 years of age.[1] The cause is unknown. Obesity is a contributing factor. From an exercise standpoint, maintenance of range of motion is the major concern.

Rheumatoid arthritis usually involves many joints of the body, including those of the hand.[1] Radiographs typically show unequivocal bone decalcification in the hand and wrist. Blood tests will reveal the presence of serum rheumatoid factors. Depression and anxiety are common due to the pain and loss of functional capacity. The disease seems to be progressive, with periods of flare-up and periods of quiescence. The pain reduces activity levels, which in turn weakens muscles, reduces bone calcification, and lowers functional capacity. The disease may also affect the heart and lungs, further lowering physical performance.

The effect of exercise on the disease process is not known, but diseased individuals should attempt some form of exercise in an effort to forestall the debilitating effects of the disease. Individuals with mild symptoms (Class 1 and 2) may be able to perform any type of exercise.[1] However, running, court games, and competitive sports may place too much stress on the knees.[1] Bicycling, low-impact aerobics, swimming, and walking are the exercises of choice. Also, exercise in heated pools is enjoyable and can include swimming, aerobics, and running in the water. Stretching to maintain range of motion becomes important.[2] High-intensity exercise programs may not be beneficial. As the disease progresses, an individual's ability to perform those exercises becomes limited. Medical assistance is needed to determine what exercises are best for this individual.

The functional capacity of a person with arthritis may be limited. Exercise testing of those with the least disease (Class 1 and 2) can be completed on a cycle ergometer, but step tests and distance runs should be avoided.[1] Flexibility and range of motion testing should be completed. The instructor must remember that there may be some pain or discomfort (this occurs in about 85% of the patients). But if the discomfort persists for 24 hours, the person should consult his physician. Physical training with the Class 1 and 2 individuals may reduce discomfort in the long run and does improve functional capacity.

These individuals should first be evaluated by a physician. Some authorities also suggest that patients' attitudes toward the disease and exercise also need to be explored by a therapist or medical professional.[1] It may be best to consult those professionals when designing the exercise prescription. Generally, Class 1 and 2 individuals can exercise on their own. If the person is not used to exercise, the increased risk of joint sprains and dislocations also exists. The intensity should be low, less than 50% of maximum. The duration depends on the state of the disease — anywhere from 15 to 60 minutes. Intermittent exercise, such as interval training, seems to work best (3 minutes of exercise, 3 minutes of rest, repeat 5 times). Individuals with more advanced disease should exercise in supervised programs.

ASTHMA

Asthma is a disease in which the air passages in the lungs narrow, thus not allowing for sufficient airflow to the lungs.[1] A variety of stimuli, ranging from pollutants to stress, can cause it to occur. Exercise can evoke an asthmatic response. In fact, almost all asthmatics develop a response to exercise at one time or another. Some individuals develop asthma only during exercise. The exact mechanism for the occurrence of exercise-induced asthma is not known, but it is believed to be related to a loss of fluids in the air passages.[2] Persons with suspected exercise-induced asthma should consult a physician as there are medications that can be used to alleviate the symptoms.

Paradoxically, although exercise can induce an asthmatic episode, exercise is an important component in the management of asthma, due to its beneficial effects on the respiratory and cardiovascular systems.[1] Exercise training will improve the aerobic capacities and can make the person with asthma more productive.

Persons with asthma can participate in a regular exercise program with a minimum of restrictions.[2] The response to exercise is individual. Furthermore, the same person can complete similar exercise regimens two days in a row and not have an episode on the first day but have an episode on the second day. Generally, swimming and walking seem to cause the least response, while running and cycling cause the most response. The inhalation of moist air seems to reduce the response. Thus, to keep the air being breathed moist and warm, some exercisers with asthma use nose and mouth masks. They also use those masks when exercising in the cold because cold aggravates asthma.

Prior to entry in any fitness program, a person with asthma should be evaluated by a physician and a respiratory specialist to determine if there are limitations. The safety and best interest of the patient may be served by starting this individual in a medically supervised program until the condition is controlled. The fitness instructor should be made aware that a person with asthma is in the class and know how to respond during an asthma episode. Exercising asthmatics should keep their medication with them at all times. The fitness levels of people with asthma can best be assessed by using a submaximal test that can include bench stepping or cycle ergometry. The person can then complete a normal exercise program without limitation or within the limitations of the condition.

There are some general considerations for exercise:[1]

1. The exerciser should consult a physician to best determine the medication and dose needed to prevent the symptoms.
2. The person should exercise during the warmest part of the day or indoors on very cold days.
3. The person should avoid exercising with high pollen counts, in dusty rooms, or in smoke-filled rooms.
4. The person should swim in heated pools rather than cold pools.
5. The exerciser should warm-up thoroughly. Allowing a rest period after the warm-up will give the person time to recover from any episode before strenuous exercise.
6. The exercising asthmatic should use medications as required.
7. If the exerciser has taken medication and is still exhibiting signs, it is wise to stop the exercise.

CANCER

In the past decade there has been considerable improvement in the detection and treatment of cancer. As a result, there are now millions of cancer survivors.[2] Many of those survivors have a very poor quality of life, exhibiting both psychological and physiological impairment. Recent evidence indicates that exercise can improve their lives by increasing their functional capacities and improving their mental status.

Entry of a cancer patient into an exercise program should be evaluated from two viewpoints: 1) the acute, postsurgery or postchemo/radiation therapy and 2) the prolonged recovery or remission phase. During the acute phase, there are a number of limitations and special considerations. Thus, the cancer patient should be screened before exercising and receive clearance from the physician. A medically supervised program is best if this is the person's first attempt at exercise postdiagnosis. If the disease is in remission and there are no limitations of oxygen delivery (lungs or blood) or risk of anemia or bleeding and the person has a physician's approval, then exercise can be prescribed in an unsupervised or a nonmedically supervised program.

CHRONIC OBSTRUCTIVE PULMONARY DISEASE

Chronic obstructive pulmonary disease (COPD) is actually several disease states in which the ability to get air into the lungs (obstructive disease) or to get air from the lungs into circulation (restrictive disease) is reduced.[1] Typically, COPD refers to disorders of air exchange within the lungs. That limits the person's ability to get oxygen into circulation or to eliminate carbon dioxide. The disease seems to be progressive. Individuals with COPD should exercise in medically supervised programs.

CARDIOVASCULAR DISEASE

Cardiovascular disease usually refers to three general categories of disease: coronary disease, congestive heart failure, and stroke.[1,2] Coronary disease is usually a result of advanced atherosclerosis. This condition reduces the ability of the heart to obtain oxygen, reducing the ability of the heart to pump. Congestive heart failure is a progressive loss of the ability of the heart to pump blood. Individuals with cardiovascular disease can benefit from a regular exercise program. They can improve cardiac, respiratory, and muscular functioning. But because of the high risk of death and debilitation, those individuals should exercise in a medically supervised program. There is also considerable controversy concerning whether those individuals should be allowed to exercise in unsupervised programs even years after their diagnosis.[1-3]

DIABETES MELLITUS

Diabetes mellitus is one of the oldest diseases known to man.[1,4] The hormone insulin is necessary for the cells to sequester glucose. Without insulin, blood glucose levels can rise to the point that a person becomes unconscious and even dies. Diabetes is a result of a defect in the insulin secretion mechanism. The defect may cause insulin not to be secreted, thus reducing cell glucose uptake. That is referred to as the Type I, juvenile-onset diabetes. The defect may also occur in the way the cells react to insulin, such that glucose uptake is limited. That is the Type II, or adult-onset diabetes. In most cases, the disease can be controlled with insulin injections, diet, and exercise. Acute complications include ketosis (diabetic coma), hypoglycemia (diabetic shock), and shin infections. The disease has the long-term complications of obesity, cardiovascular disease, retinopathy (lesions in the eye), renal disease, and neuropathy (nerve damage).

Type I diabetes is usually genetic in origin and is characterized by low or no blood insulin and a tendency to become acidotic.[4] Individuals with this type require insulin therapy. The form of therapy (dosages of fast-, intermediate-, and prolonged-acting insulin) should be developed by the patient and the physician. If the patient exercises regularly, he may have to search to find a physician that will take the time to work out the most appropriate combinations of fast-, intermediate-, and prolonged-acting insulin that will be necessary to complement an exercise program. These individuals should start their exercise program in a supervised atmosphere. Once the situation is stabilized, then they can exercise in an unsupervised program. However, it is not in their best interest to exercise alone. Also, they should notify the fitness instructor that they are diabetic and how to proceed if they have an acute reaction (Table 12.1).

TABLE 12.1
General Guidelines for a Person with Juvenile-Onset Diabetes[1]

1. Avoid strenuous exercise until the diabetes is controlled.
2. Avoid insulin administration to active limbs within an hour of exercise.
3. Reduce insulin dosage or increase food intake when increasing the exercise regimen.
4. Avoid exercise during peak insulin activity. A physician can determine the appropriate times.
5. Monitor blood glucose frequently.
6. Ingest carbohydrate snacks before, during, and after prolonged workouts.
7. Try to keep the day-to-day exercise regimen at the same time each day and similar in intensity and duration.
8. Wear proper fitting footwear and use proper hygiene to reduce the possibility of infections and gangrene.

Type II diabetes occurs later in life, around age 40 or possibly after a pregnancy.[4] The onset is gradual. The disease is characterized by normal or high levels of circulating insulin and high levels of blood glucose. Over 90% of Type II diabetics are obese. Those individuals need dietary counseling. A diet high in complex carbohydrates and low in fat seems to work best. Exercise can be a benefit to the Type II diabetic. It will increase the muscle cell's sensitivity to insulin and cellular uptake of glucose (lowering blood glucose levels) and help the person lose weight. Exercise training can reduce the risk of cardiovascular disease, improve circulation, and generally improve the diabetic's outlook on life. Many Type II diabetics find that when they exercise and control their diet, their weight is decreased and insulin therapy can be reduced.

TABLE 12.2
Type II Diabetic Exercise Guidelines[1]

1. Find a physician that understands the relationship between exercise and diabetes and is willing to take the time to formulate the proper forms of treatment.
2. Avoid strenuous exercise until the diabetes is controlled.
3. Diabetics with retinopathy should avoid strenuous exercise, including weight lifting.
4. Monitor blood glucose levels frequently.
5. Eat a carbohydrate snack before exercise.
6. Eat a carbohydrate snack before, during, and after prolonged exercise.
7. Try to keep the day-to-day exercise regimen similar and at the same time of day. That makes it easier to control diet and insulin.
8. Drink fluids during exercise sessions.
9. Keep the exercise program regular and use it as an adjunct to insulin. The reason is that the effects of exercise last only about 48 hours.
10. Wear proper fitting footwear and use proper hygiene to reduce the possibility of gangrene.

Type II diabetics can participate in regular exercise programs without restrictions. In fact, there are successful professional and world-class athletes who are diabetics. The following guidelines should be followed (Table 12.2).

The decision to allow a diabetic into an unsupervised exercise program is difficult. If an instructor decides to allow the person to participate, the instructor should obtain medical clearance before the individual exercises. Exercisers and instructors need to know when a diabetic is under their supervision or exercising with them. An emergency plan needs to be developed in conjunction with the diabetic and his physician. The instructor should know the signs and symptoms of diabetic-induced coma (hyperglycemia) and shock (hypoglycemia). The instructor should keep a sugar or a glucose solution on hand, especially when the person is exercising away from a supervised area.

HYPERTENSION

Hypertension, like cardiovascular disease, has been discussed in some detail in earlier chapters. The problem with a person with hypertension exercising is that abnormally high blood pressures can be attained during high-intensity exercise, which can cause small or weakened blood vessels to burst. Conversely, exercise can benefit the individual with hypertension by helping to reduce blood pressure.[1,3] This effect is best seen in individuals with borderline hypertension. In fact, several studies note the importance of exercise as part of the treatment for hypertension. Aerobic exercises seem to be best, because the rhythmicity of the activity improves circulation, resulting in lower blood pressures than would occur during weight lifting or sprinting. However, individuals with hypertension need to be evaluated by a physician before they take part in any exercise program. Part of that evaluation should include a stress test. Individuals with pressures at or above 150/95 mmHg should exercise in medically supervised programs. Those with borderline pressures

(135–145 over 85–95 mmHg and no ventricular hypertrophy) can exercise in supervised or unsupervised programs. Their blood pressure should be routinely checked, and if any unusual pressures are found, the participant should be removed from the program and obtain medical clearance to re-enter.

The fitness instructor needs to be aware of participants with hypertension and their medications. Some medications used for hypertension increase urine output. Increased urine output, if uncontrolled, can lead to dehydration and potassium imbalances and result in cardiac arrhythmias. Other medications used for hypertension lower the heart rate and blood pressure responses to exercise; thus, the person may not be able to attain normal target heart rates.

OBESITY

Obesity can be defined as a surplus of fat, usually around 25% for men and 30% for women.[1,3] Gross or morbid obesity is about 5% higher for each gender. Obesity is associated with other health problems (Table 12.3). The loss of weight can contribute to the general health and well being of the obese individual. Exercise can be used to control weight and positively influence many of the complications of obesity.

TABLE 12.3
Related Complications of Obesity

Respiratory abnormalities	Hypertension	Gout
Congestive heart failure	Atherosclerosis	Ulcers
Cirrhosis of the liver	Certain cancers	Arthritis
Gall bladder diseases	Renal problems	Accidents
Menstrual dysfunction	Appendicitis	Diabetes

Obese persons present a significant problem to the fitness instructor. They may not feel they have any limitations and may not want to be treated any differently than normal, but they will need special consideration. Those individuals should receive medical clearance before participating in an unsupervised program. The screening process should include stress testing.

Submaximal exercise testing may best be completed using a cycle ergometer.[1] Bench stepping is not recommended for morbid obese persons, nor is running a specific distance. A 12-minute walk could be used. The exercise program can include any aerobic activity. However, activities such as court (basketball or racquetball) and field (softball or football) games or high impact aerobic dance may lead to injury. Fast walking may be the best exercise to begin with. Other activities that work well include swimming, low-impact aerobic dance, cycling and even a walk/jog program. The surfaces used for the exercise program should be fairly smooth, because an uneven surface presents an easy way to injure a foot or leg. Weight lifting will not help on obese person lose weight. Also, keep in mind that these individuals can heat up quickly, so exercise in the heat may be difficult for them to tolerate.

CONCLUSION

Even in apparently healthy populations there are those who are at high health risk for exercise. Many of those individuals can and should exercise. In fact, considerable evidence suggests that exercise is good for most of those special cases. It may not help them recover from their diseased state, but it can improve their psychological well-being. These individuals are *not* served best by unsupervised or nonmedically supervised programs and should be screened from those programs. It is the obligation of a fitness instructor to direct these individuals to the appropriate program. Further, the fitness instructor should work with the consulting physician to determine when and if those individuals can return to an unsupervised or nonmedically supervised program and to what extent they can safely exercise.

REFERENCES

1. Skinner, J.S., *Exercise Testing and Exercise Prescription for Special Cases,* Lea & Febiger, Philadelphia, 1993.
2. Watson, R.R. and Eisinger, M., *Exercise and Disease,* CRC Press, Boca Raton, FL, 1992.
3. Stone, W.J., *Adult Fitness Programs: Planning, Designing, Managing, and Improving Fitness Programs,* Scott Foresman and Company, Glenview, 1987.
4. Cantu, R.C., *Diabetes and Exercise,* E.P. Dutton Inc., New York, 1982.

13 Medications and Exercise

Purpose: To give the reader a basic understanding of how drugs can affect the exercise response.

Objectives: To obtain the following:

1. An understanding of how the basic categories of drugs interact with exercise.
2. An understanding of which medicated individuals should not participate in an unsupervised exercise program.

INTRODUCTION

The management of many diseases has undergone significant changes during the past three decades. The greatest change for many of these diseases is the greater reliance on medication therapies. Simultaneously, there has been an increased effort to incorporate exercise into the lifestyle of individuals who have these diseases. Most drugs taken for various maladies permit normal exercise. However, there are as many exceptions as there are drugs that support this rule. Some medications limit the exercise capacity by restricting heart rate, cardiac output, blood pressure, or even reducing the ability of the heart to contract. Other medications affect metabolism.

Most medications have dose-related effects, with small dosages causing minimal or no effect and large dosages bringing about very significant therapeutic effects. However, many drugs can cause toxic responses, even death, when given in too large a dosage or for prolonged periods of time. Some medications increase or decrease their potency when administered in combination with other medications. Some medications can induce other clinical problems. For example, the use of diuretics can cause the loss of too much blood volume (hypovolemia), which increases the potential for orthostatic hypotension or dizziness when standing up quickly. Thus, there is a need to know some of the basic effects of these drugs in order to improve the safety of the exerciser. Fitness instructors also need to know this information to determine whether the individual should be exercising in an unsupervised program. The following discussion will introduce the major categories of drugs that could affect the ability to exercise, explain when they are normally prescribed, clarify how they affect exercise, and give any other information that might be needed to make informed decisions about participation in exercise programs. For further information on drugs, consult a local pharmacist.

ALPHA ADRENERGIC BLOCKERS

Alpha blockers are used for hypertension and congestive heart failure in some instances.[1-3] Recently, these drugs have been found to be useful for enlarged prostate in men. The drug lowers blood pressure by reducing blocking norepinephrine receptors (one type of adrenaline) that control the diameter of the blood vessels.[2] Some of these drugs cause a reflex tachycardia (fast heart rate).[2]

Alpha blockers reduce resting and exercise blood pressure; the effect is most pronounced with the diastolic pressure.[2] They do not seem to affect cardiovascular responses to exercise. Persons using these drugs should be tested by a qualified physician and initially participate in a supervised monitored exercise program until released by a physician.[1,3,4]

Generic Name	Brand Name
Doxazosin	Cardura
Prazosin	Minipress
Terazosin	Hytrin

BETA BLOCKERS

Beta blockers are among the most prescribed medications.[1,2] They are commonly prescribed for post heart attack patients, post coronary artery bypass patients, hypertension, tachycardia, cardiac arrhythmias, angina, tremors, migraine headaches, and even psychological disturbances. There are subcategories of these drugs that selectively affect specific receptors.[2,4] For example, Tenormin and Lopressor have effects on the heart but do not cause vasodilation.[3] Visken will not lower resting heart rate and blood pressure as much as the others.[3-5] Thus, the side effects may vary.

In general, beta blockers suppress resting heart rate and blood pressure.[1-4] The effect on blood pressure could be due to the reduced heart rate and contractility of the heart, or vasodilation. Some beta blockers also reduce renin release from the kidney, which causes greater urine output and reduces the presence of the vasoconstrictor, angiotensin.[4] The combined effect is to lower blood pressure. Beta blockers also inhibit the synthesis of thromboxine, a potent vasoconstrictor.[4] The effect helps lower blood pressure. Beta blockers in general have the capacity to reduce platelet aggregation, reducing potential for clotting. Beta blockers are not without side effects. The have the potential to worsen coronary artery spasms, worsen claudication in individuals with vascular disease, and increase the risk of congestive heart failure (because of the depressed heart functioning). They also cause weight gain in some individuals and depress sex drive in others.

Beta blockers also suppress both submaximal and maximal exercise heart rate and blood pressure, limiting the capacity of the individual to exercise. Beta blockers will reduce ischemia in the heart by reducing the oxygen demand of the heart muscle. That effect will increase the exercise capacity of some angina patients. Because the heart rate is affected, normal target heart rates cannot be used for defining exercise intensities when individuals are taking this medication. Individuals taking any of these medications should be exercise-tested by a qualified physician before starting any exercise program and should initially exercise in a supervised, monitored program until released by a physician.[1,4]

Generic Name	Brand Name
Acebutolol	Sectral
Atenolol	Tenormin
Betaxolol	Kerlone
Bisoprolol	Zebeta
Carteolol	Cartrol
Esmolol	Brevibloc
Metoprolol	Lopressor, Toprol
Nadolol	Corgard
Penbutolol	Levatrol
Pindolol	Visken
Propranolol	Inderal
Sotalol	Betapace
Timolol	Blocadren
Labetalol*	Trandate, Normodyne

* Both alpha and beta blocker

CENTRAL ALPHA AGONISTS

Alpha agonists are usually prescribed for hypertension.[1,2] These medications are not as frequently prescribed as they used to be. They stimulate the alpha adrenergic receptors in the brain, blocking the release of catecholamines (adrenaline). Thus, they blunt the sympathetic response to exercise and reduce blood pressure and heart rate. Individuals taking these medications should be exercise-tested by a qualified physician and obtain a physician's approval before exercising in an unsupervised program.[1]

Generic Name	Brand Name
Clonidine	Catepres (Oral or patch)
Methyldopa	Aldoclor, Aldomet, Aldoril
Guanabenz	Wytensin

NITRATES

Nitrates are medications commonly used in individuals that have angina, coronary spasms, and possibly hypertension.[1,2,4] They work by causing the vascular system to relax. That increases the venous return to the heart and increases blood flow to the coronary arteries. The combined effect decreases myocardial oxygen demand, reducing angina. Nitrites have the potential to cause orthostatic hypotension. This occurs because the nitrates keep blood vessels dilated. Reclining or sitting for extended periods causes the blood to pool in the lower extremities. Then when the person stands abruptly, the pooled blood cannot get back to the heart fast enough, and the person feels light-headed, dizzy, or passes out. Because the blood pressure is low, some individuals get headaches. Flushed sensations from the vasodilation are also common side effects. Some of these side effects disappear with time or reduced dosage.

Nitrates and nitroglycerin will increase the resting and exercise heart rate and usually reduce the blood pressure.[1,2,4] By improving myocardial oxygen perfusion, the exercise capacity will be improved over the nonmedicated state. The incidence of angina will also be reduced. Nitrates will improve the exercise capacity of individuals with congestive heart failure. They also cause venous pooling, which reduces venous return and lowers blood pressure. Individuals taking nitrates should complete an active cool down to avoid further venous pooling and lower the risk of syncope after exercise. Individuals taking nitrates should be initially exercise-tested by a qualified physician and start their exercise program (6 to 12 months) in a supervised, monitored exercise program.[1,4]

Generic Name	Brand Name
Isosorbide dinitrate	Isordil, Dilatrate, Sorbitrate
Isosorbide mononitrate	Ismo, Monoket
Nitroglycerin	Nitrostat, Nitrolingual spray
Nitroglycerin ointment	Nitrol ointment (Hospital use)
Nitroglycerin patches	Transderm Nitro, Nitro-Dur II, Nitrodisc
Pentaerythritol tetranitrate	Cardilate

CALCIUM CHANNEL BLOCKERS

Calcium channel blockers are used for cardiac patients who suffer from angina, coronary artery spasms, hypertension, and some cardiac arrhythmias.[1,2,4] The drugs inhibit the outflow of calcium in the cardiac and smooth muscle, thus causing the blood vessels to dilate. These drugs may also slow the electrical conduction between the atria and ventricles of the heart, slowing heart rate. The combined effect is to lower the oxygen demands of the heart and improve the oxygen supply to the heart. The effects of these drugs vary. Nifedipine will increase resting and exercise heart rate but lower the blood pressure.[3] Diltiazem and Verapamil will lower the resting and exercise heart rate and blood pressure.[3] In general, all channel blockers will improve the angina patient's ability to exercise but have no effect in patients without angina.[2]

Some of these drugs can cause significant side effects, including headache, flushing, orthostatic hypotension, dizziness, syncope, and constipation.[4] Peripheral edema can occur with Nifedipine. Some cases of death have been recently reported that were believed to have been related to prolonged use of calcium channel blockers.

Generic Name	Brand Name
Amlodipine	Norvasc
Bepridil	Vascor
Diltiazem	Cardizem, Dilacor, Tiazac
Felodipine	Plendil
Isradipine	DynaCirc
Nicardipine	Cardene
Nifedipine	Procardia, Adalat
Nimodipine	Nimotop
Nisoldipine	Sular
Nitrendipine	Baypress
Verapamil	Calan, Covera, Isoptin, Verelan

DIGITALIS

Digitalis is commonly used for patients experiencing heart failure or certain atrial arrhythmias.[2,4] It has been used for over 200 years.[4] Digitalis works by altering the sodium/potassium exchange across the cardiac muscle cell, which causes an increased contractility of the heart. The drug also reduces the conduction of electrical impulses through the AV node, thereby reducing the ventricular response to the atrial arrhythmia. Side effects are almost nonexistent unless toxic limits are reached.[4] The cardiac arrhythmias are common.

Digitalis will decrease the resting and exercise heart rate, but it does not affect the blood pressure response. It will improve the exercise capacity of patients with atrial arrhythmias and/or congestive heart failure. Digitalis causes an abnormal ECG. Hence, individuals taking that drug should not be considered for exercise-testing by anyone other than a qualified physician and should exercise in a supervised program.[1,2]

Generic Name	Brand Name
Digoxin	Lanoxin
Digitoxin	Crystodigin

ACE INHIBITORS

Angiotensin-Converting Enzyme (ACE) Inhibitors, like digitalis, are used for congestive heart failure and hypertension.[2,4] They work to reduce blood pressure by suppressing the renin-angiotensin-aldosterone system, a hormonal system regulating urine output, sodium retention and vasoconstriction. The drug is usually used for patients that do not respond to less severe treatment. The side effects include orthostatic hypotension, depression, fatigue, and a decreased desire to exercise.[4] ACE inhibitors affect the exercise responses similarly to digitalis. Exercisers using ACE inhibitors should always complete an active cool down after exercise due to the increased possibility of hypotension and fainting.

Generic Name	Brand Name
Benazepril	Lotensin
Captopril	Capoten
Enalapril	Vasotec
Fosinopril	Monopril
Lisinopril	Prinivil, Zestril
Moexipril	Univasc
Quinapril	Accupril
Ramipril	Altace
Trandolapril	Mavik

PERIPHERAL VASODILATORS

These medications are prescribed for hypertension and in some cases, congestive heart failure.[1,4] Certain vasodilators work by producing vasodilation, like the alpha blockers, while others restrain the regulation of sympathetic outflow by the central nervous system and cause vasodilation. The nonadrenergic vasodilators directly produce dilation of smooth muscle located in the vessels.[4] The dilation decreases blood pressure, which in turn, reduces the work of the heart. and potentially hypotension. The anti-adrenergic agents suppress central nervous system sympathetic nerve activity, which causes vasodilation and lower blood pressure.[4]

Peripheral vasodilators generally do not have any effect on resting and exercise heart rates, but some can cause the heart rate to increase and others may cause it to decrease. The nonadrenergic vasodilators can cause reflex tachycardia (fast heart rate). All result in a decrease in blood pressure, which may cause post-exercise hypotension, although some forms cause a transient hyperglycemia. The antiadrenergic agents may or may not decrease resting heart rate and blood pressure. They can also cause depression, fatigue, and a reduced desire for exercise.

In general, the exercise capacity of individuals taking vasodilators is unchanged, but the capacity could be increased for patients with congestive heart failure. Active cool down should be an important part of an exercise program for those individuals taking vasodilators. It is best for those individuals to be exercise-tested by a qualified physician before starting an exercise program and to be supervised when exercising.[1,4]

Nonadrenergic Vasodilators[3]

Generic Name	Brand Name
Epoprostenol	Fiolan
Hydralazine	Apresoline
Minoxidil	Loniten
Pinacidil	Pindac

Anti-adrenergic Agents Without Selective Blockade[3]

Generic Name	Brand Name
Clonidine	Catapres
Guanadrel	Hylorel
Guanabenz	Wytensin
Guanethidine	Ismelin
Guanfacine	Tenex
Methyldopa	Aldomet
Reserpine	Serapasil, Ser-Ap-Es

DIURETICS

Diuretics are commonly used for the treatment of hypertension, congestive heart failure, and peripheral edema.[1,2,4] They work by blocking the reabsorption of sodium in the kidney, increasing renal excretion of sodium and extra-cellular fluid (water). That reduces arteriolar sodium content and decreases resistance to blood flow, thus reducing blood pressure. Some diuretics can also cause loss of potassium, and others cause potassium retention. Diuretics can cause considerable loss of electrolytes: sodium, potassium, and magnesium, which can result in fatigue, weakness, and potential for cardiac arrhythmias. These medications may also increase blood levels of glucose, uric acid, LDL cholesterol, and triglycerides. Indiscriminate use of diuretics can lead to dehydration.

These drugs have no effect on the resting or exercise heart rate but may lower the blood pressure response to exercise. They do not affect the exercise capacity, but they increase the potential for hypovolemia and low blood potassium, which can cause cardiac arrhythmias. It is highly recommended that individuals taking any of these medications and wishing to exercise be first placed under direct supervision until the dosages have been stabilized. These individuals, with the consent of their physician, could then exercise in an unsupervised program.[1,4]

Generic Name	Brand Name
Bendroflumethiazide	Naturetin
Benzthiazide	Exna
Chlorothiazide	Diuril
Cyclothiazide	Anhydron
Dichlorphenamide	Daramide
Hydrochlorothiazide (HCTZ)	Esidrix, Hydrodiural, Oretic
Hydroflumethiazide	Saluron, Diucardin
Methyclothiazide	Enduron, Aquatensen
Metolazone	Mykrox
Polythiazide	Renese
Trichlormethizide	Naqua
Chlorthalidone	Hygroton, Thalitone
Loop Furosemide	Lasix
Loop Bumetanide	Bumex
Loop Ethacrynic Acid	Edecrin

Generic Name	Brand Name
Potassium-Sparing	
Amiloride	Midamor
Spironolactone	Aldactone, Aldactazide
Triamterene	Dyrenium
Combinations	
Amiloride and hydrochlorothiazide	Moduretic
Spironolactone and hydrochlorothiazide	Alactadize
Triamterene and hydrochlorothiazide	Dyazide, Maxzide
Other	
Metolazone	Zaroxolyn
Quinethazone	Hydromox
Indapamide	Lozol

ANTI-ARRHYTHMIC AGENTS

Anti-arrhythmic drugs are used for heart patients with cardiac arrhythmias, post heart surgery patients in which there is an increased risk of arrhythmias, and patients with congestive heart failure.[1,2,4] Class I of these drugs (Quinidine, Procanamide) works by slowing the electrical activity through the heart, thereby the automatic rhythm of the heart and excitability. And another class works like an anesthetic.[4] Class III agents inhibit the sympathetic activity within the heart, thereby decreasing excitability of the heart and heart rate.[4] Both beta blockers (Class II) and calcium blockers (Class IV) are considered anti-arrhythmics.

These drugs have various effects on the resting and exercise heart rate and blood pressure. Some have no effects, and others can decrease or increase the heart rate responses. Some of these medications can cause congestive heart failure by depressing heart function.[4] In some individuals, these anti-arrhythmic drugs can result in reflex arrhythmias.[4] Generally, the exercise capacity is unchanged. Individuals taking these medications should not exercise in an unsupervised program. In fact, many of these individuals should not be exercise-tested. Only a qualified physician can make these determinations.[1]

Generic Name	Brand Name
Class I	
Disopyramide	Norpace
Encainise	Enkaid
Ethmozine	Moricizine
Flecainide	Tambocor
Lidocaine	Xylocaine, Xylocard
Mexiletine	Mexitil
Moricizine	Ethmozine
Propafenone	Rythmol
Procanamide	Pronestyl, Procan SR, Procanbid
Quinidine	Quinidex, Quinaglute
Tocainide	Tonocard

Generic Name	Brand Name

Class II
All Beta Blockers

Class III

Amiodarone	Cordarone
Bretylium	Bretylol
Ibutilide Fumarate	Corvert
Sotalol	Betapace

Class IV
All Calcium Channel Blockers

SYMPATHETIC AGENTS

Sympathetic agents are medications that mimic the effects of adrenaline. They speed up heart rate, increase cardiac output, cause generalized vasoconstriction, and dilate the respiratory passageways. The are useful for asthma or other forms of pulmonary disease where bronchospasm occurs.

Generic Name	Brand Name
Albuterol	Bronkosol
Cromolyn Sodium	Intal
Ephedrine	Adrenalin
Epinephrine	Alupent
Isoetharine	Brethine
Metaproterenol	Proventil, Ventolin

BRONCHODILATORS

Bronchodilators are prescribed for individuals with asthma, exercise-induced asthma, or other patients to prevent or reverse bronchospasm.[1,4] Bronchodilators increase the size of the airways, thus increasing the person's ability to breathe. They have a beneficial effect in allowing a person to exercise who would normally have a limited capacity to breathe. These medications may be taken routinely; however, some are specifically designed to be only used when needed. These medications work in many ways. Some work by stimulating the sympathetic nervous system. That can result in tachycardia, hypertension, and arrhythmias. Other bronchodilators work by directly relaxing the smooth muscles in the pulmonary airways. They can also cause tachycardia and arrhythmias. There are over 100 various bronchodilators on the market.

Although these agents cause dilation of the airways, many are not without side effects. Many cause increased heart rates, increased blood pressure, and potentiate cardiac arrhythmias. Others may cause nausea and vomiting.

The methylzanthines and sympathomimetic agents will either have no effect or increase resting and exercise heart rate.[4] These drugs also produce various effects (increase, decrease, or no effect) on resting and exercise blood pressure. The cromolyn sodium and corticosteroids have no effect on heart rate and blood pressure.[5] All categories will increase the exercise capacity in individuals with bronchospasms.

Generic Name	Brand Name
Albuterol	Proventil, Ventolin
Aminophylline	Theo-Dur
Cromolyn sodium	Intal
Ephedrine	Mudrane, Primatene, Bronkotabs
Epinephrine	Primatine Mist
Isoetharine	Bronkosol
Isopertemol	Isuprel
Metaproterenol Sulfate	Metaprel
Metaproterenol	Alupent
Pirbuterol	Maxair
Terbutaline	Brethine
Theophylline	Elixophyllin, Somophyllin, Theophyl
Other	Airet, Atrovert, Bricanyl, Congress

HYPERLIPIDEMIC AGENTS

These medications are used to lower blood lipid levels in individuals with or without symptoms of cardiovascular disease.[1,4] They are generally administered to persons with high cholesterol and/or high triglyceride levels. Some of them work by increasing the excretion of cholesterol in the bile, decreasing the production of lipids in the liver, or enhancing the removal of lipids from the plasma.

Lipid-lowering agents do not generally affect resting or exercise heart rate of blood pressure, and have no effect on exercise capacity. However, some (Clofibrate and Dextrothyroxine) can provoke arrthymias and angina.[4] Nicotinic acid can decrease blood pressure and cause a flushing sensation.[3] Normally individuals taking hyperlipidemic agents can exercise in unsupervised programs, but the person's physician should make the ultimate decision.

Generic Name	Brand Name
Cholestyramine	Questran
Colestipol	Colestid
Clofibrate	Atromid-S
Dextrothyroxine	Choloxin
Fluvastatin	Lescol
Gemfibrozil	Lopid
Lovastatin	Mevacor
Nicotinic Acid (niacin)	Nicobid
Probucol	Lorelco
Pravastatin	Pravachol
Simvastatin	Zocor

ENDOCRINE DISORDER MEDICATIONS

Many metabolic disorders originate in the endocrine system. Examples include diabetes, goiter, thyrotoxicosis, myxedema, Cushing's syndrome, and Addison's disease.[1,4] The side effects are based upon the specific medication and are too many to list in this short summary. A pharmacist should be contacted for specific information.

An individual's exercise responses to these drugs will vary depending on the medication. Consult the individual's physician before exercise-testing or prescribing any exercise.

Generic Name	Brand Name
Levothyroxine sodium	Levothroid or Synthroid
Insulin	Humulin, Novolin

PSYCHOTROPIC MEDICATIONS

This group of medications includes anti-anxiety medications, antidepressants, and tranquilizers.[1,4] Minor tranquilizers such as Diazepam have no significant effects on the cardiovascular system.[4] Some, such as Phenothiazines and Tricyclics, can increase heart rate, cause orthostatic hypotension, cause cardiac arrhythmias, and cause significant changes to the electrocardiogram.[4,5] Others, such as Valium, will lower heart rate and blood pressure.[5] Post-exercise hypotension is a potential problem with these medications. Thus, an active cool down period should be required.[4] Still others (lithium) have no effect on exercise heart rate or blood pressure. The person's physician should be consulted to make ultimate decisions concerning exercise participation.

Generic Name	Brand Name
Amatriptyline	Elavil (ECG: prolong QRS & QT)
Benzodiazepine	Librium
Diazepam	Valium
Fluoxatine	Prozac (no cardiac effects)
Sertraline	Zoloft (no cardiac effects)
Lithium	Eskalith, Lithane, Lithobid
Phenothiazines	Compazine, Phenergan, Thorazine, Temaril
Nortriptyline	Pamelor, Aventyl

Other Notable Medications[5]

Generic Name	Brand Name	Effects
Astemizole	Hismanal (sedating antihistamine)	Can affect ECG
Dipyridamole	Persantine (chronic angina)	Will improve exercise tolerance in patients with angina
Codeine	Empracet (pain killer)	Can lower heart rate and blood pressure responses to exercise
	Can improve exercise tolerance	
Loratidine	Claritin (sedating antihistamine)	Can affect ECG

Other Notable Medications[5]

Generic Name	Brand Name	Effects
Pentoxifylline	Trental (reduces viscosity)	Will improve exercise tolerance in patients with claudications
Terfinidine	Seldane (sedating antihistamine)	Can affect ECG
Warfarin	Coumadin (anti-coagulant)	Does not affect exercise

MISCELLANEOUS FACTS

It is important to keep in mind that some of these drugs can be taken in combination with others, which can result in altering or magnifying the effects on exercise.[5] A pharmacist or physician is best qualified to answer questions regarding drug interactions.

Although the above medications are all prescription drugs, it is important to keep in mind that some nonprescription drugs can have effects on exercise tolerance and capacity. For example, some nasal sprays can cause tachycardia in certain individuals; antihistamines can cause fatigue and reduce exercise tolerance; cold medications can produce the same effect as sympathomimetic agents, but usually the magnitude of effect is diminished. When in doubt, consult a pharmacist.

CONCLUSION

Knowledge concerning medications and their interactions with exercise is important to the fitness instructor. A basic understanding improves the safety of the program participant and reduces the liability of the instructor. Because new medications are continuously being marketed, it is not so important to know all the drugs as it is to know where to get help understanding the implications of the use of these medications. The drugs included in this unit are the more commonly prescribed and should serve as an initial source on which to base decisions concerning exercise. When in doubt, do not hesitate to consult a physician or pharmacist.

REFERENCES

1. American College of Sports Medicine, *Guidelines for Exercise Testing and Prescription*, Lea & Febiger, Philadelphia, 1995.
2. Lowenthal, D.T., Kendrick, Z.V., Chase, R., Paran, E., and Perlmutter, G., Cardiovascular drugs and exercise, *Exer. Sports Sci. Rev.*, 15, 67-94, 1985.
3. Pollock, M.L. and Wilmore, J.H., *Exercise in Health and Disease*, W.B. Saunders Company, Philadelphia, 1990.
4. American College of Sports Medicine, *Resource Manual for Guidelines for Exercise Testing and Prescription*, 3rd ed., Williams & Wilkins, Baltimore, 1998, pp.672-673.
5. *Physician's Desk Reference* (51st ed.), Medical Economics Company, Montvale, 1997.

14 Care and Prevention of Exercise-Related Injuries

Purpose: To understand factors that will minimize injury to the exerciser, maximize the exerciser's performance, and potentially reduce legal liability for instructor of exercise programs.

Objectives: Upon completion of this chapter, the reader will be able to do the following:

1. Calculate heart rates, blood pressures, and respiration rates.
2. Know the methods used in evaluating the conscious and unconscious injured exerciser.
3. Understand the use of rest, cold, compression, and elevation in the initial treatment of athletic injuries.
4. Identify and treat four heat-related illnesses.
5. Identify and treat the following common athletic injuries:

Anterior Compartment Syndrome	Patello-femoral Pain
Blisters	Plantar Fasciitis
Bursitis	Shin Splints
Heat Illness	Shock
Hematoma	Simple and Compound Fractures
Joint Sprains	Stress Fracture
Muscle Strains	Tendentious

INTRODUCTION

It is common knowledge that with increased movement comes increased potential of injury. In fitness programs, the frequency of injuries increases dramatically as the person exercises more often and at higher intensities (the higher end of the target heart rate range). Individuals need to know that certain inherent risks are associated with physical activity and the necessary steps to control the factors that may contribute to possible injuries.

This chapter has two foci: how to best reduce injuries that can occur with exercise and how to respond to injuries and medical emergencies that can occur during exercise programs. The chapter gives a thumbnail sketch of injury prevention, as well as the possible causes, symptoms, and treatment of exercise-related injuries. The material presented here was not designed to replace or substitute a formal medical education but serves as a foundation. Remember that even fitness instructors are not qualified to practice medicine and should not exceed the scope of their responsibility and training. Not only is it a misdemeanor to practice medicine without a license in some states, but also the practitioner may be held responsible for any damages when actions exceed training. The primary intent of this chapter then is to prepare the individual to respond effectively to a medical emergency during exercise. Minor injuries can simply require self-treatment. However, if a significant injury occurs, the injured should always be referred to a medical physician for formal diagnosis and treatment.

PREVENTION OF EXERCISE-RELATED INJURIES

EXERCISE-RELATED ISSUES

To reduce the chances of a major problem, all middle-age or older adults should be screened by a physician before participating in any fitness activity.[1] The screening should highlight the areas that could contribute to an increased health risk. That information must be made available to the exerciser and if necessary to the exerciser's fitness instructor for review. Conducting proper assessments and designing an individual exercise program with proper progression are other important factors involved in reducing the risks associated with an exercise program.[1] In addition, there are exercises that should be avoided and those that need to be part of any exercise routine.

Stretching: Stretching exercise should be used as part of the warm-up at the beginning of an exercise program. Stretching can possibly reduce the chances of "pulled" muscles and joint pain. Stretching can also be used after a workout to reduce muscle soreness. Proper stretching techniques include the following:

1. Using static stretching, holding the position for at least a 10-count, not bouncing
2. Not using another person's assistance to stretch the muscle
3. Including stretching exercises as part of both a warm-up before and cool down after exercise
4. Including hamstring, calf, groin, and Achilles tendon stretching exercises
5. Watching for exercises that hyperextend any joint

Exercises to avoid: Avoid any exercise that overstresses the joints, particularly knees, back, neck, and shoulders. The following are examples of exercises to avoid and their potential risk. A full description of these exercises can be found in Chapter 9.

1. Duck walk — knee trouble
2. Straight leg sit-ups — related to low back injuries
3. Cobra (back hyperextension) — related to low back injuries
4. Plow (bring legs over the head and touch the floor with the toes) — related to low back and neck injuries
5. Hurdler's stretch with the knee to the side — related to knee trouble

6. Straight-leg leg lifts — related to low back pain
7. Neck circles — potential damage to cervical vertebrae

Exercises to do: The following exercises should be part of a standard exercise routine:

1. Bent knee sit-ups
2. Hamstring, shoulder, Achilles, and groin stretches
3. Butterfly exercises for the low back

Use *proper progression* of exercises: Start slowly in distance, time, repetitions or intensity, and increase as the body adapts. The philosophy of "no pain, no gain" can lead to serious injuries and lifelong complications. Participants should be encouraged to progress slowly and avoid doing too much too soon. When designing a fitness program, the rate of progression should be based on the participant's age, gender, body structure, and fitness level. Failure to consider these factors can lead to chronic overuse injuries, extreme muscle soreness, and undue fatigue. This philosophy should be used when planning a workout session as well as planning the long-term goals of the fitness program.

EQUIPMENT CONSIDERATIONS

The use of sports equipment presents many problems that the exerciser may not even be aware of. The use of wrong size, shape or type of equipment can result in injuries. Some of those injuries are slow to materialize and can become chronic problems. For example, the wrong size grip on a tennis racquet can lead to tendentious in the elbow. Similarly, the wrong size weight machine could cause sprains or strains.

Shoes need to fit properly. Keep in mind that not all shoes can be used for all sports. Today's athletic shoes were designed for specific activities. Basketball shoes are not made for running, running shoes are not made for basketball, and cross-training shoes are not made for long-distance running. In addition, unless the individual has been diagnosed as a pronator or supinator, avoid shoes for pronators or supinators. In general, shoes will last only about four to six months or roughly 200 miles of walking or running (which ever comes first). The characteristics of a good shoe are as follows:

1. Firm heel counter and built-in heel cup (stabilizer)
2. Cushioning in the heel
3. Flexible mid-sole made of variable-density materials
4. Arch support
5. Built-in cushioning in the sole, both forefoot and heel
6. Well-padded tongue

Racquets should be the right size, weight, and grip size. That will avoid many cases of tennis elbow.

Be careful of *broken weight equipment*. It can cause a multitude of injuries.

Dress properly for the activity. That is not to say that the exerciser must wear *only* biking shirts and shorts for cycling or a tennis outfit for playing tennis. The important factor is that the exerciser should dress appropriately for the sport, e.g., long, loose pants can get caught in the sprocket of a cycle and flip the rider. Proper dress also includes keeping in mind the environmental conditions (see the following section on environmental considerations).

Exercise environment: Watch out for slippery or uneven workout surfaces that can lead to sprains or strains. Also be aware of trees, shrubs, fences, or poles that can inflict considerable damage for the unsuspecting exerciser.

ENVIRONMENTAL CONSIDERATIONS

Although considerable information was presented in the physiology section on exercising in the cold and heat, this section presents more specifics on how to exercise in the environmental extremes.[1]

Cold Exposure

Prevention: The exerciser should wear multiple thin layers of clothing. That way if the person heats up, a layer can be removed. Wet clothing conducts heat 25 times faster and thus should be removed as soon as possible during cold exposure to reduce the potential for cold injuries. The best layering method includes the following:

1. Cotton or polypropylene next to the body
2. Down or insulation in the middle
3. Real windbreaker on the outside
4. Avoid nylon pants or shorts

Warm-up inside. That will reduce the layers of clothing needed to maintain warmth.

Acclimatize to the cold by working out throughout seasonal changes.

Avoid drinking alcohol before exercise. It will cause increased heat loss from the skin.

Cold Maladies[1,2]

Frostbite normally occurs in fingers, toes, ears, nose, or any body part that has poor circulation. Symptoms are numbness and white, translucent skin. Treatment: Warm in 100 to 108°F (38 to 42°C) water. DO NOT MASSAGE.

Hypothermia (progressive loss of body temperature) can happen during an acute exposure (e.g., cold water immersion) or can have a more gradual onset (e.g., skiing).

Symptoms are slowed mental or physical functioning, loss of manipulative functioning (using a zipper), and even hallucinations. Treatment: Treat for shock and warm. If the person is conscious, a water bath about 105°F (40°C) can be used. If unconscious, use warm moist towels; CPR may be needed.

Heat Expsoure[1,2]

Prevention: Dress appropriately: no heavy sweat suits; use materials that breathe like cotton or polypropylene.

Watch for sunburns. The use of sunscreen is justified. Watch out because some of the heavy, thick sunscreens can reduce sweating. Also, sweating may cause the screen to drip off the body. A hat is recommended.

Weigh before and after exercise to monitor for dehydration.

Stop for fluid breaks every 15 minutes and "prehydrate" before exercise.

Acclimatize to the heat by exercising throughout the seasonal change. If starting a new program, reduce the intensity to compensate for the heat. Regularly check heart rates; keep near target zone.

Heat-related Illness

Poor physical condition, although a contributing factor, is not the primary cause of heat-related illness.[1,3] Even the most highly conditioned person can suffer a heat-related disorder. The exercise load and/or the environment can place a large heat load on an individual. Severe sweating can lead to possible dehydration, reducing the body's ability to lose heat and increasing the likelihood of heat-related illness. There is a need for education to recognize symptoms of overexertion: nausea or vomiting, extreme breathlessness, dizziness, unusual fatigue, and headache.

Heat Syncope

Symptoms are fainting, headache, and nausea. Treatment: Stop exercising and move to a cool environment, increase fluid intake.

Heat Cramps

Symptoms are muscle cramping (calf is very common) and multiple cramping (very serious).

Treatment: For isolated cramps, try to slowly and carefully stretch and relax the muscle. Ice massage will also help. Ingest water, fruit juices, or electrolyte drinks. Multiple cramps increase the danger of heat stroke. The person should be treated the same as heat exhaustion (see below).

Heat Exhaustion

Symptoms are profuse sweating, paleness, cold clammy skin, dizziness, nausea, headache, shallow breathing, and/or weak, rapid pulse. Temperature may be normal or slightly elevated.

Treatment: Move individual out of sun to a well-ventilated area. Take off wet clothing and replace with dry clothes. Wipe off sweat. Wipe forehead, neck, and torso with cool towels to prevent shivering. Place in shock position (feet elevated 12–18 in.). Prevent heat loss or gain. Force fluids in small sips.

The instructor should also reassure the patient, monitor body temperature and other vital signs, and seek referral for medical assistance. If the person will not ingest fluids or vomiting occurs, call an ambulance.

Heat Stroke

Symptoms include no perspiration (generally), dry skin, very hot to the touch. The person would also have labored breathing, a core temperature as high as 106°F, skin color bright red or flushed (African Americans — ashen). And the person may be semi-unconscious or unconscious.

Treatment: This is an extreme medical emergency — transport to hospital quickly!

Remove as much clothing as possible without exposing the individual. Cool the person quickly, starting at the head and continuing down the body; use any means possible — fan, hose down, alcohol sponges. NO ICE WATER or TOTAL BODY IMMERSION. Wrap in cool, wet sheets for transport. Treat for shock. If the patient's breathing is labored, place him in a semireclining or side-lying with knees flexed position. Watch for convulsions!

INJURY EVALUATION: A PLAN

An instructor should have an emergency plan and/or procedures in case any injury occurs to a participant in the fitness program. Obviously, the most life-threatening emergencies are the coronary, breathing and bleeding problems.[1,2] Those should be considered first, and a plan to deal with those should be in place in your facility. However, most of the injuries you will be concerned with are usually of a minor, non-life-threatening nature, but they will still need a plan to evaluate the injury: what to check first, second, and so on. A plan is important because some exercise-related injuries have origins that may not be obvious at the anatomical sight of injury, and the cause could be easily missed.

The first part of the plan is to do an immediate assessment of the injury to determine if it is life-threatening. That would include an analysis of vital signs and acute signs and symptoms of the injury. Unless necessary, it is always best not to move the injured until the basic assessment is complete and the extent of the injuries is known. As part of the initial assessment it is also important to determine exactly what happened. The circumstances of the accident can give clues as to the extent of the injuries or the severity of the medical emergency.

VITAL SIGNS

Vital signs include heart rate, blood pressure, breathing, body temperature, and skin color.[1,2] *Heart rate*: The normal pulse rate for adults at rest is 60 to 100 bt/min.; for children, 70 to 100 bt/min. The best method for calculating heart rate is to put the index and middle fingers against the radial artery (thumb side of the wrist) or, if the radial artery pulse cannot be felt, the carotid artery (between muscle and larynx on throat) can be used. Count the number of beats for 10 seconds. Then multiply the number of beats by 6. If the count is for 15 seconds, then multiply the number of beats by 4.

Analysis:

Is there a pulse?
Is the pulse rapid or slow or does it appear to be normal?
Is the pulse regular in rhythm?
Is it strong or weak? A rapid, weak pulse is one indicator of shock.
Remember: Pulse rate will increase with exercise.

Blood pressure: Normal blood pressure for adults varies. The first number (systolic pressure) ranges from 100 to 135, and the second number (diastolic) may vary from 60 to 85. Pressures above the upper limits of those numbers are considered hypertension, and pressures below are hypotension. Hypotension may be a result of shock or other medical emergencies.

Breathing: Normal respiration rate will vary, but it will usually be between 10 to 16 breaths/min. To evaluate this function, you may need to get close to the mouth and nose. Listen for the respiration and/or feel the exhalation on the cheek.

Analysis:

Are respirations present?
Are they slow or fast?
Are they shallow or deep?
Are they easy or gasping, choking or labored?
Look for cyanosis — grayish blue discoloration of skin membranes due to
    lack of oxygen.

Temperature: Normal body temperature at rest is 97.5 to 99.2°F, or 36.1 to 37.2°C. Evaluation of this vital sign is important when hypothermia or heat maladies are expected. Skin temperature should be warm, but not hot or cold to the touch.

Skin color: Skin color may suggest a variety of medical problems.

Analysis:

Is the skin red? (Possible high blood pressure, heat illness, fever)
Is the skin white? (Possible shock, heart attack, anemia, fainting)
Is the skin blue? (Possible asphyxia, heart attack, cold maladies)
Is the skin black and blue? (Possible bruising, injury to tissues)
Has the skin lost it sheen? (Many potential problems)

CARE OF MUSCULO-SKELETAL INJURIES

Participants should be educated about the signs and symptoms of overuse and the difference between simple muscle soreness and an injury. Overuse injuries tend to be localized within specific body parts and "nag" the exerciser. They may not be evident at the onset of exercise, but as the person fatigues, the pain increases. Delayed onset exercise muscle soreness is usually more generalized and tends to peak 24 to 48 hours postexercise and dissipate with use and time. Usually that type of soreness occurs after a particularly hard workout or at the beginning of an exercise program. Delayed onset muscle soreness can be minimized by using proper progression of exercises and proper warm-up.

General signs and symptoms of musculo-skeletal injury include the following: [1-4]

1. Point tenderness
2. Pain that persists even when the body part is at rest
3. Joint pain
4. Pain that persists after warming up
5. Swelling and/or discoloration
6. Increased pain upon weight-bearing or active movement
7. Changes in normal bodily functions

The initial concerns in any musculo-skeletal injury are the control of hemorrhage, early inflammations, muscle spasm, and pain. The acronym for the treatment process is P.R.I.C.E. (Protect, Restricted activity/Rest, Ice, Compression, and Elevation).[1,4]

Protect: Protect the person from further injury by using padding, strapping, slings, splints, or other ambulatory devices.

Restricted activity/Rest: For persons with serious injury, this may indicate complete rest. However, prolonged rest can lead to reduced functional length of the musculotendinous tissue. Thus, some activity, within the pain-free range of motion, is recommended. Movement will reduce atrophy (loss of muscle mass). Judgments regarding immobilization should be made by a physician. In general, if pain or disability prevents individuals from performing their daily routine for more than 24 hours, medical attention is warranted.

Ice/cold application: Cold applied for 5 to 10 minutes decreases the swelling that usually occurs 4 to 6 hours following injury. It also minimizes pain and muscle spasms. Cold also initially decreases the blood flow to the injured area. Prolonged application of cold can cause frostbite.

For best results, ice packs (crushed ice and towel) should be applied directly to the skin. Frozen gel packs should not be used directly against the skin because they reach much lower temperatures than ice packs. A good rule of thumb is to apply a cold pack to a recent injury for 20 minutes and repeat every 1 to 1 1/2 hours throughout the day. Depending on the severity and site of the injury, cold may be applied intermittently 1 to 72 hours after injury. For example, a mild strain will probably require one or two 20-minute periods of cold application, and a severe knee or ankle sprain might need three days of intermittent treatment. The use of cold sprays may not be advisable because improper use can lead to frostbite.

Compression: Immediate compression of the injured area is considered an important adjunct to cold and elevation, and in some cases may be superior to them. Placing external pressure on an injury assists in decreasing hemorrhage and hematoma. Fluid seepage into interstitial spaces (edema) is retarded by compression, and absorption is facilitated. An elastic wrap is generally recommended. Apply the wrap 4 to 6 in. above and below the injury. Pads can be cut from felt or foam rubber to fit difficult-to-compress body areas. A horseshoe-shape pad, for example, placed around the malleolus (bones on the side of the foot) in combination with an elastic wrap and tape, provides an excellent way to prevent or reduce ankle edema. Although cold is applied intermittently, compression should be maintained throughout the day. At night, rather than removing the wrap completely, it should be loosened to avoid the pooling of fluids when the body processes slow down. When possible, allow some skin to be visible below the compression to ensure proper blood flow; the skin should not be blue.

Elevation: Along with cold and compression, elevation reduces internal bleeding. By elevating the affected part above the level of the heart, bleeding is reduced and venous return is encouraged, further reducing swelling.

Typical schedule for treatment of minor musculo-skeletal injuries:

1. Evaluate the extent of injury.
2. Apply an ice pack on the injury using an elastic wrap.
3. Elevate injured part above the level of the heart.
4. After 20 minutes, remove ice pack.
5. Replace ice pack with a compression wrap and pad the injury.
6. Keep injured part elevated.
7. Reapply ice pack in 1 to 1½ hours, and depending on degree of injury, continue these procedures until injury resolution has taken place and healing has begun. The ice should not be left on a body part overnight, as it can lead to frostbite.
8. Wear a compress bandage and pad at night that is applied looser than during the day.
9. Elevate injured part above the heart.
10. Elevate injured part above the heart the next day.
11. Continue this same process for three or five days.

SPECIFIC INJURIES

This part of the chapter focuses on specific exercise-related injuries. The injuries are presented in basically an outline form, giving a brief description of the injury, the signs and symptoms, and treatment. Some of these injuries are minor, such as contusions, bruises or blisters, and can be easily treated by nonmedical personal. However, some of the injuries are major, such as fractures, or chronic, such as tendentious. These injuries require recognition so that proper medical treatment can be obtained. For the exercising individual, treatment of chronic injuries such as tendentious, plantar fasciitis, bursitis, or tennis and pitcher's elbow are best treated by a sports medicine specialist.

Acute Injuries

Contusions and hematomas: Bruising of the skin and pooling of blood within damaged tissue.[1,2]

Signs and symptoms: Local discoloration of the skin, localized pain.

Treatment: Ice, compression, elevation and rest.

Blisters: Fluid filled sac on the surface of the skin causes by friction.

Signs and symptoms: Fluid filled sac near the surface of the skin, usually at friction points.

Treatment: Do not evacuate (pop) unless necessary. Cover with compression and protect from further damage.

If necessary to evacuate (e.g., when activity must continue, such as overnight hikes) position drainage opening so that blister will continue to drain. Use a disinfected needle, not pin. Use a general disinfectant in the immediate area, cover and keep compression on the area of the reduced bubble, and watch for infection.

Muscle strains: Damage to musculo-tendinous unit. Strains are classified as Grade 1, 2, or 3.[1-3]

Signs and symptoms:

Grade 1 — Microtears (small tears) in muscle tissue, spasm, swelling, point tenderness.

Grade 2 — Microtears in muscle accompanied by swelling, point tenderness, spasm, decreased range of motion and strength.

Grade 3 — Nearly complete or complete tearing, swelling, point tenderness, deformity in muscle, decreased range of motion and strength.

Treatment: P.R.I.C.E. (Protect, Rest, Ice, Compression, and Elevation)

Crutches if necessary.

Refer for medical evaluation.

Joint sprains: Damage to ligamentous structures. Sprains are classified as Grade 1, 2, or 3. [1-3]

Signs and symptoms:

Grade 1 — Microtears in the ligament with point tenderness, little swelling, no instability in the joint.

Grade 2 — Partial tearing of the ligament with point tenderness, swelling, some joint laxity (increased movement), decreased range of motion, and strength.

Grade 3 — Nearly complete or complete tearing accompanied by swelling, point tenderness, significant joint laxity, decreased range of motion, and strength.

Treatment: P.R.I.C.E. (Protect, Rest, Ice, Compression, and Elevation)

Splint and crutches if necessary.

Refer for medical evaluation.

Simple fracture: Interruption in the normal continuity of a bone.[3]
> Signs and symptoms: Point tenderness, obvious deformity in bone, sharp, radiating pain, crepitus, limited movement or weight bearing by the limb.
> Treatment: Immobilize, seek medical treatment.

Compound fracture: The normal continuity of a bone is interrupted with a segment of the bone protruding through the skin causing an open wound. Such injuries are rarely seen in an exercise program. They are more evident in competitive, contact sports.
> Signs and symptoms: Bleeding, deformity, bone protruding through skin, and shock.
> Treatment: Immobilize and control bleeding by using the pressure point above injury.
>> Cover with a clean or sterile dressing to prevent further contamination. Seek medical treatment.

Shock: A failure of the cardiovascular system to provide an adequate blood supply to the body.[1,2] Because shock can occur with most major injuries, treatment for shock usually accompanies treatment for most major acute injuries.
> Signs and symptoms:
>> *Acute*: Restlessness, anxiety, weak rapid pulse, cold clammy skin and/or profuse sweating, pale skin color, later cyanotic.
>> *Prolonged or severe*: Shallow labored respiration, dull eyes, dilated pupils, thirst, nausea and possible vomiting, below normal blood pressure, possible cyanosis.
> Treatment: Maintain an open airway, control bleeding, and avoid further trauma.
>> Elevate lower extremities approximately 12 inches off the ground. (Exceptions: heart problems, head injury, head or torso bleeding, breathing difficulty. For these cases place in comfortable position usually semireclining unless spinal injury is suspected, in which case DO NOT MOVE.)
>> Maintain normal body temperature, cover above and below if necessary.
>>> Monitor vital signs and record at regular intervals every five minutes.
>> Do not feed or give any liquids.
>> Medical treatment is required.

Overexertion, heat stress, and kidney failure: This condition is also referred to as exertional rhabdomyolysis.[1,3,4] It is extremely rare but has been related to death in some instances. The condition is usually caused by repetitive, excessive novel exercises such as 100 push-ups, squat thrusts, or over-zealous weight lifting, accompanied by heat stress and dehydration or a lack of physical conditioning for specific exercises.
> Signs and symptoms: Muscle weakness, muscle pain, swelling of the limbs, and dark urine (hematuria).
> Treatment: Immediate hospitalization.
> Prevention: Avoid repetitive, excessive exercises during the first few days of a new training program. Avoid strenuous recreational activity unless properly conditioned. Drink plenty of fluids. Avoid diuretics before strenuous exercise. If there is dark urine one to two days after exercise, consult a physician.

CHRONIC INJURIES

Shin splints: This is a catch-all term for most anterior and posterior, medial pain in the lower leg.[1,3] Pain usually increases with continued exercise. Shin splints are generally caused by pronated feet, or flat feet; running on crowned, hard roads, indoor tracks with banked turns, uneven ground or unusually soft surfaces such as beaches. They can also be caused by improper shoes or heavily worn shoes over 8 months old, or overtraining.

>   Signs and symptoms: Pain in the front of the lower leg and increased pain with active plantar flexion and inversion or with active dorsi-flexion; some point tenderness; tightness or swelling in the area.

>   Treatment: Ice, compression, rest, use of anti-inflammatory medication like aspirin or ibuprofin; arch supports (orthodics); special taping by qualified personnel.

Anterior compartment syndrome: Pain in the front of the lower leg.[1,3,4] Could be acute onset or exercise-induced. The exercise-induced form is often confused with shin splints.

Acute compartment syndrome: Caused by some trauma such as a direct blow to the front of the lower leg. It is the less common of the two forms, but it is a medical emergency.

>   Signs and symptoms: Pain in the front of the lower leg, weakness of the foot when flexing and extending, pain when trying to evert the foot.

>   Treatment: Requires medical attention (surgery)

Exercise-induced compartment syndrome: This is the most common form, resembling a severe contusion to the front of the lower leg.[1,3] Found in individuals who run a lot: soccer, lacrosse, and basketball players, and runners. The swelling of the tissue compresses the blood vessels, reducing blood flow and causing pain. It can lead to permanent damage.

>   Causes: Changing the training intensity (low to high); wearing shoes that are too flexible; starting uphill or stairs training.

>   Signs and symptoms: Pain increases during exercise and subsides after exercise; weakness of the foot and possible numbness of the top of the foot.

>   Treatment: Ice immediately. A physician is required to properly diagnose and treat.

Tendonitis: Inflammation of a tendon.[1-4] A tendon is enclosed within a sheath that contains enough fluid so the tendon can slide easily. Repetitive overextension of the tendon may cause the sheath to become inflamed and thickened. Tendentious usually occurs with overuse, thus a gradual onset of pain. The Achilles tendon is most often involved.

>   Causes: Hill running, running on uneven surfaces, sudden large increases in mileage; tight hamstrings, high arches in the foot, tight muscles of the lower leg (gastroc-soleus complex); hard shoes, no heel stabilization in shoes; and failure to complete stretching exercises.

Treatment: Ice. Exercise should be decreased or stopped depending on the degree of swelling. Crepitus (feeling of grating or grinding) signals the stopping of all exercises using that joint. Inflamed tendons are prone to rupture if exercise is continued.

Refer to a physician. Heel lifts should be inserted to reduce Achilles tension, use of stretching during warm up can help.

Tennis and pitcher's elbow: This is usually due to overuse of the joint, or using an implement that is the wrong size or weight.

Signs and symptoms: Pain on inside or outside of the elbow. Loss of grip strength. Inability to shake hands or turn a doorknob without pain.

Treatment: Ice, massage, rest. Possible heat and ultrasound after five days of ice. Once symptoms lessen, strengthen muscles, improve the techniques, and get the right-sized equipment. If symptoms persist, a physician's assistance is necessary.

Plantar fasciitis (Heel Bruise, Stone Bruise): Partial or complete tear of the fascia on the bottom of the foot, usually due to trauma to underlying tissues.[1,3,4] Fasciitis may develop into a chronic inflammatory condition of the periosteum.

Causes: Inadequate arch support, poorly fitted shoes with stiff soles; weak ankles, all chronic exercise involving sudden turns or stops.

Signs and symptoms: Severe pain on the heel radiating toward the sole of the foot. In some cases, the only symptom is the pain that occurs when getting out of bed in the morning or when trying to walk after sitting for a long time.

Treatment: P.R.I.C.E. Arch support and pad for comfort when weight bearing is resumed. Refer to physician.

Patello-femoral pain: Generalized pain on the front of the knee or on the kneecap (patella).[1,3,4] The most common runners complaint. It usually occurs when mileage increases and has a slow onset.

Signs and symptoms: Pain and soreness under and around the kneecap. Increase in pain during the first few walking steps after a period of rest. Pain aggravated when climbing stairs or hills.

Treatment: Ice and rest; refer to physician. Once pain-free, quadriceps strengthening exercises are suggested.

Bursitis: Inflammation of a bursa within a joint.[1,3] A bursa is a fluid-filled sac placed where there are structures moving over one another causing friction. An excessive amount of fluid is secreted into the sac, causing swelling. Normal sites include knee, shoulder, elbow, and hip.

Signs and symptoms: Slow onset of symptoms, including pain in joint, tenderness, excessive swelling, localized redness, and limited range of motion in the joint.

Treatment: Ice massage*, massage, elevation, and possible immobilization if needed. Possible use of heat if it feels better than cold; refer to physician.

An alternate form/type of exercise is recommended until the inflammation subsides.

* Ice can be used to attempt to control inflammation as an adjunct to anti-inflammatory medication.

Stress fracture: Caused by an overused or overstressed bone.[1,3] It is most frequently seen in lower leg and metatarsal (foot). The causes include, change in shoes or running surface, increase in intensity or distance, compensatory change as a result of some other condition, a high-arched (pes cavus) or severely pronated foot.

>   Signs and symptoms: Point tenderness, swelling, achiness at all times, even during rest; weight bearing exercise significantly increases pain; and muscle spasm.

>   X-rays may be negative initially, but callus formation is seen in 1 to 14 days.

>   Treatment: Stop exercise and consult a physician. Correct underlying causes. An alternate non-weightbearing exercise program can be used, such as weight training, cycling, water running, or swimming.

EMERGENCY EVALUATION OF THE UNCONSCIOUS EXERCISER

An unconscious exerciser can pose a serious problem. Unconsciousness can be brought about by a blow to the head, shock, heat stroke, or even cardiac arrest. It is very difficult to determine the exact cause of the unconsciousness. To recognize and evaluate the injury sustained by an unconscious exerciser, use the following procedures:

1. The unconscious exerciser should not be moved until a thorough examination has been made. Check breathing, pulse, and any bleeding. Call for medical assistance. Once the life-threatening possibilities have been eliminated, try to understand the sequence of the accident by talking to anyone who may have witnessed the event or questioning bystanders.
2. After learning how the accident occurred, decide what part of the body was most affected. Often no one is fully aware of just how or when the exerciser was hurt. Because it is normal for a person to pull away from an injuring force and grasp at the painful area, the position or attitude in which the unconscious exerciser was found may present an important key as to how the injury took place.
3. Conduct the examination. Start with the head and determine first whether there is bleeding or if there is a straw-colored fluid coming from the nose, eyes, ears, or mouth. If there is no *major* (life-threatening) bleeding, check pulse and respiration. Then look for bumps, lacerations, or deformities that may indicate a possible concussion or skull fracture. Moving down the body, check each part for deformities and, where possible, make a bilateral comparison. Palpate for abnormal movements and uneven surfaces. Placing ammonia under the nose of the injured exerciser will often cause arousal; however, ammonia should not be used on an unconscious exerciser because it tends to elicit a jerk reflex.[1,4] If for example, a cervical spine injury is present, such action could result in greater injury. The aid-giver should be completely satisfied that no serious injury is present before moving the injured exerciser. To avoid possible aggravation of an injury, transportation of the person must be directed by emergency medical personnel. When such

transportation is necessary, it should always be carried out in the manner used for moving a person with a fractured spine.

4. Complete a secondary emergency evaluation by looking for possible head injury, spinal injury, deformity, loss of function, and range of motion.

An unconscious exerciser with unknown causes occurs very rarely. The typical injuries are not life-threatening and usually are of a musculo-skeletal nature. The usual cause of unconsciousness after or during exercise is a heart attack, but that is also very rare. However, it is in the best interest of exercisers to be aware of the potential problems that can exist and how to treat the situation in an emergency.

REHABILITATIVE EXERCISES

After an injury has occurred, one of the most therapeutic tools available is exercise.[4] Although it is often overlooked, a carefully applied exercise program in conjunction with other therapies as directed by a physician can assist the injured person in returning to an exercise program safely and quickly. It should be understood that the rehabilitation program must be started as soon as possible after an injury. Failure to do so results in loss of range of motion and muscle strength and other complications. The implication here is not that the injury should be "run off," or "worked through," but a proper balance between resting and exercise should be maintained. The severity and type of injury will determine the appropriate therapeutic treatment and exercises. The fitness instructor's role in rehabilitation should be limited. Those exercises and procedures are best prescribed and directed by a sports medicine specialist or a physical therapist.

CONCLUSION

It is important to understand that physical fitness instructors should not attempt to take the place of qualified medical personnel in diagnosing and treating athletic injuries. They should however, be able to relate to the students a knowledge of possible injuries that can occur and the recognized treatment for those injuries. Medical hazards exist with exercise, and the instructor must be prepared to respond to medical emergencies as they arise.

REFERENCES

1. Howley, E.T. and Franks, D.B., *Health/Fitness Instructor's Handbook*, Human Kinetics Publishers Inc., Champaign, 1996.
2. Griffith, H.W., *Complete Guide to Sports Injuries*, The Body Press, Tucson, 1986.
3. Arnheim, D.D. and Prentice, W.E., *Principle of Athletic Training*, Mosby Year Book, St. Louis, 1993.
4. Prentice, W.E., *Rehabilitation Techniques in Sports Medicine*, Times Mirror/Mosby College Publishing, St. Louis, 1990.

15 Civil Liability in Fitness Programming

Purpose: To present to fitness instructors some of the key issues that will affect how they manage and administer their physical fitness programs.

Objectives: The reader will be able to do the following:

1. Describe how required fitness training differs legally from voluntary fitness training in terms of injuries to employees.
2. Define "disparate treatment" in a physical fitness program for Title VII purposes.
3. Define "disparate impact" in a physical fitness program for Title VII purposes.
4. Identify the principal legal requirement of the Americans with Disabilities Act and Protection of the Handicapped Statute for physical fitness requirements.
5. Describe two differences between civil liability under state tort law and federal constitutional law concerning inadequate training.

INTRODUCTION

Two separate aspects of physical fitness are important. One aspect is general wellness. The employee that follows recognized good health practices (exercise, diet, regular medical checkups) benefits from reduced sick leave, decreased disability claims, and lowered health costs. That is true even for purely sedentary jobs. A second aspect of fitness is maintaining the physical ability to perform the specific physical tasks that a job requires. Those tasks may require strength, endurance, speed, or agility.

This chapter approaches liability from two perspectives. It discusses liability from the viewpoint of participant safety and discusses legal issues associated with physical fitness standards imposed by an employer. Although the legal right of an employer to impose reasonable fitness standards cannot be denied, a multitude of legal issues should be evaluated by an employer before a fitness program is begun.

LIABILITY ISSUES OF PARTICIPANT SAFETY

NEGLIGENCE

When a person participates in an exercise program, there is an assumption of risk on his part: "known risks."[1] However, if the organization administering the program does not maintain the equipment and facilities, it may be negligent: "unknown risks."[1-3] It is those unknown risks that serve as grounds for most legal claims. To reduce liability, the organization must provide trained leaders, safe facilities, and an exercise program within the capabilities of the participants. The instructor should regularly inspect and provide upkeep of facilities and equipment as part of the duties. Those procedures should be documented. The instructor should see that medical screening of all participants for an exercise program occur. Also, the fitness instructor should be trained in basic first aid and rescue, including cardiopulmonary resuscitation. In the same vein, the agency should have a written emergency plan and practice it regularly.

Staff qualifications: The specific individuals who administer the fitness program must have received training to qualify to lead the program.[1] The training can come from obtaining advanced degrees in related fields (bachelor's or master's degrees in physical education, exercise physiology, fitness management), attending workshops administered by experts/organizations in the field, or being certified by a nationally recognized agency.

Knowledge of accepted practice: Not only must the fitness instructor be initially trained, but he also needs to be "updated" as to current standards of practice.[1] New information may indicate that some of the old techniques, exercises, and practices may not be appropriate. The fitness instructor must be aware of those changes through continuous retraining by attending workshops, in-service programs, or other educational experiences.

Standards of practice: The benchmark used in a court of law is the accepted standards of practice. Those standards are commonly accepted guidelines developed by professional organizations. In the area of exercise, guidelines have been developed by the American College of Sports Medicine, American Heart Association, American College of Cardiology, American Association of Cardiovascular and Pulmonary Rehabilitation, American Medical Association, National Council of YMCAs, Aerobic & Fitness Association, American Physical Therapy Association, and others. The problem is that not all those guidelines are the same, which can create confusion rather than clarity. Fitness instructors need to be aware of those guidelines and make informed decisions, in some cases with the assistance of legal council, to determine which guidelines are best to follow.

COMMON POTENTIAL AREAS OF LIABILITY

Herbert and Herbert, in the Resource Manual for Guidelines for Exercise Testing and Prescription, suggest the following main omissions as potential liability for exercise programs.[1] An accident or injury that occurs during any of these omissions could result in litigation.

1. Failure to monitor an exercise test properly.
2. Failure to stop an exercise test if deemed by professional judgment.
3. Failure to adequately evaluate the participant's physical capabilities or impairments, factors that would proscribe or limit certain types of exercise.

4. Failure to prescribe a safe exercise intensity in terms of cardiovascular, metabolic, and musculoskeletal demands.
5. Failure to adequately instruct participants as to the safe performance of the recommended physical activity or as to the proper use of exercise equipment.
6. Failure to properly supervise the participant's exercise during the program sessions or to advise individuals regarding any restriction or modifications that should be imposed in performing the conditioning activity during an unsupervised period.
7. Failure to assign participants to an exercise setting with a level of physiologic monitoring, supervision, and emergency medical support commensurate with their health status.
8. Failure to perform, or render performance in a negligent manner, in a variety of other situations.
9. Rendition of advice to a participant that is later construed to represent diagnosis of a medical condition or is deemed tantamount to medical prescription to relieve a disease condition and that subsequently and/or proximately causes injury and/or deterioration of health and/or death.
10. Failure to refer a participant to a physician or licensed professional in response to the appearance of signs or symptoms of a health problem.
11. Failure to maintain proper and confidential records documenting the informed consent process, the adequacy of participant instructions with regard to the performance of program activities, and the response to the physical activity.
12. Failure to respond adequately to an untoward event with appropriate emergency care.

OTHER ISSUES RELATED TO FITNESS IN THE WORKPLACE

IMPOSED STANDARDS

Injury-Avoidance and Worker's Compensation

Fitness programs should be designed to avoid injuries.[1-3] Specific standards should be related to nationally prevailing practices in other agencies. A multitude of scientific studies evaluate differing fitness programs. Thus, finding a suitable standard in a recognized program should not be difficult. The American College of Sports Medicine has published such standards.[1]

Before starting any physical ability test, a prior medical history, a doctor's examination, and fitness screening are generally recognized as essential. Specific "pretest" procedures may be selected from a variety of recognized sources: medical schools, schools of public health, university sports physiology experts, and similar sources of expertise as well as other agencies. The instructor or agency should document the selection process: How was a given screening program decided upon? Who recommended it? What body of scientific knowledge supports the screening program?

Standards adjusted for age and sex are common features of many physical fitness programs. For example, a 40-year-old female may have a slower acceptable time for a 2-mile run than a 30-year-old male. Such differentials are legally defensible as rationally related to the ultimate goal of improved general fitness of all employees. However, they may create legal problems under Title VII as amended by the 1991 Civil Rights Act.[3]

Injuries suffered by an employee during an agency-required fitness program are compensable under the North Carolina Worker's Compensation Act: "Controlling Liability Risks in Voluntary Work Place Health Promotion Programs," Popular Government, Summer, 1989, footnote 7, page 19.[4] In most cases, worker's compensation claims are paid by an insurance company contracted by the employer. The premium cost to the employer is directly related to the historical claim/loss experience of the employer. Injuries occurring in a physical fitness program can be costly. In one North Carolina city, a "semivoluntary" volleyball program for in-service police officers caused more "injured-on-duty" leave and compensable injury than fighting drunks and pursuit driving combined.

The worker's compensation statute prevents a lawsuit for negligence against a co-employee or the employing agency, except in cases of intentional injuries or wanton reckless injuries. An employee who is injured in a required fitness program cannot bring a negligence lawsuit against the employer, even if the program is indeed negligently administered. In addition, a co-employee cannot be found liable for simple negligence if another employee is injured in a fitness activity.

This feature of worker's compensation is termed "exclusivity of remedy."[3] The same doctrine prevents a police officer hurt in an automobile accident from suing the department for negligent maintenance of a patrol car. Although negligence lawsuits are prohibited, recovery under worker's compensation is almost guaranteed. The injured employee may have contributed to the injury (contributory negligent), but the claim is still valid.

Reasonableness of Fitness Standards is a Discretionary Issue for Agency Policy Makers[2]

An agency may adopt reasonable physical fitness standards for hiring, promotion, and continued employment so long as specific legal prohibitions, such as employment discrimination or protecting handicapped persons, are not violated. Employees who fail to comply with those standards may be fired or denied job benefits.

The exact physical fitness standards selected by an agency are largely within the discretion of agency policy makers. If a running standard is thought appropriate by the agency policy makers, the distance selected and the required time for completion is a discretionary matter. All that the law requires is that the standard is rationally related to the job and is not arbitrary. Suppose an agency decides all employees should have the strength and cardiovascular ability to run two miles in 20 minutes. No law fixes the distance at two miles or the time at 20 minutes. No law says the distance cannot be four miles and the time 32 minutes. So long as the requirement is not clearly arbitrary and beyond any rational justification, the courts decline to substitute their notion of appropriateness for the determination made by the agency policy makers. Judges do not want to decide whether two miles in 20 minutes is legal and three miles in 35 minutes is not. In a court of law, choosing a given standard is recognized by judges as an appropriate task for an agency policy maker, not a judge.

"*Arbitrary and unreasonable*" is the legal outer limit for setting a fitness standard by an employer.[2-4] The limit might be violated if the CEO suddenly turned into an exercise fanatic and decided everyone, including the janitor, must be able to run at least 20 miles in not more than two hours. Twenty miles in two hours might test the limits of rationality. Judges may follow the law to its logical conclusion, but basic common sense and fairness often are more important to a judge than a technical rule of law.

The broad legal latitude given agency policy makers in setting policy was recognized by the U.S. Supreme Court in *Kelley v. Johnson,* 425 U.S.238, 96 S.Ct. 1440 (1976), the "haircut" case. Police officers challenged a hair length regulation set by Suffolk County, New York. The court rejected the challenge and approved the right of the locality to determine how it would organize and operate its police force. The agency can have a uniformed force, with officers forced to wear specified clothing as a condition of employment. Thus, hair length is only one aspect of that local power.

In another case, *Grusendorf v. City of Oklahoma City,* 816 F.2d 539 (10th Cir. 1987), the court approved the firing of a trainee fire fighter who violated a no-smoking policy that required no use of tobacco on or off duty for one year after employment. Mr. Grusendorf took three puffs of a cigarette while on his lunch break. He lost his lawsuit, which he based on a claimed right of privacy and liberty. Regulations adopted by a local agency are entitled to a presumption of validity. The danger to good health posed by cigarette smoking has been recognized by the U.S. Surgeon General with the support of the health community. "We take notice that good health and physical conditioning are essential requirements for fire fighters," the court observed, page 543 of 816 F.2d.

Any fitness program that is created or administered in an unfair manner will trouble a conscientious judge, who may then seek reasons to invalidate it. In addition to the legal issues, unfairness, or a questionable justification, may also jeopardize the "political" support of a program. Political consequences may come through the city council or mayor, and no city administrator can safely ignore political problems created by a decision to fire, or not hire, because of physical fitness standards.

Title VII — Federal Protection Against Discrimination on Account of Race, Color, Sex, Religion, or National Origin[4]

The Civil Rights Act of 1964, Title 42, United States Code, Section 2000(e), created the Equal Employment Opportunity Commission to enforce a prohibition against any employment practice that discriminated on the basis of race, color, sex, religion, or national origin.[5]

A physical fitness program may be illegal under this statute because it produces a "disparate impact" on a group or because a protected group is treated differently during the training, a practice called "disparate treatment." Once either disparate impact or disparate treatment is shown by the employee, the burden shifts to the employer to justify the job-necessity for that standard. If the employer cannot do that, the employee prevails.

Disparate treatment means that a member of a group defined by race, color, religion, sex, or national origin is treated differently from other group members. That occurs most often in sex or gender discrimination cases. For example, a new female employee is harassed or given special attention in an apparent effort to provoke a resignation. Males do not suffer the same harassment. Disparate treatment can be blatant, such as a rule that says women cannot be assigned to hazardous duties.

Disparate impact may not expressly focus on a particular group. However, the use of a neutral standard may cause one group to be excluded at a higher rate than other groups. The classic illustration is a minimum height requirement. It excludes short males and short females alike. But the average female is shorter than the average male, so more females than males are excluded by a minimum height rule. If the disparity between male and female rejection rates exceeds 20%, a "prima facie" case of disparate impact is proven.

Other physical fitness standards that produce a disparate impact on females are tasks that depend on upper body strength or percentage of body fat. Tasks dependent on height for success — scaling a wall or jumping a ditch — may discriminate against Hispanic and Asian males as well as females.[3,5]

With respect to fitness standards, Title VII does not make all tests of upper body strength illegal. The courts have indicated that an employer can still use that standard if it can be validated, even if a given fitness standard produces a disparate impact as to females. Thus, a carefully designed and fairly administered fitness program can be fully effective and also perfectly legal under Title VII. Requirements that depend on height or upper body strength must be strictly tied to a clear necessity of the job, e.g., lifting a spare tire from a jacked-up car and then lifting it back onto the hub (a task used by police).

Validation of a discriminatory standard is not easy. Regulations issued by the Equal Employment Opportunity Commission require that validation studies comply with rigid scientific standards. Trained personnel must be employed to analyze job tasks and relate a particular fitness test to successful completion of a job task. These validation methods are discussed in *Zamen v. City of Cleveland,* 686 F.Supp. 631 (E.D.Ohio 1988). An inadequate attempt at validation is described in *Thomas v. City of Evanston,* 610 F.Supp.422 (N.D.Ill.1985).

The best strategy for avoiding an illegal physical fitness standard under Title VII is selection of tasks that do not unduly emphasize upper body strength or height. A carefully designed test will avoid creating disparate impact; women will be equally capable of passing the test. Use of sex/age differentiated standards further reduce the chance of disparate impact. If disparate impact is avoided, validation difficulties will also be avoided.

An example of a physical ability test that passed Title VII requirements appears in *U.S. v. Maine State Police,* (U.S. District Court, Maine, FP # 4725 J, 1983). The

Civil Rights Division of the U.S. Department of Justice approved a new applicant's physical ability test. The test included 1) Pushing a standard vehicle a distance of 12 feet, 2) Simulating a rescue of an injured child from a school bus, 3) Carrying one end of a stretcher holding a 175-lb dummy for 200 ft, 4) Climbing a flat-bed truck, 5) Doing 45 sit-ups in 2 minutes, and 6) Running one and a half miles in 15 minutes.

Two cases, *Richardson v. City of Albuquerque,* 857 F.2d 727 (1989), (attached) and *Burney v. City of Providence,* 563 F.Supp. 1088 (D.R.I.1983), (attached) demonstrate that physical fitness and officer defense training can be rigorous and stressful and not be illegally discriminatory against women. In both cases, female rookie officers failed physical training or defensive tactics and were fired. Both lost their lawsuits.

Protection of the Handicapped and Americans with Disability Act

This statute treats handicapped persons, as defined in the statute, much like the "protected" category under Title VII of federal law. Employment practices that discriminate against a handicapped person, including the obese, are prohibited unless successful job performance justifies use of the particular practice. Employers are required to make "reasonable accommodation" for a handicapped person.

Care should be given to the interpretation of the definitions of "handicapped person," and "qualified handicapped person" in Section 168A-3. Those definitions are crucial to an understanding of prohibited discriminatory practices. A handicapped person is qualified if that person is able to satisfactorily perform the duties of the job with or without reasonable accommodation by the employer.

If a handicapped person is "qualified," failure to hire, promote, or to discharge because of the handicap, constitutes illegal discrimination. Pre-employment tests are allowed, but only if job-related abilities are measured in an accurate manner. That may be difficult to prove in court.

The handicapped protection statute has not been in effect long enough for a clear interpretation of all its controversial provisions. Its definitions are broad and may be difficult to apply, particularly for older police officers who must participate in a mandated in-service fitness program.

CONCLUSION

Assuming legal prohibitions and basic fairness are taken into account in its design, a physical fitness program can be mandated for new and veteran employees. The long-term benefits to the agency are clear: Better employee health is conducive to better job performance and lowers the cost to the agency of illness and disability. Some legal assumptions must be made in adopting any fitness program. We cannot be absolutely sure how handicap protection statutes will impact a fitness program for older employees, who suffer a greater frequency of back and knee infirmities. Fitness programs cannot be used as a subterfuge against employment of women in traditional male jobs, and sensitivity is required in this regard.

TABLE 15.1
Selected Court Cases

Berkman v. City of New York, 812 F.2d 52 (2nd Cir., 1987)
Brunet v. City of Columbus, 642 F.Supp. 1214 (S.D., Ohio, 1986)
Burney v. Pawtucket, 559 F. Supp. 1089 (1983)
Donoghue v. County of Orange, 828 F. 2d 1432 (9th Cir., 1987)
Griffin v. City of Omaha, 785 F 2d 620 (8th Cir., 1986)
McDonnell Douglas Corp. v. Green, 411 U.S. 792, 93 S.Ct. 1817, 36 L.Ed.2d 668 (1973)
N. C. Department of Corrections v. Gibson, 308 N.C. 131, 301 S.E.2d 78 (1983)
Thomas v. Evanston, 610 F.Supp. 422 (1985)

REFERENCES

1. Herbert, D.L. and Herbert, W.G., Legal Considerations, in *Resource Manual for Guidelines for Exercise Testing and Exercise Prescription*, American College of Sports Medicine Eds., Williams & Wilkins, Baltimore, 1998, pp. 610-615.
2. Carter, R.W., Legal Aspects of Maintaining Physical Fitness, *Police Chief*, January, 39-41, 1984.
3. More, H.W. and Kenney, J.P., *The Police Executive Handbook*, Charles C Thomas Publisher, Springfield, 1986.
4. Summers, W.C., Title VII Challenges to Physical Fitness Requirements, *Police Chief*, February 13, 1985.
5. Yuille, J.C., *Police Selection and Training*, Martinius Nijhoff Publishers, Boston, 1986.
6. Hogan, J. and Quigley, A.M., Physical Standards for Employment and the Courts, *Am. Psychol.*, 41, 1193-1217.

Section IV

Lifestyle Considerations

16 Cardiovascular Disease: Etiology and Risk Reduction

Purpose: To provide medically sound information on the issues of fitness and disease prevention.

Objectives: At the end of this chapter, the reader will be able to do the following:

1. Identify heart and vascular disease as the most common fatal disease of adult Americans.
2. Define "atherosclerosis" and explain how it contributes to heart disease.
3. Know the four primary risk factors for coronary heart disease.
4. Obtain some ideas for reducing risk factors for cardiovascular disease.

INTRODUCTION

Heart disease, cardiovascular disease, and stroke combine to be the major cause of death in the U.S. adult population. Furthermore, they are the most common fatal diseases in adults.[1] Although death rates have declined by about 40 to 50% in the past 40 years,[2] heart disease and stroke still cause more deaths in men than women and in more African Americans than Caucasians.[2] Studies report that the incidence of heart disease is higher in lawyers,[3] individuals that exhibit Type A behavior pattern,[4] and diabetics.[1] Law enforcement officers and fire fighters may also be at slightly higher risk than normal.[5] For example, in North Carolina, of all disabilities for law enforcement officers and firemen, 37.8% have been diagnosed as heart disease.[6]

HEART DISEASE

Heart and vascular disease is the most common fatal disease of adult Americans. Fifty-four percent of deaths of adult Americans are caused by heart and vascular disease.[1] The total number of deaths from heart disease each year is about 1 million. Approximately half of those deaths occur outside hospitals, many of them suddenly. Most of those deaths are caused by inadequate blood supply (and oxygen) to the heart's muscle, which results in a localized malfunction or death of the muscle cells. The inadequate blood supply is caused by a blood clot (*thrombosis*) lodging in a narrowed area, blocking flow beyond that point. The coronary thrombosis is a more frequent cause of heart attacks (*myocardial infarctions*) than a gradually narrowing vessel due to atherosclerosis.[7]

TABLE 16.1
Health Concerns of Adult Men and Women*

Men	Women
1. **Heart attack**	1. Breast cancer
2. Lung cancer	2. **Heart attack**
3. Auto accidents	3. **Arteriosclerosis**
4. Liver disease	4. Auto accidents
5. **Arteriosclerosis** (hardening of the arteries)	5. Liver disease and lung cancer

* In order of their occurrence

ATHEROSCLEROSIS

Coronary heart disease is caused by atherosclerosis or "hardening of the arteries."[1,4] Atherosclerosis is a build-up of fatty substances (including cholesterol) and other tissue (smooth muscle cells) in the lining of arteries. That material is called plaque and generally takes on the appearance of fatty tumors or *atheromas*.[7] Later, scar tissue can be deposited in and around the plaque formations, and calcium deposits accumulate causing hardening of the artery. Plaque build-up creates a rough surface on the inside of an artery, which creates a tendency for the blood to clot and obstruct flow. There is also the likelihood that the artery may have a transient occlusion or spasm at the site of the atheroma, where narrowing has occurred. The spasm can lead to heart attack-like symptoms.

The sites more prone to buildup are the points where major arteries originate or branch, where blood flow must make a turn; coronary arteries, carotid arteries in the neck, the abdominal artery, and the bifurcation of the abdominal artery into the iliac arteries in the pelvis. The force of the blood against the wall causes microtears or injuries, which creates a site for the plaque to develop. High blood pressure, smoking, and high levels of low-density lipoproteins (LDLs) promote the injury and accelerate the build-up of plaque.[7] At the site of the injury, blood platelets accumulate and scavenger cells congregate. The scavenger cells tend to collect lipids and calcium and make up the bulk of the plaque. The platelet aggregation can result in the formation of clots that can then break off and lodge in narrower arteries. The platelets also release substances that can cause the artery to constrict (spasm), further reducing blood flow below the constriction.

Atherosclerotic plaque build-up can lead to closure of the artery and resultant restriction of blood flow. Atherosclerosis also diminishes the ability of the blood vessel to dilate, thus reducing the potential to increase blood flow when the heart is working harder. Plaque build-up may accumulate for years without causing trouble. It takes about 70% obstruction of an artery's cross-sectional area before blood flow is significantly reduced.[7,8] High demands for blood flow to the heart occur during exertion. If that demand cannot be met because of reduced blood supply through diseased and narrow vessels, angina (chest pain), heart attack, and even sudden death can occur.

There is evidence that atherosclerosis begins early in life. Young American soldiers killed in Korea and Vietnam showed plaque build-up in one or more coronary arteries. Some had advanced atherosclerosis in at least one coronary artery.[7] Thus, prevention needs to begin early.

Atherosclerotic Plaque Causes Several Disease Conditions or Syndromes

Angina pectoris: This is chest pain that occurs when a person exercises or is stressed.[8] When a major amount of plaque accumulates in the coronary arteries, the blood supply through those arteries may be sufficient for normal, light activities. However, when the work load on the heart is increased because the heart is beating faster or the blood pressure is elevated and additional blood flow is required to deliver the needed oxygen, the plaque formation can limit the extra blood flow that the heart muscle needs. This under-oxygenation of the heart causes chest pain or angina pectoris. The pain is normally characterized as pressure under the sternum (breast bone), but it can also be located in the left shoulder, neck, jaw, back, or radiate down the left arm.[7] Angina is brought on by exertion, stress, and overeating, and it goes away with rest. It never occurs without provocation. The muscle is generally not permanently damaged by the occurrence of the pain. Many people have angina pectoris for many years without having other problems. They may use a nitroglycerin patch or sublingual (below the tongue) to improve the oxygenation and reduce the pain.

Unstable angina pectoris: Unstable angina is characterized by worsening severity of pain at progressively lower levels of exertion.[4,7,8] The pain may even occur at rest, and nitroglycerin may not help. Unstable angina is probably caused by temporary clogging of coronary arteries by blood clots at the plaque site. At that point, there is usually little or no loss of heart muscle cells (necrosis). However, the unstable angina usually indicates increasing severity of coronary heart disease, which in some patients will precede a heart attack (myocardial infarction) or sudden death.[7] Many of those individuals will have a bypass operation or a balloon procedure to relieve the pain.

Myocardial infarction (MI): This is death of a portion of the heart muscle caused by deprivation of blood supply for a prolonged period of time.[4,7,8] MI is commonly caused by formation of a blood clot, or *thrombosis*, due to the atherosclerotic plaque in a coronary artery. The pain of a heart attack resembles that of angina, but it spreads and becomes more severe as the attack persists. Unlike angina, pain from an MI will last more than 30 minutes and can be accompanied by sweating, nausea, shortness of breath, and weakness.[7] The MI should be confirmed by electrocardiogram and blood enzyme testing. Ultimately, the dead heart muscle is replaced by scar tissue if the patient survives. That leaves the heart in a permanently weakened state, and it will probably never be able to pump as much blood as a normal heart.

An MI is frequently the first sign of coronary heart disease (CHD) in about 25 to 33% of the cases.[7] About half of those who suffer myocardial infarction die, most before they reach the hospital. About 90% of the victims who reach the hospital will survive, and a lesser proportion will recover without incident. Of those discharged, 15 to 20% will have more trouble or die within the following year.[4,7] The remainder may have various complications, including abnormal heart rhythms, inadequate pumping function of the heart, congestive heart disease, and increased risk for another heart attack and chest pain.

Sudden coronary death: This is instantaneous collapse and death, or death within one hour of the onset of chest pain or other symptoms.[1,8] This is the most common way 60 to 70% of the people with known CHD die.[7] In addition, in about 30% of heart disease cases, sudden death is the first sign of CHD; there is no angina pectoris or previous MI. Ninety-five percent of the people who die suddenly have major coronary artery obstruction by atherosclerotic plaque build-up. The immediate cause of death is a total disturbance in the way the heart beats. Rather than having the entire atriums and ventricles of the heart pumping rhythmically, individual muscle cells contract on their own. On an electrocardiogram this is what is called ventricular fibrillation; the electrical impulses become completely disorganized.

In some cases, the heart can be "shocked" back into a normal rhythm by the use of a defibrillator. The defibrillator applies an electrical current to the heart that causes it to recycle back to a normal pattern. In some cases, physicians and other health care workers can recognize the development of a disturbance in the pattern of contraction of the heart before fibrillation occurs. They can then administer anti-arrhythmia medications that reduce the chances of fibrillation. That is why it is so important for heart attack victims to seek medical attention *early*, rather than "tough it out."

Chronic heart failure: Chronic heart failure, or congestive heart failure, is a slow degeneration of the heart's ability to pump blood. Chronic heart failure occurs when an MI or other heart disease destroys so much heart muscle that the heart cannot pump adequate blood to supply the body's needs.[4] Because the heart cannot pump blood effectively, the blood collects in the chambers of the heart and venous blood starts to accumulate. Swelling occurs in the extremities — legs and ankles. Fluids also accumulate in the lungs, making breathing difficult. The result is fatigue and shortness of breath, especially when the patient tries to be active. In addition, long-term fluid retention can damage kidney function. Chronic heart failure left unattended will become a downward spiral and is fatal. But if it is diagnosed early, chronic heart failure is treatable through a combination of drugs and lifestyle changes.

Many, if not most, adult Americans have some degree of CHD in the forming stage and probably do not know about it. There is no practical test that will reliably indicate the presence of coronary atherosclerotic plaque build-up in a person who has no symptoms (chest pain, former heart attack, etc.). Exercise testing has been used, but it is not reliable if the person does not have chest pain during exercises. It is also less reliable in women than men. Cardiac catheterization, or coronary angiogram, can be used to show an outline of the plaque, but the test is invasive, expensive and not without health risk. Thus, the best approach is to practice methods of prevention of heart disease, reducing the risk factors for CHD.

CHD RISK FACTORS

Risk factors are characteristics or habits associated with heart disease in large groups of people. Some risk factors are modifiable and some are not. Nonmodifiable risk factors for cardiovascular disease (CVD) include family history, gender, age, and race.[1,4,7,8] Having an immediate relative, brother, sister, father, or mother less than 55 years of age with diagnosed CVD increases the chances of CVD.[8] Men are more at risk than women; further, men with early-onset male pattern baldness are at higher risk than normal males.[1] Older individuals are more likely candidates of heart disease than younger people or females.[8] With regard to race, African Americans are at greater risk than Caucasians. Thus, an African American man with a father who had a heart attack or some other form of heart disease at age 45 is at higher risk than a Caucasian female with no family history of heart disease.

It is important to understand that having one or more of those risk factors does not mean that one has or will develop heart disease. Those risk factors have been identified through studies on very large groups of people. Longitudinal (also called follow-up or cohort) studies have been most important in defining the risk factors. Those studies pick a group of people and measure the presence or prevalence of disease and risk factors. Usually people who already have the disease are excluded from follow-up. The people who were free from disease are followed and measured periodically for one year, five years, 20 years, and longer, depending on the study design. After the follow-up period, researchers look at the people with disease and the people without disease to see if there are characteristics that are different between the groups.

MAJOR RISK FACTORS

With regard to studies of cardiovascular disease, in general, the people in the diseased group had higher cholesterol, smoked, had higher blood pressure and were less physically active than the people without disease.[1,4,7,8] For example, at the individual level there are people with high cholesterol with and without documented CVD, but there are more people with high cholesterol in the CVD diseased group. Researchers have also examined the number of people with disease among smokers as compared to nonsmokers. The phrase "smoking a pack a day doubles your chance of having heart disease" means that in a group of smokers and a group of nonsmokers there would be twice as many cases of heart disease in those smoking a pack a day as in the nonsmokers. When interpreting those results, one must remember that there were smokers that did not have heart disease and there were nonsmokers that had heart disease. It is very difficult to predict which individual will get heart disease, but risk factors are one way to try to predict risk in an individual. The following is a synopsis of the four major CVD risk factors.

High blood cholesterol: Pure cholesterol is an odorless, white, waxy substance. It cannot be tasted or seen in foods. It is found in all foods of animal origin and is part of every animal cell. The body uses cholesterol to make essential body substances such as cell walls, enzymes, and hormones. The liver manufactures enough cholesterol to meet the body's needs, even when consuming a cholesterol-free diet. In fact, the liver generally produces about 1,000 mg per day.[1] But in individuals with familial hypercholestemia, the liver can produce much larger quantities of cholesterol.

The role cholesterol plays in the formation of heart disease is complex and not well understood. However, cholesterol is one of the major components in the atherosclerotic plaque found on the inside of the arterial walls. High levels of circulating cholesterol can also damage the inner lining of blood vessels, which allows for cellular debris, platelets, fats and calcium to be deposited in the artery wall, resulting in eventual blockage.

The 10% of people with the highest cholesterol levels (240 mg/dl or higher [>6.2 mmol/L]) have three times the rate of CHD compared to the people with levels below 200 mg/dl (5.17 mmol/L), or the 50% of American people with the lowest cholesterol levels.[1,7,8] Even cholesterol levels from 200 to 239 mg/dl can have increased risk when other risk factors are present.[7] In addition, there are subcomponents of total cholesterol that are important.

The cholesterol is carried on a large molecule called a lipoprotein that also contains phospholipids (a form of fat), proteins, and triglycerides (another form of fat used for energy or stored in adipose tissue). Lipoproteins are broken down into three categories: very low-density (VLDL), low-density (LDL), and high-density lipoproteins (HDL). VLDLs serve as a reservoir for triglycerides and a precursor for other lipid-based molecules. They are not typically related to cardiovascular disease. LDLs carry the most cholesterol and are associated with an increased risk of cardiovascular disease. Diets high in saturated fats result in high levels of LDLs. LDL levels above 160 mg/dl (>4.13 mmol/L) are considered high risk, and levels below 130 mg/dl (<3.36 mmol/L) are considered low risk.[1,7] HDLs are a cholesterol fragment that help clear cholesterol and fats from the blood. Individuals with HDL levels above 50 mg/dl (1.3 mmol/L) have reduced risk of CVD. In addition, individuals with the ratio of HDL to total cholesterol above 1:4.5 are also at increased risk for CVD.

Blood levels of cholesterol are determined both by diet and by inherited differences in metabolism. With regard to diet, eating a large portion of meals at fast food restaurants contributes because those meals are usually high in saturated fats (hamburgers, French fries, and milk shakes). Saturated fats encourage the liver to produce more LDL cholesterol. Also, sedentary occupations or the lack of physical activity can result in weight gain, which also is associated with higher levels of cholesterol. Generally, a reduction of dietary intake of cholesterol and saturated fat can cause a 10 to 15% decrease in blood cholesterol levels.[8]

Cigarette smoking: Smokers have two to three times the rate of CHD than nonsmokers.[1,7,8] The inhalation of cigarette smoke forces the heart to work harder due to the nicotine increasing heart rate and raising blood pressure. At the same time, the smoke contains carbon monoxide, which reduces the amount of oxygen blood carries to the heart and other muscles. Cigarette smoking enhances the formation of blood clots, which can completely block small blood vessels and cause a coronary thrombosis and stroke. Further, nicotine is believed to cause injury to the artery wall, allowing for atherosclerotic plaque to form. In addition to cardiovascular disease and stroke, cigarette smokers are 12 times more likely to die of lung cancer than nonsmokers, 10 times as likely to die of cancer of the larynx, five times as likely to die of cancer of the pancreas, and twice as likely to die of cancer of the bladder.[9]

In general, the number of years a person smokes is directly related to CVD risk.[7] That suggests that early prevention is important. In addition, there is accumulating evidence that nonsmokers living with smokers also increases the risk of CVD.[7] The

TABLE 16.2
Benefits When One Quits Smoking

1. Energy levels rise within the first 48 hours.
2. Cough and phlegm production due to chronic bronchitis and emphysema disappear during the first few weeks.
3. Respiratory function improves, and breathing becomes easier in the first 2 to 12 weeks.
4. Circulation improves in the first 2 to 12 weeks.
5. Smoker's cough will lessen or disappear in the first 1 to 9 months
6. Self-esteem improves in the first 1 to 9 months.

benefits of smoking cessation start to accumulate within the first three days. It had been suggested that the risk of a sudden MI decreases 24 hours after stopping, and the risk of early MI is reduced by 50% a year after quitting smoking. There is some evidence that shows that by cutting out smoking entirely, a person can reduce the risk of having a heart attack to the level of the nonsmoker in as short a period of time as 10 to 12 weeks.[8] The damage to the lungs may still be present, but at least the coronary risk profile is significantly improved. Other studies have shown that 10 to 15 years after quitting, the life expectancy of a former smoker is similar to a nonsmoker. However, in some long-time smokers, people who have smoked for decades, it appears that the risk is never as low as in nonsmokers.[7]

High blood pressure: High blood pressure, or *hypertension*, is defined as systolic blood pressure at or above 150 mmHg and/or a diastolic pressure above 90 mmHg.[1,8] However, some believe that a systolic blood pressure above 140 or a diastolic blood pressure above 90 is indicative of hypertension.[7] People with blood pressure above 160/110 have two to three times the risk of heart disease as do those with blood pressure below 140/90.[1] Proper treatment of high blood pressure reduces the rate of death from stroke by 40 to 50%.

Hypertension contributes to CVD by accelerating the damage to the arteries, particularly at the branching points, and promotes the deposit of cholesterol at the sites of injury. Hypertension also increases the work of the heart to pump the blood against the resistance. Years of hypertension can lead to a pathological enlarged heart (*cardiac hypertrophy*) which further increases the need for oxygen. However, cardiac hypertrophy may not be accompanied by increased blood flow. Thus, in stressful situations the need for more oxygen may not be met and the threshold for ischemia (possible angina) is lowered.[7,8] Hypertension is not only a risk factor but a disease itself. According to the American Heart Association, over 61 million people have hypertension.[1] About 47% are not aware of the hypertension, and only 11% are receiving adequate therapy.

Some occupations, such as law enforcement officers or accountants, may be at higher risk for developing hypertension. The long hours, sedentary activities, rotating shifts, and dietary habits are contributing factors. The long hours and rotating shifts make regular exercise difficult. Eating a large portion of meals at fast food restaurants makes it easy to overeat and indulge in too much fat and sodium. Mental stress, either arousal or boredom, also affects blood pressure. The body responds to mental stress with the "fight or flight" mechanism, which causes blood vessels to constrict and increases heart rate, thereby elevating blood pressure. Boredom can increase anxiety, which can elevate blood pressure. In addition, obesity, low-calcium diets, high-sodium diets, lack of exercise, and alcohol are also factors that increase blood pressure.

Physical inactivity: Data from the Centers for Disease Control indicated that 59% of the people who died of cardiovascular disease were physically inactive.[10] People who exercise at a relatively high level (running 15 or more miles per week) have 30 to 50% lower CHD rates than people who do not exercise. In fact, people who regularly perform exercise, such as jogging or swimming, for a minimum of 30 minutes three times per week have half the heart disease of those who are not active.[11,12] Finally, physical inactivity increases the likelihood of sudden death during stress or strenuous activity.[12]

The recent NIH Consensus Committee noted that 54% of adults reported little or no regular physical activity.[13] Conversely, only 30% of young women and 42% of young men report vigorous physical activity. The trend starts in the teenage years, as 70% of the 12-year-olds report regular physical activity, but only 50% of high school-age youth take physical education classes and an even greater proportion do not perform regular physical activity.[13] Today, most jobs in America are sedentary, which also contributes to the inactive lifestyle.

Regular physical activity has many benefits.[7,13] It helps improve the balance between oxygen demand and supply of the heart by increasing coronary blood flow. The heart becomes stronger and more efficient. In people with elevated blood pressure, exercise can lower the pressure by about 10 mmHg. Total cholesterol may be lower, and HDL cholesterol may elevate with regular exercise. Thus, exercise promotes a good blood lipid profile. Exercise reduces the risk of obesity and improves insulin resistance. Exercise reduces the adhesiveness of platelets, decreasing the possibility of thrombosis. Exercise may also help slow the formation of atherosclerotic plaque. Finally, exercise can be an effective stress-reduction method. Thus, exercise can have a positive impact on all other risk factors for CVD.

SECONDARY RISK FACTORS

Although not as significant as the four main risk factors, other characteristics have been shown to be related to CVD. These factors are considered secondary risk factors:

Obesity: Percent of body fat greater than 35% for adult women and 30% for adult men increase the risk of CVD.[8] A direct relationship between body weight or body mass index and CVD has also been reported.[7] Obesity has been shown to cause elevated blood pressure, cause abnormal lipid profiles (cholesterol and tryglycerides), cause insulin resistance, and reduce physical activity. The relationships to these other major risk factors is why an independent relationship between obesity and CVD has not been accepted. In addition, there is little evidence suggesting that treatment of obesity alone can prevent CVD.[7] However, reducing body fat does appear to have a positive impact on the major CVD risk factors as well as reducing insulin resistance.

There is a theory that two subtypes of obesity exist. Those subtypes of obesity have been called the "apple-shaped," or male-pattern, and the "pear-shaped," or female pattern. Apple-shaped persons retain fat in the abdominal and waist areas, whereas pear-shaped persons retain fat in the thighs, buttocks, and hips. It appears that the apple-shaped individuals of either gender are more at risk than the pear-shaped individuals of either gender. [7]

Diabetes or glucose intolerance: Maintenance of a consistent blood glucose level is important for the health of an individual. Too little or too much blood glucose will cause the body to go into coma or shock. Blood glucose is maintained in a fairly narrow range with the help of the hormone insulin from the pancreas. When blood glucose goes too high, as occurs right after eating, insulin increases and causes the cells of the body, particularly muscle cells, to increase uptake of glucose. Some individuals have defects in the insulin system and have difficulty controlling blood glucose. Those individuals have the syndrome diabetes mellitus. Diabetes is a syndrome in which the body fails to produce insulin or cells of the body become resistant to insulin. Failure of the pancreatic cells to produce insulin is referred to as Type I diabetes. That type is usually diagnosed in children and as such, may be referred to as "juvenile onset" diabetes. Failure of the cells of the body to respond to insulin is called Type II diabetes. Type II diabetics produce insulin, but the insulin does not bind at the target cells or there is a defect in the target cells that does not allow insulin to have its effect on glucose uptake. Type II diabetes accounts for about 80% of all cases in the U.S.

The presence of insulin-dependent or noninsulin-dependent diabetes increases the risk of CVD.[1,7,8] For a diabetic, the risk of CVD is double that of a nondiabetic.[7] Although specific mechanisms are unknown, diabetes accelerates the rate of atherosclerosis and stroke. Also, many diabetics, as many as 80%, are extremely overweight, which contributes to elevated blood pressure, abnormal lipid profiles, and increased blood coaguability.

Stress: Typically, for stress to be a risk factor the stress must cause a physiological or psychological response to the "stressor" beyond what is needed to accomplish a task.[7] In addition, the stress must be prolonged — years. Stress elevates catecholamine (adrenaline) levels, which makes the heart more susceptible to arrhythmias. Stress elevates blood pressure and increases heart rate. Those two results combine to increase the work of the heart, but blood flow may not be increased. As with hypertension, prolonged elevation of blood pressure can cause hypertrophy. Stress causes the release of stored lipids into the blood. In physical stress (exercise), those lipids would be used for energy; however, with mental stress the increased lipids may adversely affect myocardial functioning.[7] The increased lipids may also circulate to the liver and be converted to LDLs. Stress increases the coagulation of blood, thus increasing the risk of coronary thrombosis or sudden MI. Therefore, there appears to be a number of ways stress can acerbate cardiovascular disease. Certain individuals that present abnormal hostility appear to be at risk for stress-induced CVD.

Abnormal resting ECG: An ECG (electrocardiogram) is a graphic record of electrical activity and heart beat patterns. This test must be conducted by a physician.[8] An ECG has the capacity to determine ischemia even when overt signs and symptoms are not present. That is sometimes referred to as "silent ischemia." ECGs can also pick up abnormal rhythms that alert physicians of impending problems, such as ventricular rhythms that can lead to flutter and fibrillation. They can also diagnose abnormal electrical patterns in the heart that suggest that the heart may not be functioning adequately.

In general, the effect of accumulating risk factors is not additive. That is to say that the presence of two risk factors doubles the risk, whereas the presence of three risk factors triples the risk. Actually, each risk factor magnifies each other. In 1,000 men aged 30 to 57 who have a low cholesterol, do not smoke, and have normal blood pressure, there will be 1.6 CHD-related deaths over 6 years.[1] Smoking doubles the risk (3.2 per 1,000).[1] However, high blood pressure and smoking together make the risk 6.3 per 1,000.[1] In men with cholesterol 245 mg/dl who smoke and have high blood pressure, the risk is 21.4 per 1,000.[1] Thus, the presence of multiple risk factors increases the risk of CVD geometrically.

OTHER METABOLIC RISK FACTORS

Scientific and epidemiological studies in the last decade have brought to light other metabolic markers for risk of CVD that are found in the blood. Those include homocysteinemia, small LDL trait, elevated lipoprotein little a [Lp(a)], abnormal apolipoprotein E, and the ratio of apoprotein A to B.[14] With the exception of homocysteinemia, the other metabolic factors are derived from a closer examination of the lipoproteins. Thus, determination of those metabolic risk factors requires much more sophisticated blood testing than simply measuring blood cholesterol or lipoproteins.

Small LDL trait is determined by measuring the size of the LDL molecules. In most individuals, the large or buoyant-size LDL molecules are present in large amounts and the small particles are relatively sparse. A preponderance of the small molecules is associated with increased risk of CVD. Small LDL trait increases risk of CVD three- to five-fold and is found in 50% of men with CVD.[14] The small LDL trait may be inherited, but it is also associated with increased adiposity. Effective therapies appear to include exercise, weight loss, and the use of large dosages of niacin.[14]

Elevated Lp(a) is also associated with increased risk of CVD. Levels of Lp(a) above 25 to 30 mg/dl is related to a high incidence of CVD and acute myocardial infarction, independent of other risk factors.[15] Elevated Lp(a) is found in about one-third of the population with CVD. Lp(a) is similar to LDL but has a slightly different molecular structure. The variance in structure leads to an impaired ability to break-down clots (thromboses) and at the same time allows the molecule to behave similar to the normal LDL in that it can deposit its cholesterol into the arterial wall.

Each type of the lipoprotein contains specific proteins, called apoproteins. For example, the LDL contains only apoprotein **B**, whereas the HDL contains apoprotein A and no **B**. Thus, a high B to A ratio is also indicative of CVD, as would be a high ratio of LDLs to HDLs. Another apoprotein that appears to be associated with CVD is apoprotein **E**. However, at this time more research is needed to solidify this relationship.

Homocysteine is an amino acid derived from methionine. Studies have indicated that the blood levels of homocysteine above 14 μM/L increase the risk of CVD death by 50 to 115%; however, all the research is not in agreement.[16] The homocysteine appears to accumulate in the arterial wall, exacerbating the plaque formation. This appears to be particularly true in individuals with low vitamin B status. Thus, the recommendation for people with homocysteinemia is to increase vitamin B_6, vitamin B_{12}, and folate intake.[16]

PREVENTIVE MEASURES

There are a number of lifestyle changes and preventive measures that can be taken to reduce the risk of cardiovascular disease. Making those lifestyle changes will not *insure* against CVD; however, they will reduce the potential risk. For some individuals, a very few, maximizing those lifestyle changes may be sufficient to reverse early signs and symptoms of CVD.

CHOLESTEROL

Every person should have his blood level measured. Because both inheritance and diet affect cholesterol levels, it is impossible to just estimate the blood level. Individuals with fasting cholesterol levels above 240 mg/dl need further testing and may be treated with special diets or possibly medication. Individuals with measures above 200 mg/dl should have the test repeated for accuracy and to differentiate between the "good" (HDL) from the "bad" (LDL) cholesterol levels to determine if special medical treatment is needed.

Diet is very important in lowering cholesterol and maintaining normal cholesterol levels.[7,8] Lowering cholesterol intake by reducing the consumption of meat, organ meat, eggs, and whole milk products can help reduce cholesterol (Table 16.3). Cholesterol is synthesized in the liver from saturated fat in the diet. The more saturated fat consumed, the more cholesterol produced. Saturated fats are found in meats, bacon, under the skin of poultry, cheeses (especially the hard cheeses), tropical oils (palm, palm kernel, coconut, and cocoa butter), whole milk, chocolate candy, and baked goods. Studies show that the intake of saturated fats is more directly related to blood cholesterol than the intake of cholesterol! In addition, the ingestion of transfatty acids increases circulating cholesterol. Transfatty acids are man-made from unsaturated fats. They are easily recognizable on food labels as "partially hydrogenated" or "hydrogenated" oils.

Diet may also be important to reducing some of the newer metabolic risk factors. The most important nutrients appear to be the B vitamins.[16] Niacin (B_3) is used to reduce total cholesterol. It also has a positive impact on LDL cholesterol, small LDL particle trait, and Lp(a). Adding vitamin B_6, vitamin B_{12}, and folate can improve homocyteine status. Vitamin E, an antioxidant, may also protect against CVD, but the relationship is still in need of further research.[16] Therefore, to reduce the risk of CVD, diets should not only lower fat and cholesterol intake but also increase the intake of food containing the B vitamins and vitamin E.

TABLE 16.3

Suggested Dietary Changes to Lower Cholesterol

A. Eat less than 6 oz. of meat or poultry per day.

B. Limit eggs to three per week.

C. Avoid organ meats, sausage, bacon, hot dogs, and canned meats.

D. Use low-fat dairy products: 1% milk or less, low-fat sour cream and cream cheese.

E. Avoid saturated fats, especially lard, butter, coconut oil, palm oil, cocoa butter, and hydrogenated vegetable oils.

F. Avoid commercial baked goods, as they are usually made with saturated fats.

G. Eat more vegetables, fruits, whole grains, and cereals to increase dietary fiber, which also has a positive effect on lowering cholesterol.

H. Consume fewer cream or Alfredo sauces.

I. Exercise regularly to help maintain weight and raise HDL cholesterol levels.

J. Achieve and maintain ideal or recommended body weight.

K. If all else fails, medications are available. These medications do have side effects. Thus, they should be used as a last resort.

HYPERTENSION

High blood pressure should be treated by a physician. However, there are a number of ways to help lower blood pressure. Most doctors first attempt lifestyle changes when trying to reduce mild to moderate hypertension. Overweight individuals with hypertension can reduce their blood pressure simply by losing weight. Regular aerobic exercise can help normalize blood pressure in many people. The reduction may be a result of the exercise or any weight loss that occurs due to the exercise. About one-third of people with hypertension can reduce their blood pressure by limiting sodium intake to less than 1,000 mg per day.[7] Alcohol intake also has been related to hypertension. Therefore, limiting the consumption of alcoholic beverages in heavy drinkers may help reduce blood pressure. Relaxation therapies may also be effective in reducing blood pressure. Those therapies include meditation, progressive relaxation, and biofeedback, and are administered by a professional during 20- to 30-minute sessions. Finally, counseling for stress management may also have an impact on lowering blood pressure.

If an individual with hypertension does not respond to those lifestyle changes or if the hypertension is severe, then medications such as diuretics, beta blockers, vasodilators, and others can lower blood pressure.[7] Those drugs can have serious side effects, such as sluggishness, light headedness, impotence, and liver problems. Many people with hypertension (about 50%) discontinue their medication without the permission of their doctor due to the side effects. However, failure to comply with the prescription can increase the risk of a cardiovascular event during any strenuous activity. Because there are many choices of medications and because the medication helps protect the heart from the damage caused by hypertension, the patient should consult his physician when side effects occur. It is possible a medication change will bring about the desired blood pressure response without the debilitating side effects. In general, most people can prevent high blood pressure by maintaining an ideal body weight, limiting sodium intake to 3,000 mg or less per day, exercising regularly, not drinking more than 3 beverages containing alcohol per day, and finding positive ways to cope with or reduce mental stress.

EXERCISE

Every person should be on an exercise program that involves activity such as running, walking, swimming, or biking.[4,7,8,12] Many people feel they do not have the time to exercise. It does take planning and dedication to organize exercise time, but there are many options. Home fitness equipment may be more convenient for those who have child-care responsibilities. Exercising as a family activity can help develop a healthy lifestyle. Walking, cycling, and hiking are appropriate activities for every age group. Jogging and running are other options that require only a good pair of shoes. Joining a health club, community recreation center, or YMCA may reduce the dislike for exercising alone. Even if leisure activity seems impossible, a person can make work time more active by walking more, taking stairs more often, or using breaks to exercise.

SMOKING

Smoking is one of the most difficult habits to break. That is why it is important that no one should begin smoking cigarettes or using smokeless tobacco, especially youngsters. Many smokers want to quit, but the strength of the addiction counters any attempt. The longer one smokes, the harder it is to quit. No one single method works for all. Some individuals try many methods before finding one that works for them.

In general, a smoker who is trying to quit may want to avoid situations that trigger smoking behavior, such as bars, drinking alcohol, or coffee. At first the smoker should write down those situations so that an awareness is developed. Increased consumption of water and fruit juices may help for two reasons. Also, the liquid increases the removal of nicotine from the body. The sugar in the juices has a tendency to reduce hunger, and it is known that increased eating occurs during smoking cessation.

Some individuals can quit "cold turkey;" however, for many individuals, cutting back more and more as time progresses or switching brands with less nicotine works best. That is the idea behind some of the graded filters used for quitting. Some individuals find that nicotine gum or the nicotine patch help them quit smoking. However, the nicotine gum may simply switch from one source (the cigarette) to another (the gum). Finally, some individuals have used hypnotism and acupuncture.

The initial success rate for smoking cessation programs is not good: 30 to 50%. And the long-term rate is very poor: 20 to 30%.[7] Thus, it appears that eliminating smoking is an ongoing process and relapses are common. A relapse program may also be needed to defeat this addiction.

CONCLUSION

CHD is the most common killer of adult Americans. Presently the best way to reduce the risk of CVD is to reduce blood cholesterol levels, avoid cigarette smoking, treat high blood pressure, and engage in regular, vigorous exercise. Diets low in cholesterol and saturated fats can help, as can diets rich in the B vitamins and vitamin E. Improved physical condition may help prevent heart attacks that could occur when a person has to react to a sudden crisis. Physical conditioning can also help people better understand their strengths and weaknesses, which improves self-confidence and lowers stress levels. Reducing cholesterol, blood pressure, and smoking while increasing regular physical activity may or may not add years to your life, but it will add life to your years.

REFERENCES

1. American Heart Association, *1991 Heart and Stroke Facts*, AHA National Center, Dallas, 1991.
2. *HeartMemo*, National Heart, Lung, Blood Institute Information Center, Bethesda, MD, fall 1997.
3. Buring, J.E., Evans, D.A., Flore, M., Rosner, B., and Hennekens, C.H., Occupation and risk of death from coronary heart disease, *J. Am. Med. Assoc.*, 258, 791-792, 1987.
4. Pollock, M.J. and Wilmore, J.H., *Exercise in Health and Disease*, W.B. Saunders, Philadelphia, 1990.
5. Sparrow, D., Thomas, H.E., and Weiss, S.T., Coronary heart disease in police officers participating in the normative aging study, *Am. J. Epidemiol.*, 118, 508-513, 1983.
6. Surles, K.B., Johnson, P.W.C., Buescher, P.A., and Kaufman, K.P., *Occupational Mortality Among North Carolina Males 1984–1986: A Death Rate Analysis*, State Center for Health Statistics, North Carolina Department of Human Resources, Raleigh, NC, 1988.
7. Smith T.W. and Leon, A.S., *Coronary Heart Disease: A Behavioral Perspective*, Research Press, Champaign, 1992.
8. Fraser, G.E., *Preventive Cardiology*, Oxford University Press, New York, 1986.
9. *HeartMemo*, National Heart, Lung, Blood Institute Information Center, Bethesda, MD, winter 1993.
10. Powell, K.E., Thompson, P.D., Casperson, C.J., and Kendrick, J.S., Physical activity and the incidence of coronary heart disease, *Ann. Rev. Public Health*, 8, 253-287, 1987.
11. Blair, S.N., Kohl, H.W., Paffenbarger, R.S., Clark, D.G., Cooper, K.H., and Gibbons, L.W., Physical fitness and all-cause mortality: a prospective study of healthy men and women, *J. Am. Med. Assoc.*, 262, 2395-2401, 1989.
12. Blair, S.N., Kohl, H.W., and Gorden, N.F., How much physical activity is good for health? *Ann. Rev. Public Health*, 13, 99-126, 1992.
13. National Institute of Health, *NIH Consensus Statement: Physical Activity and Cardiovascular Health*, National Institute of Health, Bethesda, MD, 1995.
14. Superko, H.R., The most common cause of coronary heart disease can be successfully treated by the least expensive therapy — exercise, *Certified News*, American College of Sports Medicine, Indianapolis, April 1998.
15. Scanu, A.M., Lipoprotein(a). A genetic risk factor for premature coronary heart disease, *J. Am. Med. Assoc.*, 267, 3326-3329, 1992.
16. Council on Epidemiology and Prevention of the American Heart Association, *Abstracts of the 38th Annual Conference on Cardiovascular Disease Epidemiology and Prevention*, Santa Fe, NM, March 18-20, 1998.

17 Nutrition for Optimal Health and Performance

Purpose: To explain what is required in a healthy diet and outline components of nutrition that are of special interest for physically active people.

Objectives:

1. Know the composition of and reasons for a healthy diet.
2. Know the importance of a high carbohydrate diet.
3. Know protein requirements and be able to describe the difference between complete and incomplete protein. The reader will be able to explain how incomplete proteins can be combined to form complete proteins.
4. Be able to describe the functions of fats, types of fat, and know why unsaturated fats are "better" than saturated fats.
5. Understand the importance of micronutrients and know the micronutrients that are important for physically active people. Understand the dangers of over-supplementation and deficiency.
6. Be aware of ergogenic aids and their potential dangers.

INTRODUCTION

A healthy diet should provide the body with 1. adequate fuel to meet metabolic and daily activity needs, 2. eight essential amino acids so the body can make proteins, 3. adequate amounts of the essential vitamins and minerals, 4. adequate amounts of the essential fatty acids, 5. adequate amounts of fiber, and 6. adequate amounts of fluids.[1] To ensure those requirements are met is difficult in a world full of food choices. In fact, it takes a nutritionist to fully understand proper dieting. However, many national health organizations and even governments have attempted to simplify and specify foods that provide those six requirements.

Many of us grew up learning to choose foods based on the four food groups: meats, dairy products, fruits and vegetables, and cereals and breads. We learned that we should have at least one serving from each group at each meal. Getting adequate amounts of "complete protein" was emphasized. The *Basic Four Food Groups* were developed to help Americans get adequate levels of nutrients. However, applying the basic four food groups to a diet can cause overnutrition because calories and fat content are not considered. Thus, the high calorie value of hidden fats in meats and dairy products are not taken into consideration. A serving of fish, which is low in fat, has the same value as a serving of beef, which is typically high in fat content (and has considerable cholesterol). In addition, diets based on the basic four can result in undernutrition because

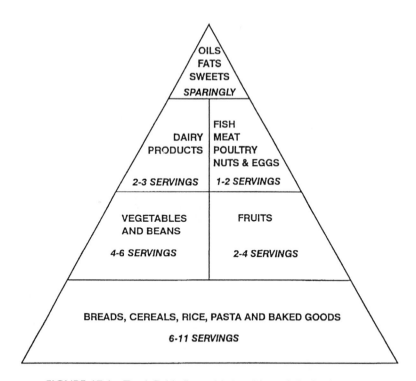

FIGURE 17.1   Food Guide Pyramid: A guide to daily food choices.

they can be low in vitamin B_6, vitamin E, and magnesium. In addition, many foods do not fit into the basic four food groups: butter, margarine, sour cream, jams, jellies, mayonnaise, coffee, tea, salad dressings, alcohol, or synthetics.

The present dietary recommendations are based on the *Food Guide Pyramid* developed by the U.S. Department of Agriculture.[2] The *Food Guide Pyramid* focuses on eating a high complex-carbohydrate, high-fiber, low-fat, and low-cholesterol diet (Figure 17.1). The change in recommendation is a response to the scientific evidence that shows that high-fat diets increase the risk for obesity, hypertension, and high cholesterol, which are risk factors for heart disease and/or cancer. The base of the pyramid is composed of the carbohydrates, as these should make up at least 55% of the diet. In contrast, fats and oils are located at the tip of pyramid because they should be used sparingly. Once again, the pyramid provides a general guideline, but not all foods within the same grouping have equal nutritional and caloric value. For example, fish may be a better source of protein than beef because of its lower fat content. Skim milk would also be a better dairy choice than whole milk because of its lower fat content. The pyramid is basically a high carbohydrate diet that is most appropriate for an athlete. The pyramid also has the benefit of incorporating adequate vitamin and mineral consumption.

In the U.S. food choices are basically unlimited. Although Americans eat a wide variety of foods, some nutrient problems are evident. The composition of the average

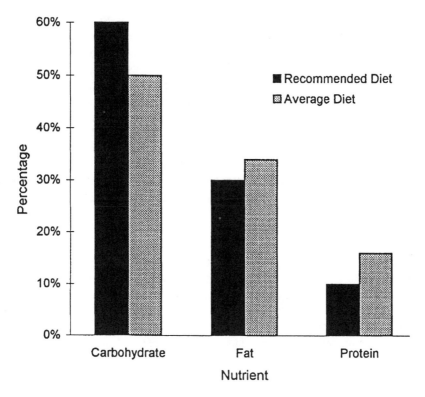

FIGURE 17.2 Composition of the average U.S. and recommended diet.

American diet is shown in Figure 17.2. The average American obtains about 34% of the calories from fat, 16% of the calories from protein, and 50% of the calories from carbohydrates.[3] In comparison, the composition of the optimal diet appears to be 55 to 60% carbohydrates, 25 to 30% fats, and 10 to 15% protein.[1] The diet seems to be improved since the early 1980s during which the fat and carbohydrate contents were approximately 40%. However, total calorie content is increasing. Thus, there is still a need for improvement. Reports also suggest that the American diet could be improved by adding foods that contain iron, vitamin B_6, vitamin C, folate, magnesium, zinc, and fiber.[4,5] If overnutrition exists, it is usually related to a high fat intake and an excess alcohol intake.[6] Overnutrition may also relate to portion size. In the U.S., a typical serving is much larger than in the rest of the world. A steak in France is about 6 oz. (170 g), and in the U.S. it is 8 to 12 oz., or 226 to 340 g.[7] Most soft drinks are sold in 16- or 20-oz. (450 to 570 ml) size in the U.S. but are 10- to 12-oz. (280 to 340 ml) size elsewhere.

Snacking has become an integral part of the American diet. The Nationwide Food Consumption Survey[4] has indicated that the most popular snacks seem to be soft drinks, bakery products, and desserts. However, salty snacks, candy, fruit, and meat have also been widely reported. Snacking does not seem to be related to obesity. In fact, a report suggests that slender individuals eat more snacks than obese persons!

The fast pace of westernized culture has forced people to look for convenience meals, many of which are higher in fats, sugar, and sodium. On a typical day in the U.S., 134 million people eat out, including 16 million at McDonalds.[8] Twenty five million hot dogs are eaten, and 525 million colas are consumed. About $14 million is spent on potato chips and tortilla chips. Although nutritious modern microwave or oven-ready meals can be purchased, those convenience foods are limited in choices. While $203 million is spent on low-calorie food, $22 million is spent on snack foods. For example, 100 million packages of M&M's and 2 million Hershey's Kisses® are sold daily. Those figures do not even consider the multimillion dollar nutritional supplement industry that is utilized by many athletes. Such feeding patterns may create difficulties for the individuals who are attempting to control weight and simultaneously keep energy stores supplied for training.

CARBOHYDRATES

The major function of carbohydrates (CHOs) in the diet is to provide energy.[9,10] A gram of CHO supplies about 4 calories. There are two kinds of carbohydrates, simple and complex. *Simple carbohydrates* (also called monosaccharides and disaccharides) make foods taste sweet. Table sugar (also called sucrose) is an example of a simple carbohydrate or sugar. Sources typically do not have many other nutrients, such as vitamins and minerals. In addition, many foods high in simple sugars, such as candy, often come packaged with a lot of fat. The most important simple sugar is glucose. The body uses glucose as its main energy source for many functions, including exercise.[9,10] All carbohydrates are eventually converted by the body into glucose.

Generally, no more than 10% of total daily calories should come from simple carbohydrates.[6,11] Unfortunately, simple carbohydrates from pastries, doughnuts, cakes, cookies, sweetened cereals, etc., account for 20% of the average American's total carbohydrates intake.[12] Those foods contribute nutritionally "empty" calories to the diet. However, during extended periods of exercise, simple carbohydrates (typically sports drinks) can provide a quick source of much needed energy.

Complex carbohydrates (also called polysaccharides) are the most important part of our diet.[1,6] Although they provide energy, they also contain many other nutrients. For example, a potato contains about 220 calories, but it also has protein, iron, potassium, niacin, folate, and vitamin C. Complex carbohydrates are found in fruits, vegetables, seeds, nuts, grains, breads, cereals, pasta, rice, dairy products, and dried beans or legumes. Meats have only trace amounts of carbohydrates. Most complex carbohydrates are high in nutrients and fiber and low in fat.

The body breaks down (metabolizes) all complex carbohydrates into glucose. Some of those complex carbohydrates metabolize to glucose quite quickly; others metabolize more slowly. The classification of the speed of metabolism is called the Glycemic Index.[13] Those that metabolize quickly have a high glycemic index, which brings about a swift insulin reaction. Thus, blood glucose levels rise quickly and then fall quickly. The complex carbohydrates that metabolize more slowly, have a low glycemic index because they release glucose into the blood more slowly which does not cause as great an insulin reaction. That prevents large fluctuations in blood sugar and reduces the possibility of rebound hypoglycemia (low blood sugar), which

TABLE 17.1
Glycemic Index of Some Common Foods[13,15]

Maltose	105	Sweet corn	59
Glucose	100	Sucrose	59
Carrots	92	Orange juice	57
Rice (instant)	91	Popcorn	55
Honey	87	Oatmeal cookies	55
Potatoes (baked)	83	Sweet potatoes	54
Potatoes (instant)	83	Grapes	52
Rice Krispies	82	All Bran cereal	51
Rice cakes	82	Peas	51
Cornflakes	80	Yams	51
Mashed potatoes	80	Potato chips	51
Grape Nuts Flakes	80	Spaghetti	50
Jelly beans	80	Baked beans	48
Waffles	76	Bulgur	48
Doughnuts	76	Banana cake	47
Cheerios	74	Lactose	46
Graham crackers	74	Wheat kernels	41
Corn chips	73	Apple juice	41
Bread (whole-wheat)	72	Oranges	40
Bagels	72	Apples	39
White rice	72	Fish sticks	38
Watermelon	72	Spaghetti (whole-wheat)	37
Life Savers	70	Ice cream	36
Bread (white)	69	Pears	36
Cornmeal	68	Yogurt	36
Soft drinks	68	Beans (butter)	36
Grape Nuts	67	Milk (whole)	34
Shredded Wheat	67	Chick peas	33
Angel food cake	67	Milk (skim)	32
Wheat crackers	67	Beans (navy)	31
Rice (brown)	66	Beans (kidney)	29
Life cereal	66	Lentils	29
Pineapple	66	Barley	25
Raisins	64	Fructose	20
Sugar beets	64	Beans (soy)	18
Bananas	62	Peanuts	13
Oatmeal	61		
Bran muffins	60		

Index is expressed as a percent in comparison to 50 g of glucose.

occurs when large amounts of simple carbohydrates are consumed. Examples of the glycemic index of food can be found in Table 17.1.

The glycemic effect is influenced by the interaction of the carbohydrate with simultaneously ingested protein, the kind of carbohydrate ingested, the form of the food source (dry, paste, liquid), and the presence of molecules that may bind the starch, e.g., pectin fiber.[13,14] The presence of either fats or proteins in the food source of carbohydrate causes a lower glycemic index. For example, lactose is a sugar found in milk. The glycemic index of lactose by itself is twice that of the lactose found in whole milk due to the fat and protein content of the milk. It is also known that food preparation techniques can influence the glycemic index. The glycemic index of mashed potatoes is higher than a raw potato. A common misconception is that starches have a lower glycemic index than simple sugars. On the contrary, mashed potatoes (a starch) has a high glycemic index, while fructose, a simple sugar, has a lower glycemic index than most starches. Therefore, the true benefit of complex carbohydrates is that they contain other important nutrients than just energy. In addition, there is some suggestion that high glycemic index foods cause faster weight gain, but there is presently no proof of that.

NUTRIENT DENSITY

Complex carbohydrates contain lots of micronutrients (vitamins and minerals) and few calories, so they are nutrient-dense. For example, a baked potato has 220 calories and 6% protein, 8% folate, phosphorus, magnesium, 10% of iron, niacin, copper, 15% iodine, 20% vitamin B$_6$, and 35% vitamin C of the U.S. Recommended Daily Allowances[6] (USRDA) and virtually no fat (unless it is added). However, two Pepperidge Farm Nantucket Chocolate Chunk Cookies® have 240 calories, of which 45% are from fat, and contain only 2% of the USRDA for calcium and less than 2% of the USRDA for protein, vitamin A, vitamin C, thiamin, riboflavin, niacin, and iron. Thus, in terms of nutrient density, the potato is a more "nutritious" food than the cookies. When food choices are made, the concept of nutrient density should be taken into consideration. The information needed to compare nutrient density is usually found on the food label.

CARBOHYDRATE REQUIREMENTS

Carbohydrates in the form of glucose are needed for most bodily functions. In fact, the brain can use only glucose for energy. Most other energy needs can be met by a combination of carbohydrate (glucose), proteins, and fats. Carbohydrates are stored in the body in two forms: blood glucose and glycogen (a chain of glucose molecules). The total stores of blood glucose amount to about 20 calories, whereas the muscle and liver stores of glycogen amount to about 2,000 calories.

To meet the need for carbohydrates, each person should eat 6 to 11 servings of grains, pasta, cereals, and breads; 3 to 5 servings of vegetables; and 2 to 4 servings of fruits daily (Table 17.2). Thus, carbohydrates should make up the majority of each meal. That may represent a big change in eating habits for many Americans because traditionally meat has been the main focus of the meal. The sources of carbohydrates should be chosen from a wide variety of foods. Variety will improve the chance of meeting the daily requirements for micronutrients.

CARBOHYDRATES AND EXERCISE

Carbohydrates are an important source of energy at rest and especially during exercise. At rest, about 40% of the energy comes from carbohydrates.[9] During exercise carbohydrates (mostly glycogen) can account for up to 95% of the energy, depending on the intensity. The higher the intensity of exercise, the higher the proportion of carbohydrates burned for energy. Carbohydrates are necessary even to burn fats: "Fat burns in a carbohydrate flame." Thus, even during dieting it is best to consume carbohydrates. The human body cannot store large amounts of carbohydrates, only enough for about 90 minutes of exercise in a normal person.[9,10] Thus, the more physically active the person, the more carbohydrates that person needs to consume. When marathon runners or long-distance cyclists deplete their carbohydrates, fatigue sets in very quickly. Long bouts of exercise (1.5 hours and longer) can lead to hypoglycemia or low blood sugar. That leads to fatigue and dizziness, so it is important to consume carbohydrates during and immediately after prolonged exercise.

Exercise of any type or duration will decrease glycogen stores in the muscle. It is important to replenish those stores by consuming plenty of carbohydrates in the diet. It takes about 24 hours for muscle to replenish glycogen stores when the amount of carbohydrates in the diet is adequate, 55 to 60% of the total calorie intake.[9,10] Replenishment of glycogen takes longer when there are not enough carbohydrates in the diet.[10] One result of regular aerobic exercise is that trained muscles store more glycogen than untrained muscles. However, even in trained individuals, if glycogen stores are not replenished daily, glycogen stores in the muscle will become depleted over time and that leads to chronic fatigue and burnout. Lack of glycogen severely reduces athletic performance of all types.

Carbohydrate loading is a technique used by many endurance and sport athletes to improve glycogen stores to perform longer at a high intensity of exercise.[10] Beginning about a week before a competition or race, an athlete will begin to decrease intensity and duration of training. Three days before the competition or race, the athlete will increase his intake of complex carbohydrates to 500 to 600 g per day and either rest or train very lightly. That helps to ensure the athlete's glycogen stores will be at their highest level possible.

Energy bars (PowerBars, for example) can help maintain blood glucose levels during prolonged exercise, but they take longer to break down than sport drinks (Gatorade,® PowerAde,® All Sport®). In addition, the use of solids requires that water must be taken in as well. Those energy bars sometimes contain undesirable amounts of fat. Fig Newtons® (they also come in other flavors: apple, raspberry, strawberry, cranberry) work just as well as energy bars, and they are much cheaper and are available in fat-free versions. In general, energy bars are necessary only during exercise of long (upwards of 90 minutes) duration. Also, care is needed not to confuse sport drinks and energy bars with carbohydrate "loading" drinks and bars (such as Gatorlode or Exceed High Carbohydrate Source). Those loading drinks and bars were designed to speed glycogen replacement in muscles after exercise. If they are consumed before or during exercise, they will remain in the stomach.[16,17] These

TABLE 17.2
Food Sources of Carbohydrates and Proteins with Respect to Normal Serving Sizes[19]

	Food	Serving Size
Mainly Carbohydrate	Rice, oats, other grains	½ cup cooked
	Bread	1 slice
	Cereal	¾ cup
	Pasta	½ cup cooked
	Vegetables	½ cup cooked; 1 cup raw
	Fruits	½ cup chopped; 1 medium fruit
Protein	Meat, poultry, game, fish	3 oz. cooked
	Shellfish	6 oz.
	Cheese	1 oz.
	Milk, yogurt	1 cup
	Nuts, seeds	1 oz.
	Eggs	1 egg
	Dark green leafy vegetables	1 cup
	Tofu	4 oz.
Both	Dry beans, legumes, peas	½ cup cooked

"loaders" should be consumed within two hours after a triathalon, marathon, or other long intense exercise.[18]

PROTEINS

Protein is an essential nutrient and is used by the body to build and repair tissue and bone. Protein is found in varying amounts in most foods, including meats, dairy products, fruits, vegetables, seeds, beans, and grains (Table 17.2). Meats and dairy products are very high in protein. Grains, seeds, and beans have moderate amounts of protein, and fruits and vegetables generally contain very little. Proteins are made up of different combinations of 20 amino acids, eight of which are called essential amino acids because they cannot be manufactured by the body.[20] Foods that have adequate amounts of all eight essential amino acids are considered complete proteins. The egg is considered the best source of complete protein and is used as the "reference" for which the nutrient density of all other protein sources are compared.[20]

Animal-based foods usually contain complete proteins. Meat, poultry, seafood, eggs, cheese, yogurt, and milk are all examples of complete proteins. Although high in protein, animal sources are usually high in saturated fats. Plant-based foods also contain protein, but most are considered incomplete proteins because many of those sources do not have all eight essential amino acids. Plant foods are usually eaten in combination to ensure that all amino acids are present in adequate amounts. Many of these food combinations are common in other countries. They include beans and corn tortillas, red beans and rice, lentils and rice, chickpeas and sesame seeds (humus or falafel), beans and pasta, stir-fried vegetables with tofu and rice, stir-fried vegetables

TABLE 17.3

Example of the Computation of Protein Needs and a Sample Menu of How Those Needs Can Be Obtained

Example: 150-lb person

Number of grams of protein needed daily = 150 × 0.36 g

Number of grams of protein needed daily = 54 g or less than 2 oz.

* The conversion from pounds to kilograms: 1 lb = .4536 kg or 1 kg = 2.2 lb

* The conversion for ounces to grams: 1 oz. ≈ 29 g

Based on the USRDA for protein, a 150-lb. person can meet his needs by eating the following:

2 oz. of Quaker Oat Squares and a cup of skim milk	300 calories, 24 g protein, 4 g fat, 96 g carbohydrates
3-oz. grilled chicken breast	115 calories, 20 g protein, 2 g fat, and 0 carbohydrates
1½ cups of red beans and rice	313 calories, 14 g protein, 1 g fat, 45 g carbohydrates
Total*	728 calories, 58 g protein, 7 g fat, 141 g carbohydrates

* The total protein intake of some of the above choices may be higher than necessary, but the total calories are fewer than half of that required for this person and the amount of fat is very low.

with almonds and rice, and peanut butter on whole grain bread or crackers. The advantage of those combinations is that protein requirements can be obtained with less fat than is present in many animal products and lots of carbohydrates. Another way to complement the protein in plant foods is to add a small amount of animal protein. A common example is cereal with milk; other examples are macaroni and cheese, pancakes, potatoes au gratin, vegetable and meat stir fry, pizza with vegetables and cheese, chicken and rice soup, and rice pudding.

PROTEIN REQUIREMENTS

The need for protein is based on weight and can be calculated as shown in Table 17.3. The USRDA for protein for most adults is 0.8 g of protein per kilogram body weight or 0.36 g of protein per pound of body weight.[6] Although the USRDA contains sufficient protein to meet the needs of over 95% of the general population, it may not be adequate for those who exercise for extended periods of time or are building muscle. For individuals exercising an hour or more a day, the protein recommendation is raised to 1.5 g/d, and for weight lifters and body builders the recommendation is approximately 2 g/kg. The majority of people in America eat more than twice the amount of protein that they actually need.[8,11] Because the body recycles a large percentage of the protein that it uses, our daily requirement for protein is very small. Eating too much protein is associated with kidney problems, loss of bone mass, and dehydration.[10,20] Extra protein cannot be stored as protein to some extent. Most is either broken down and excreted or stored as fat.

Extra protein in the diet has three possible destinies: metabolized and excreted in the urine, converted to carbohydrate, or converted to fat. The majority is excreted in the urine. That converted to carbohydrate can be used for energy or stored as glycogen. If glycogen stores are filled, the carbohydrate is converted to adipose (fat) stores. In addition, the typical sources of protein foods in the Americans diet (meat and dairy products) have considerable fat content,[21] thus contributing to weight gain. For example, a 3-oz. hamburger by itself has 245 calories with 21 g of protein and 17 g of fat. Each gram of fat has 9 calories, so 153 (or 63%) of the 245 calories come from fat, and that is before you add the cheese (70% fat). Hot dogs are even worse: for 7 g of protein, they have 15 g of fat. That means that of 180 calories, 75% come from fat, 23% from protein, and 2% from carbohydrate. Broiled or grilled chicken eaten without the skin is a much better choice (see Table 17.3); only 16% of the calories come from fat. Seafood has a make up similar to chicken, and some types of seafood have even less fat than chicken. Vegetable sources of protein can be very low in fat. For example, one serving with 3/4 cup cooked beans and 3/4 cup cooked white rice has only 1 g of fat, which means only 3% of the calories come from fat, plus there are lots of carbohydrates. It has been suggested that to keep fat intake low, one should limit meat and poultry intake to 6 oz. or less per day.[2] See Table 17.3 for serving sizes for protein.

PROTEIN AND EXERCISE

Regular physical activity does not automatically increase the requirement for protein. In general, individuals exercising three times per week for 30 to 40 minutes do not need extra protein. Because protein accounts for less than 10% of energy used during exercise and because a small amount of protein is lost in sweat,[10] only endurance athletes who exercise for long periods of time (upwards of 1.5 hours) daily burn significant amounts of protein for energy. Research suggests that weight lifters may need more protein than a sedentary person (up to 2 g/kg body weight); however, the typical diet contains sufficient protein to meet the needs of the weight lifter.

Those individuals who exercise often and hard must eat more calories than people who are sedentary. That increase in caloric intake usually means the active person eats more protein. Most people already consume two times the protein they need, so they already get extra protein. The only people at risk for inadequate protein are those who are on low-calorie diets (<1,200 kcal) or exercise very strenuously for long periods of time.[10]

High-protein diets have been promoted by coaches and athletes of all levels as being necessary for building muscle. Promoters of amino acid and protein supplements have gone as far as saying those substances increase muscle mass. That is a myth; only training builds muscle. There is no valid scientific research that supports the claim that exaggerated protein or amino acid supplements will increase muscle mass or performance.[10] In fact, excessive intake of a particular amino acid may block uptake of other important amino acids and prevent the body from getting enough protein. Also, the body can process only a certain amount of protein per day; intakes above this level are excreted in the urine or stored as glycogen or fat. Because it takes large amounts of water for the kidneys to process extra protein, excessive intake can lead to dehydration, a very serious and debilitating condition.

FATS

In the past few decades, fat has been recognized as a contributor to the development of lifestyle diseases. Studies show that eating excess fat increases the risk of heart disease, several types of cancer, and obesity.[11,22] It is important to recognize that fat in itself is not bad. In fact, it has several important functions, but excess fat intakes are bad for your health. Body fat cushions the internal organs, provides energy for activity, and helps regulate body temperature. Fats are used by the body to manufacture hormones, neurotransmitters, and cell membranes. Fat contributes to a feeling of fullness.[23] Fat also adds flavor to food. Many recipes begin with hot oil or butter. The flavors in the ingredients are retained by the heated fat. Thus, the food tastes better. That is why many very low-fat foods seem bland.

THREE TYPES OF FAT

Triglycerides are generally what are thought of as fats. They are made up of a glycerol molecule and three fatty acids.[9] There are basically three types of triglycerides: saturated, monounsaturated, and polyunsaturated. The classification of the fat is dependent upon the chemical bonds between the carbon and hydrogen atoms that make up the long chain of the fatty acid molecules. Figure 17.3 shows the general structure of these three triglycerides. A saturated fat has each carbon atom on the fatty acid molecule surrounded on all sides by either a hydrogen atom or a carbon atom. The atoms are bonded together by what is referred to as single bonds (both atoms share one electron). Those bonds are very stable and do not break down easily. Saturated fats solidify at room temperature. Monounsaturated fats have fatty acids that have one double bond (two shared electrons) in the chain of carbon atoms, so two carbons are not bonded to a hydrogen on each side (unsaturated with hydrogen). Polyunsaturated fats have two or more of those double bonds, so at least four carbons are unsaturated or not bonded to hydrogen on each side. Double bonds are less stable than single bonds, so unsaturated fats break down more easily than saturated fats.

Of the three types of fats, saturated fats are most harmful.[11] Intake of saturated fat is directly related to blood levels of LDL cholesterol. LDLs are the harmful type of cholesterol that can end up as atherosclerotic plaque inside the arteries of the heart.[22] Thus, in general, the more saturated fat a person eats, the higher his blood cholesterol. The mechanism is not completely understood, but basically saturated fats are transported to the liver and cause the liver to increase production of LDL cholesterol. One way to reduce blood cholesterol is to reduce the total amount of saturated fat in the diet.

Saturated fats are found almost exclusively in animal sources with a few exceptions, coconut oil, palm kernel, and palm oil. Those vegetable fats are highly saturated and contribute to elevated blood cholesterol. Coconut oil and palm oil are used in manufactured cakes, cookies, snack crackers, pie crusts, and candy because they are inexpensive and have a long shelf life. Many food manufacturers have replaced those fats with healthier unsaturated fats in response to consumer demand for healthier products. The top sources of saturated fats in the American diet are red

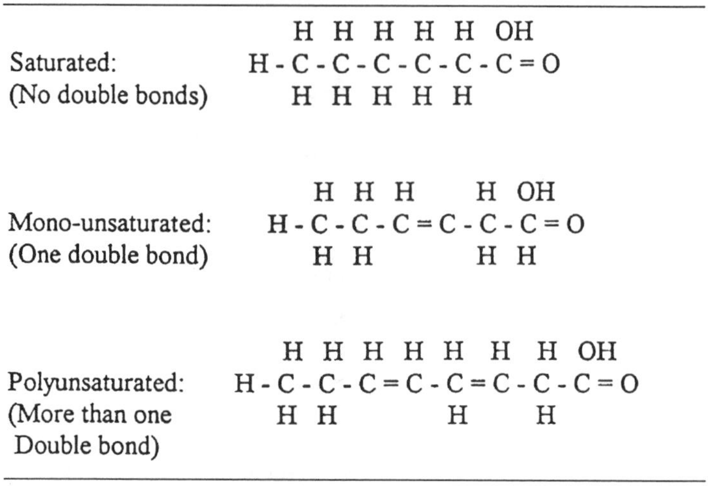

```
                        H  H  H  H  H  OH
Saturated:              H - C - C - C - C - C - C = O
(No double bonds)       H  H  H  H  H


                        H  H  H      H  OH
Mono-unsaturated:       H - C - C - C = C - C - C = O
(One double bond)       H  H          H  H


                        H  H  H  H  H  H  H  OH
Polyunsaturated:        H - C - C - C = C - C = C - C - C = O
(More than one          H  H          H      H
Double bond)
```

FIGURE 17.3   Schematic of the three types of fatty acids found on the triglyceride molecules. Each triglyceride molecule is made up of a glycerol component and three fatty acids.[8]

meat (especially hamburgers), whole milk, cheeses, hot dogs, lunch meats, doughnuts, cookies, cakes, eggs, butter, and ice cream.[8,21] Saturated fat should be limited to 10% of total calories per day or less. The most effective way to reduce saturated fat is to limit the intake of animal products. That can easily be accomplished by 1) reducing meat intake to less than 6 oz. per day; 2) avoiding sausage, bacon, organ meats, and processed meats (such as hot dogs and lunch meats); 3) avoiding whole milk and dairy products made with whole milk; 4) limiting intake of doughnuts, cookies, and cakes; 5) avoiding processed foods made with lard, palm oil, butter or coconut oil; and 6) cooking with liquid oils instead of solid fat.

Mono-unsaturated fats and polyunsaturated fats are both liquid at room temperature.[24] They are found in seeds, nuts, grains, and vegetables. Corn oil, sunflower oil, safflower oil, soybean oil, and cottonseed oil are polyunsaturated fats. Wesson® oil, Puritan® oil, and Mazola® oil are also examples of polyunsaturated oils. Early studies on polyunsaturated fats showed that people with high cholesterol who began using polyunsaturated fats in place of saturated fats lowered their cholesterol significantly. The mono-unsaturated fats are olive oil, peanut oil, canola oil, and avocado oil. Mono-unsaturated fats are more closely related to a reduced risk of CVD than polyunsaturated fats. Research has found that people in Mediterranean countries (Italy, Greece, and others) who used mono-unsaturated fats had lower rates of heart disease than other European and North American countries that used predominantly saturated and polyunsaturated fats. Diets of people in Mediterranean countries are not lower in total fat, but most of the fat comes from olive oil rather than saturated animal fat. Typical meals of Mediterranean countries are based on bread or pasta and vegetables; meat is used more as a side dish, than a main dish and olive oil is used extensively.[23]

Stick margarines are made from polyunsaturated fat that has been chemically altered to make it solid by the process of hydrogenation. Recent evidence suggests that the hydrogenated fats found in margarine are almost as harmful to the heart and arteries as saturated fats. Those hydrogenated fats, sometimes called "trans fatty acids," elevate cholesterol similar to saturated fats. Furthermore, trans fatty acids have just as many calories as saturated fats. Thus, eating a lot of margarine will make you just as fat as eating a lot of butter; excess fat is still excess fat!

The healthier types of fat may not contribute to an increase in blood cholesterol, but they do contribute extra calories, which can lead to weight gain. In a normal diet, no more than 30% of the total calories should come from fats. In addition, no more than one-third of total fat intake should come from saturated fats, with one-third or less from polyunsaturated fats and the balance from mono-unsaturated fats.[1,6] Polyunsaturated fats should not exceed one-third of total fat intake because a high intake of polyunsaturates appears to be associated with an increased risk for cancer. However, the data is not conclusive.

To increase mono-unsaturated fats in your diet, use peanut or olive oil to stir-fry vegetables. Peanut oil is ideal for stir-frying because it can be heated to a very high temperature before burning. That makes it possible to cook vegetables and meats in a very short time (1 to 3 minutes) and have them come out hot, still crisp, and very tasty. Oriental food restaurants cook almost exclusively in peanut oil. Olive oil can be used for home cooking. It is great for sautéing vegetables such as tomatoes, mushrooms, garlic, and onions to serve over pasta. Vegetables such as tomatoes, potatoes, zucchini, or eggplant brushed with a little olive oil, sprinkled with salt and pepper, and cooked on the grill are easy to prepare yet flavorful and healthy.

FAT REQUIREMENT

Our nutritional requirement for fat can be satisfied by 1 tablespoon (13 to 14 g) of fat per day.[23] A small amount of fat goes a long way. There are nine calories in one gram of fat. That is more than twice as many calories per gram as protein or carbohydrate, which both have 4 calories per gram. The average American gets 34 to 37% of total daily calories from fat. Individuals who eat more than one meal per day in a fast food restaurant and are not careful about choices probably get close to 50% of their calories from fat. As stated above, no more than 30% of total calories per day should come from fat, and no more than 10% of calories should come from saturated fat.[6] Figure 17.4 shows the basic breakdown of the sources of total fat in the American diet (A) and the breakdown of sources of saturated fat (B).

Red meat and dairy products contribute almost half of the total fat and more than half of the saturated fat in the American diet. Eating chicken and fish and using nonfat dairy products could lower fat intake considerably. Sweets and snacks, such as candy bars and doughnuts, also contribute a hefty 15% of total and saturated fat. There are also "hidden" fats in the diet in the form of processed foods and baked goods. People may not consider them high in fat because the fat is not in the form of oil or butter.

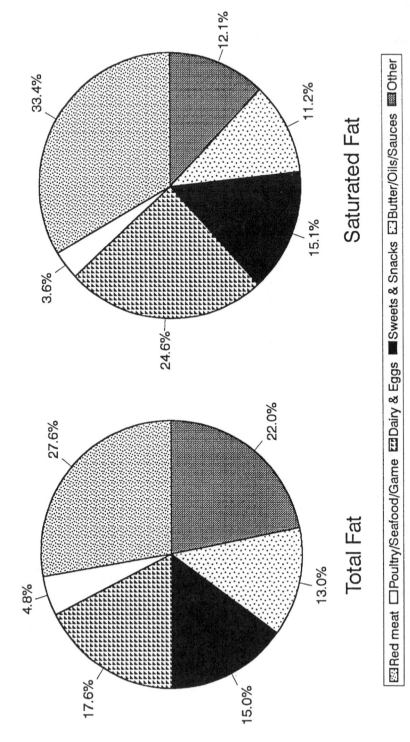

Saturated Fat

Total Fat

☒ Red meat ☐ Poultry/Seafood/Game ☷ Dairy & Eggs ■ Sweets & Snacks ⊞ Butter/Oils/Sauces ▨ Other

FIGURE 17.4 Basic breakdown of the sources of total fat in the American diet and the breakdown of sources of saturated fat.

FATS AND EXERCISE

Those who exercise regularly do not need extra fat in their diet. The only exception is elite ultra-endurance athletes who train upwards of four or more hours per day. At that level of training, it is difficult to obtain adequate calories by eating just carbohydrates. A diet with 30 to 35% of the calories from fat could be beneficial. In addition, aerobic exercise does not "neutralize" the effects of saturated fats or trans-fatty acids on cholesterol. Thus, the best choices of foods are those that contain polyunsaturated and monounsaturated fats.

FIBER

Fiber is the part of plant that is not digestible. Fiber contributes to feeling full and satisfied. It also helps to bind cholesterol and fat for elimination from the body. Fiber from oats and kidney beans are considered the most effective in lowering cholesterol. Fiber helps to reduce the amount of time that food spends in the intestine. Many studies have supported the idea that fiber helps to reduce the risk for colon (large intestine) cancer and diverticulosis. Each person should consume at least 25 g of fiber per day.[1,6] Ideally, each person should consume about 5 g of fiber for every 400 calories.[24] That means that a woman who eats 2,000 calories per day should take in about 25 g of fiber, and a man who takes in 2,500 calories per day should take in about 30 g of fiber per day. Dried beans and peas supply on the average 6 to 8 g of fiber per serving. Black-eyed peas have the highest amount of fiber. Products made from unrefined grains such as whole wheat bread and oatmeal are a little higher in fiber than beans and peas. Vegetables and fruits that are especially high in fiber include apples, beets, berries, broccoli, cabbage, carrots, cauliflower, corn, dates, eggplant, figs, grapes, kale, lettuce, mangoes, okra, onions, peppers, prunes, raisins, rhubarb, spinach, and sprouts.

MICRONUTRIENTS: VITAMINS AND MINERALS

Vitamins and minerals are called micronutrients because they are required in very small amounts. These substances are used in a variety of metabolic functions throughout the body. The USRDAs sources and functions for all the essential vitamins and minerals are shown in Tables 17.4 and 17.5. There is concern that people do not get enough vitamins and minerals from their diets. Thus, many people turn toward supplementation. Still supplementation is a very controversial subject. Some experts recommend that everyone take a multivitamin and mineral supplement "just to be sure they are getting all the micronutrients." Other nutritionists say people should try to eat a balanced diet so they get the necessary nutrients from their food; a vitamin and mineral supplement cannot make up for poor eating habits. The research is not clear, and the results seem to be very individualized. However, the research does show some trends. Smokers and people who drink more than three alcoholic drinks per day should take a multivitamin and mineral supplement. Nicotine and alcohol block absorption of several vitamins and minerals. In addition, people on diets less than about 1,500 kcal per day could benefit from supplementation, as could women who are pregnant or lactating. The levels of micronutrients in a multivitamin and mineral supplement should not exceed 100% of the USRDA because high intakes of certain vitamins and minerals can detrimental to health.[9,10]

VITAMINS

There are two types of vitamins: *fat soluble* and *water soluble* (Table 17.4). The *fat soluble* vitamins are A, D, E, and K. Those vitamins can be stored in the body in the liver or fat cells.[6] Excessive supplementation with vitamins A, D, and K is dangerous.[6] When large amounts of those vitamins accumulate in the body, they become toxic or poisonous. Symptoms of excess consumption of vitamin A include nausea, headache, fatigue, liver and spleen damage, skin peeling, and pain in the joints; for vitamin D they include loss of appetite, nausea, irritability, joint pain, and calcium deposits in soft tissues such as the kidney; for vitamin K they include clot formation and possible vomiting. Vitamin E does not seem to be toxic even in large doses.[25] Getting adequate amounts of A, D, and E may help to reduce the risk of certain types of cancer. See Table 17.4 for the recommended daily requirements and foods that are high in fat-soluble vitamins.

The *water soluble* vitamins include all the B vitamins (thiamin, riboflavin, niacin, folate, B_6, B_{12}, biotin, and pantothenic acid) and vitamin C. These vitamins are not stored in large quantities by the body; thus, they need to be ingested daily.[6] These vitamins are more easily destroyed during cooking and storage than fat-soluble vitamins.[23] Although water-soluble vitamins are generally safe even in high dosages, some can cause significant side effects. Excessive intake of niacin is associated with headache, nausea, burning, and itching skin and flushing of the face. Too much vitamin B_6 is associated with loss of nerve sensation and impaired gait. Taking too much vitamin C is associated with diarrhea, possible kidney stones, and rebound scurvy.

MINERALS

Minerals are divided into *major minerals* and *trace minerals*. Sources, functions, and RDAs are given for the most important minerals in Table 17.5. The *major minerals* include calcium, phosphorus, magnesium, potassium, sodium, and chloride. Deficiencies of those minerals are rare, except in those individuals whose job or exercise program causes them to routinely sweat for prolonged periods of time. As with vitamins, excessive supplementation is to be avoided. Too much calcium can lead to kidney stones and reduced absorption of iron and zinc. Phosphorus intake highly exceeding calcium intake will cause calcium to be lost from the bones. That makes the bones brittle and more likely to break. (Processed foods and sodas are especially high in phosphorus.) Excessive intake of magnesium contributes to diarrhea.

The *trace minerals* are needed in levels of 100 mg or less. The most important trace minerals are iron, zinc, copper, selenium, and chromium. Once again, care should be taken if a person decides to supplement. Iron supplements of 25 to 75 mg per day are considered safe for adults. However, too much can cause iron to be stored in the liver, which results in symptoms similar to cirrhosis of the liver. Zinc supplementation may aid an exerciser, yet quantities greater than 100 mg per day are associated with decreased absorption of copper, increased LDL (bad) cholesterol, decreased HDL (good) cholesterol, impaired immune system, nausea, and vomiting.[10] Copper, chromium, and selenium can also be toxic, even in small amounts.

MICRONUTRIENTS AND TRAINING

In general, moderately active to very active people do not need extra vitamins and minerals if they eat a well-balanced diet. If a person eats five servings of fruits and vegetables per day, plus lean meats, breads, and dairy products, vitamin and mineral intake will probably be adequate. However, many people do not eat a balanced diet. Those individuals should supplement with a one-a-day type vitamin.

There are certain vitamins that are important for more active people.[25] Research has shown that "vigorous exercise increases the production of cell-damaging free radicals in the body, which may contribute to muscle soreness and inflammation after a workout."[25] Free radicals are produced during exercise when oxygen is processed by the body to make energy. When exercising outside, increased breathing rates increase the exposure to ozone and other harmful pollutants such as carbon monoxide. Those substances also contribute to the formation of free radicals. Vitamins C and E are antioxidants that help reduce the effects of free radicals. Some preliminary research suggests that supplements of vitamins C and E may reduce the damage of those free radicals. Vitamin C is found in many fruits and vegetables. Vitamin E, on the other hand, is hard to get from food, so many scientists recommend supplements not to exceed two times the RDA.[6,25]

There are seven key minerals that are especially important for those who exercise.[25] Iron is very important because it is necessary to transport oxygen throughout the body. Heavy endurance training is more likely to lead to depletion of iron stores than other types of exercise. Women, vegetarians, and dieters are most at risk for developing exercise-induced anemia. It is best to consult a doctor before beginning iron supplementation. Use of cast iron cookware and eating foods high in vitamin C along with foods high in iron are excellent ways to maximize iron intake.[25] Sodium and potassium are important for maintaining fluid balance. There is loss of these minerals in sweat, but the loss is usually very small and the minerals are easily replaced by fruits and vegetables in the diet. It is not a good idea to take salt tablets because taking those tablets without sufficient water can lead to electrolyte imbalances and further dehydration. There is some concern that Americans do not consume enough chromium. Chromium helps to regulate blood sugar. Good sources of chromium are listed in Table 17.5.

TABLE 17.4
Sources, Functions, and Recommended Daily Allowances of Vitamins

Nutrient	Major Functions	Good Sources	Deficiencies	RDA for Adults	
		Fat Soluble			
Vitamin A	Required for healthy bones, teeth, skin, hair, neurons, immune function	Yellow, orange, or dark green vegetables, milk, eggs, cheese, liver	Night blindness, decreased growth, decreased resistance to disease, rough skin	Men

Women | 1000 µg
5000 IU
800 µg
4000 IU |
| Vitamin D | Necessary for bones, teeth, calcium and phosphorus uptake | Fortified milk, fish oils, tuna, salmon, sunshine | Rickets (bone deformities), osteomalacia | 19–24 y
25+ | 10 µg/400 IU
5 µg/200 IU |
| Vitamin E | Antioxidant, normal red cell and muscle function | Vegetable oils, wheat germ, margarine, green leafy vegetables | Breakdown of red blood cells, nerve destruction, cramps | Men
Women | 10 mg
8 mg |
| Vitamin K | Essential for normal blood clotting | Dark green leafy vegetables, liver, eggs | Hemorrhage | Men
(19–24)
25+
Women
(19–24)
25+ | 70 µg
80 µg

60 µg
65 µg |
| | | **Water Soluble** | | | |
| Thiamin (B_1) | Nerve function, carbohydrate metabolism | Whole and enriched grains, dried beans, peas, lean meats | Loss of appetite, poor coordination, muscle spasms, nausea, heart changes, confusion | Men
Women | 1.5 mg
1.1 mg |

Vitamin	Function	Sources	Deficiency Symptoms		RDA
Riboflavin (B₂)	Normal growth and development, good vision, healthy skin, carbohydrate metabolism	Eggs, milk, leafy green vegetables, whole grains, lean meats, dried beans and peas	Cracking of the corners of the mouth, skin inflammation, impaired vision	Men Women	1.7 mg 1.3 mg
Niacin (B₃)	Carbohydrate, fat and protein metabolism, normal growth and development, nerve function, hormones	Liver and organ meats, fish, poultry, whole grains, nuts, green leafy vegetables, dried beans and peas	Confusion, depression, weakness, weight loss, diarrhea	Men Women	19 mg 15 mg
Vitamin B₆	Protein and fat metabolism, red blood cell formation, nerve function	Vegetables, meats, whole grain cereals, spinach, broccoli, bananas, potatoes	Depression, muscle spasms, irritability, nausea, headache, anemia, flaky skin	Men Women	2.0 mg 1.6 mg
Vitamin B₁₂	Normal growth, red blood cell formation, nerve function	Animal meats (organ), poultry, fish, eggs, milk, cheese	Impaired balance, weakness, weight loss	Men Women	2.0 µg 2.0 µg
Folate (Folic Acid)	DNA synthesis, cell growth and reproduction, red blood cell formation	Organ meats, leafy green vegetables, dried beans, whole grains	Lower resistance to infection, diarrhea, poor growth, mental disorders	Men Women	200 µg 180 µg
Biotin	Fat synthesis, carbohydrate metabolism	Liver, eggs, milk, nuts, cheese, dark green vegetables	Inflamed skin, muscle pain, depression, weight loss	Men Women	30–100 µg 30–100 µg
Pantothenic Acid	Carbohydrate and fat metabolism, fat synthesis	All natural foods, liver, eggs, nuts, milk, dried beans and peas	Depression, fatigue, nausea, leg cramps, headaches	Men Women	4–7 mg 4–7 mg
Vitamin C	Normal teeth, bones and blood vessels, protects against infection, collagen formation	Fruits and vegetables, particularly citrus fruits, broccoli, tomatoes, strawberries	Slow healing wounds, loose teeth, rough scaly skin, irritability, hemorrhaging	Men Women	60 mg 60 mg

TABLE 17.5
Major Functions, Sources, and the Adult RDAs for the Major Minerals

Nutrient	Major Functions	Good Sources	Deficiencies	RDA for Adults	
Calcium	Teeth and bone strength, muscle contractions, nerve function	Dairy products: milk, yogurt, cheese; green leafy vegetables	Bone pain and fractures, osteoporosis, muscle cramps	Men	1200 mg
				Women (19–24)	1200 mg
				25+	800 mg
Iron	Major component of hemoglobin (carries O_2 in blood), immune function	Meat, seafood, eggs, enriched and whole grains, green leafy vegetables	Nutritional or training induced anemia, overall weakness	Men	10 mg
				Women	15 mg
Phosphorus	Teeth and bone strength, energy release regulation	Dairy products, meats, dried beans, whole grains, processed foods, fish	Bone pain and fracture, weight loss, weakness	Men (19–24)	1200 mg
				25+	800 mg
				Women (19–24)	1200 mg
				25+	800 mg
Zinc	Component of insulin, hormones and enzymes, normal growth and development	Seafood, meat, whole grains, nuts, eggs, dried beans	Loss of appetite, diarrhea, slow healing wounds, skin problems	Men	15 mg
				Women	12 mg
Magnesium	Bone strength, nerve function, carbohydrate and protein utilization	Whole grains, green leafy vegetables, nuts, seafood	Weakness, irregular heartbeat, muscle spasms, sleeplessness	Men	350 mg
				Women	280 mg
Sodium	Body fluid regulation, nerve function, heart action	Table salt, processed foods, meat	Muscle cramps, but rarely seen	No RDA	>500 mg*
Potassium	Nerve function, heart action, bone formation, energy release regulation	Legumes, whole grains, bananas, potatoes, spinach, orange juice, milk	Irregular heartbeat, nausea, loss of appetite, muscle cramps, weakness	No RDA	2000 mg*
Chromium	Blood glucose control	Egg yolks, whole grains, pork	High blood glucose levels after eating	Men	50–200 µg**
				Women	50–200 µg**

* Estimated minimum requirement[1]
** Estimated safe and adequate daily dietary intake[1]

WATER AND OTHER FLUIDS

Water is very important; it is involved in almost every chemical process in the body. The pressure it creates in the tissues even helps give structure and form to the body.[9,10] Water accounts for 55 to 70% of total body weight. A person who does not take in any fluid will die within a few days. The average fairly inactive adult requires about 2.5 l of water per day (1 l = 1.06 qt). This water is obtained from three sources: liquids, foods, and metabolism. An average adult takes in about 1.2 l, or 41 oz., of fluid per day. All foods contain water. Fruits and vegetables have the highest water content, whereas foods such as bread, cake, dried meat, butter, and chocolate contain very little water. On average, people take in about 1 l of water from foods. Water and carbon dioxide are formed when food is metabolized or broken down for energy. This metabolic water accounts for about 25% of the requirement of an average *sedentary* person.[9,10]

Water is lost from the body in four ways: in urine, through the skin, from the lungs as water vapor in exhaled air, and in feces.[9] Anywhere from 1 to 1.5 l of water are lost in urine. The amount of water lost in urine is controlled in part by the amount of waste that must be excreted by the kidneys. The more waste that must be filtered by the kidneys, the more water required for dilution.[9] For example, consumption a high-protein diet will cause more water loss because the metabolism of protein to form energy results in a larger amount of byproducts that must be diluted to be excreted. Water is continually lost at a very slow rate through the skin by a process called insensible perspiration. About 250 to 350 ml of water is lost that way each day. Water is also lost as sweat; under resting conditions at comfortable temperatures, about 500 to 750 ml is lost per day.[9] However, sweat rates can be as high as 1 l per hour when a person exercises in hot humid conditions. Under sedentary conditions, an average adult loses .2 to .25 ml water per minute in exhaled air. During heavy exercise, this water loss can increase to 2 to 5 ml per minute. In addition, 100 to 200 ml of water is lost in feces. Diseases that produce diarrhea or vomiting can increase water loss from 1.5 to 5 l per day.[9]

Present recommendations indicate that everyone should drink the equivalent of eight 8-oz. glasses of noncaffeinated fluid daily.[24] Water, seltzer water, and juices are good choices. Carbonated drinks that contain caffeine, coffee, and tea are not as effective in providing fluids for the body, because caffeine is a diuretic that increases water loss. Alcoholic beverages also act as diuretics and so do not supply the body with fluid. Those who exercise should drink extra fluids in balance with the amount of exercise they perform.

Exercise increases the requirement for water. The higher the intensity of exercise and the warmer or more humid the environment, the greater the water requirement.[18] Fluids should be consumed before, after, and during exercise. Hydration can best be maintained by drinking 12 oz. of fluid less than 15 minutes before exercise and drinking 8 oz. every 20 minutes during exercise.[18] It may not be necessary to drink "sports drinks" (such as Gatorade® or Exceed®) to hydrate before, during, or after moderate- to high-intensity exercise if the exercise lasts less than 90 minutes in a comfortable environment. For short-term exercise sessions, water may be the best choice.[17] For exercise in a hot and/or humid environment or exercise exceeding 90 minutes, sports drinks are the best choice.[18]

Properly formulated sports drinks supply glucose as well as fluid, which helps maintain blood glucose levels. When blood glucose levels stay low, the body will deplete the glycogen in the muscles and liver and fatigue will occur quickly. If blood glucose levels are maintained, then fatigue will be delayed. Glucose, sucrose, and glucose polymers are the best absorbed and quickly used sugars in sports drinks; drinks with fructose are not absorbed as quickly. Sports drinks should contain 6 to 8% carbohydrates.[17,18] Liquids containing this percentage of carbohydrates are absorbed as quickly as water and provide significant amounts of carbohydrates. Beverages containing less than 6 to 8% carbohydrates will not provide enough fuel to delay fatigue during prolonged exercise.[16] Beverages containing a higher percentage of carbohydrates slow the gastric emptying of water. Further, the high carbohydrate concentration of the beverage actually slows the absorption of the solution in the intestine.[17] To calculate the percentage of carbohydrates in a beverage, use the label information for an 8-oz. (240 ml) serving and follow the formula below:

Example: % CHO = (grams CHO per 8-oz. serving/240 ml) * 100%
            CHO% = (15 gms CHO per 8-oz. serving/240) * 100%
            15/240 = .0625
            .0625 × 100% = 6.25% CHOs

Sports drinks usually include electrolytes such as sodium and potassium. Extra electrolytes do not hurt but are only necessary for those participating in ultra long training sessions such as triathletes training for an Ironman competition. Someone who exercises four to five times a week for an hour or less will usually obtain adequate amounts of electrolytes with regular meals. Sports drinks are better for rehydration after exercise of long duration than plain water.[18] Sports drinks usually contain a small amount of sodium. That sodium helps to maintain thirst. That is important because people lose their drive to drink after a glass of water or so due to dilution of the blood. When sports drinks with sodium are consumed, the concentration of sodium in the blood is maintained and thirst is maintained. The sodium also helps prevent increased urination which is also due to blood dilution. For many individuals, sports drinks taste better than water, and it may be easier for them to drink more and rehydrate more effectively.

ALCOHOL

The role of alcohol in a healthy diet is a small one. Use of alcohol is associated with considerable death, disability, and social problems in our country. Therefore, it is not prudent to promote moderate intake of alcohol as health promoting. However, there is some evidence that moderate alcohol consumption is not harmful and may even be beneficial in reducing heart disease.[26] Moderate alcohol intake is no more than one drink per day for women and no more than two drinks per day for men.[26] Abstaining from any alcohol all week and drinking a six-pack on Friday night is not moderate drinking; it is binge drinking and should be avoided. Several large epidemiological studies have shown slightly lower rates of heart disease among moderate drinkers as compared to nondrinkers.[26] However, a heavy intake of alcohol is associated with an increased risk of heart disease above that of nondrinkers. Intake of three or more drinks per day is associated with high blood pressure. High alcohol intake is also associated with higher rates of cancer and osteoporosis. One of the most serious consequences of high alcohol intake is cirrhosis of the liver, which can be fatal.

FOOD LABELS

As of May 1994, the U.S. Food and Drug Administration requires all foods to carry labels like that pictured in Figure 17.5. The labels are supposed to help consumers evaluate the nutritional value of foods more easily and prevent food manufacturers from putting misleading information on foods.[19] Specifically, these labels were designed to help Americans avoid the things they eat too much of: fat, saturated fat, cholesterol, and sodium. The regulations also reduce the number of calculations the consumer must do to evaluate similar foods because they require standard food servings for similar foods. So for example, nutrient information for all brands of ice cream will be based on the same size serving. Serving sizes are thought to be close to actual serving sizes. The percent daily value information will help consumers figure out how a food can fit into their diet. Sodium and cholesterol limits have been set so consumers can easily know how much of their daily quota is derived from a certain food.

1. **Serving sizes** have been standardized to reflect the actual serving eaten. Serving sizes of similar foods are the same as well.
2. The **list of nutrients** has been changed to reflect the fact that most Americans are not at risk for nutrient deficiencies.
3. The **label** gives consumers an idea of how much fat, carbohydrates, fiber, and protein they should be eating based on two levels of calorie intake. It also gives limits for cholesterol, saturated fat, and sodium.
4. **Percent Daily Value** tells consumers what percent of their daily allowance for fat, carbohydrate, and protein supplied by that food based on an intake of 2,000 calories per day.
5. **Percent Daily Value** also provides information on saturated fat, cholesterol, sodium, simple carbohydrates (sugars), and fiber contained in the product.
6. The new labels list the **number of calories per gram** for protein, carbohydrate, and fat.

The daily requirements for fats, saturated fat, carbohydrates, and fiber are based on an intake of 2,000 total calories per day. Although smaller or less active people should eat less, and larger or more active should eat more, those values can at least serve as guidelines. Actually, the total daily values for two levels of calorie intake are given on the bottom of the label. That can be confusing to understand. Calories per gram of fat, carbohydrate, and protein are given at the bottom of each label, so consumers can calculate for themselves the percentage of calories from carbohydrates,

Nutrition Facts	
Serving Size 1/2 cup (114 g)	Servings per Container 4

Amount per Serving

Calories 274	Calories from Fat 90
	% Daily Value*

	% Daily Value*
Total Fat 10 g	17%
Saturated Fat 3 g	15%
Cholesterol 50 mg	17%
Sodium 300 mg	13%
Total Carbohydrate 38 g	13%
Dietary Fiber 2 g	8%
Sugars 7 g	
Protein 8g	

Vitamin A	11%	Vitamin C	5%
Calcium	20%	Iron	3%

*Percent Daily Values are based on a 2000 calorie diet. Your daily values may be higher or lower depending on your calorie needs:

	Calories	2000	2500
Total Fat	Less than	65g	80g
Sat Fat	Less than	20g	25g
Cholesterol	Less than	300mg	300mg
Sodium	Less than	2400mg	2400mg
Total Carbohydrates		300g	375g
Fiber		25g	30g

Calories per gram:

Fat 9	Carbohydrates 4	Protein 4

FIGURE 17.5 Standard Nutrition Food Label.

proteins, or fats. Another plus is that the labels give people a handle on how much of the fat in the product is saturated and an idea of how that amount fits into the total saturated fat limit. That is especially helpful for people who are trying to lower their cholesterol.

The government has also made strict laws limiting the sorts of claims manufacturers can make about foods.[19] Claims for seven food/disease relationships are allowed. The relationships that can be claimed are calcium and osteoporosis; fat and cancer; fruits and vegetables and cancer; fiber containing grain products, fruits, and vegetables and cancer; fiber containing grain products, fruits, and vegetables and coronary heart disease; saturated fat and cholesterol and coronary heart disease;

sodium and high blood pressure. Those claims can be represented by statements, symbols, or descriptions, but they cannot overstate the relationship and must point out that other factors contribute to those food/disease relationships. The regulations also strictly define descriptive words used on packaging such as "light," "low fat," or "cholesterol free." Those terms are defined in the next section.

FREQUENTLY USED DIETARY TERMS

The following is a list of the definitions for terms that may be used on food labels as set forth by the U.S. Food and Drug Administration.[19] All regulated food labels must conform to these guidelines as of May 1994.

Free — The product contains none or only negligible amounts of fat, saturated fat, cholesterol, sodium, sugar, and/or calories.

Low — The product can be eaten frequently without causing the person to exceed dietary guidelines for fat, saturated fat, cholesterol, sodium, sugar, and/or calories. Specifically:

Low fat = 3 g or fewer per serving
Low saturated fat = no more than 1 g per serving
Low sodium = fewer than 140 mg per serving
Low cholesterol = fewer than 20 mg
Low calorie = 40 calories or fewer per serving

Lean, extra lean — Describes fat content of certain meats, poultry, seafood, and game.

Lean = < 10 g fat, < 4 g of saturated fat, < 95 mg cholesterol per serving
Extra lean = < 5 g fat, < 2 g saturated fat, and < 95 mg cholesterol per serving

Reduced — Indicates that the food has been nutritionally altered and contains 25% less of a particular nutrient or substance (such as fat or cholesterol) than the regular product.

Less, fewer — These terms indicate that the product contains 25% less of nutrient or substance than comparable food. For example, pretzels contain less fat than potato chips.

Light — Indicates that the product has been nutritionally altered to reduce calories by at least one-third and/or fats and sodium by at least one-half of what they were in the regular product. Light can mean that sodium has been reduced by half, but if the product is not low-calorie or low-fat, then the label must state specify "light in sodium." The problem is that light can also refer to texture or color, but that must be specifically spelled out, e.g., "light brown sugar."

More — The product contains at least 10% of the daily requirement for a given nutrient than a comparable food.

Good source — The product contains 10 to 19% of daily requirement of nutrient described.

High — The product contains at least 20% or more of daily requirement for nutrient described.

Percent fat free — This term can be used only on foods that are low fat or fat free already; it indicates the fat content of a food based on weight.

NUTRITIONAL ERGOGENIC AIDS

Over the years, athletes of all types have looked for "aids" to improve performance. To fulfill the athletes needs, many substances have been put on the market that claim to improve physical performance. In most cases, little or no valid scientific research has been completed on those substances. In Table 17.6, substances that are commonly used as ergogenic aids are listed with their claimed benefit and the results of research done with those substances concerning performance.[10] Williams[10] gives the following list to be used as a guideline for identifying claims that are probably "too good to be true." If the answer to any of those questions is yes, then it is a good idea to try to find more information about the substance before investing any money.

- Does the product promise quick increases in physical performance?
- Does it contain some secret formula or ingredient?
- Is it advertised primarily by use of case histories or testimonials?
- Are currently popular star athletes used in its advertisement?
- Does it take a simple truth about a nutrient and exaggerate its claim relative to physical performance?
- Is it advertised in a sports magazine whose publishers also sell nutritional aids?
- Does it use the results of a single study or dated and poorly controlled research to support its claims?
- Is it expensive, especially when compared to the cost of equivalent nutrients that may be obtained from ordinary foods?

CONCLUSION

This chapter has explained the components of a healthy diet and discussed some of the special dietary needs of people who exercise. The best way to improve performance is to train wisely and eat a diet high in carbohydrates and nutrients. Yet food serves as more than just fuel for our bodies. A nourishing diet is a significant part of a healthy lifestyle. In general, most people should focus on eating more fruits, vegetables, legumes, and whole cereals and grains. However, making dietary changes from a typical American diet is not easy for most people. Cultural, emotional, and social forces have significant impacts on eating behavior. The current focus on convenience and quickness has become more important than the nutritional content of the food. Making changes to improve the diet takes time, effort, and planning. The best way to modify the diet is for the person to pick one change and work on it until it becomes natural, then move on to another modification. The important thing for the person making changes is to avoid being overwhelmed by trying to make too many changes at once.

TABLE 17.6
Common Nutritional Ergogenic Aids

Substance	Training Benefits	Does it Work?	Potential Hazards
Adenine	Decreases cholesterol; sublingual or injected improves angina	Questionable	High dosages cause renal tubular damage in dogs
Alcohol ethanol	Depressant effect may relax individual, reduce anxiety, muscle tremors for shooters, archery	No improvement in exercise performance	Too much can affect motor coordination
Amino acid supplements	Stimulates growth hormone, which causes increased muscle; leucine can be used for exercise (distance runners)	Studies have not confirmed benefits	Too much of one amino acid may block uptake of another
Bee Pollen	Mixture of various vitamins, minerals and proteins; may improve recovery and endurance performance	6 studies — no effect on endurance performance or recovery	15–20% of population allergic to the pollen (protein)
Caffeine — xanthines	May improve endurance by enhancing muscle contraction; improves availability of fatty acids; conserves glycogen	Improved cycling to exhaustion; activity must be > 90 min; effects lost with high users	Irritability, nervousness, extreme mood changes, cardiac arrhythmias, peptic ulcers, seizures
Carnitine	Increased aerobic capacity; increased power output; increased energy production from fats	Questionable	AVOID DL-carnitine: causes muscle weakness in dialysis patients
Chromium	Increases LBM; decreases body fat; lowers total cholesterol; decreases blood glucose	No effect on exercise, but lowers cholesterol and may help weight loss	No side effects reported in humans
Creatine: creatine monohydrate	Increases anaerobic energy production; increases work capacity (delays fatigue) during repeated bouts of exercise; weight gain; reduces triglycerides and VLDL-cholesterol	Studies have confirmed benefits, but other studies show no effect except significant water weight gain	Can get GI distress if taken by itself on an empty stomach — osmotic diarrhea
Coenzyme Q10 — ubiquinone	Enzyme in electron transport system; improved myocardial contractility	In cardiac patients, 4–8 weeks increased submaximal work capacity by 6% and maximal capacity by 12%. No studies on athletes.	Increased cell damage with supplementation, thus not beneficial

TABLE 17.6 (continued)
Common Nutritional Ergogenic Aids

Substance	Training Benefits	Does it Work?	Potential Hazards
Ginsing: Chinese (Panax) Russian (Red) American	Reduces fatigue; spares glycogen; increases production of DNA, RNA, and protein metabolism; elevates mood; animal studies using mega-dosages have shown increased endurance times and increased anabolic activity	Questionable; Chinese has highest content, may work best; Russian may not actually contain any ginsenoside	No side effects reported in humans
Inosine	Enhances ATP production; improves oxygenation	Questionable; oral dose probably degraded in intestine, so no effect	No side effects reported but can cause increased free radicals, uric acid, and ammonia production; exacerbates gout
Lecithin and Choline	Aids in creatine synthesis; increases muscular power and endurance times	No effect	Choline: Up to 20 g/day is safe, but no effect on exercise
Medium Chain Triglycerides	Improves endurance exercise capacity; delays fatigue	Works for some individuals	Can cause nausea and vomiting (best mixed with some sugars)
Phosphate Loading	Elevates phosphate concentrations for increased formation of ATP; may facilitate oxygen unloading from red blood cells; increases anaerobic threshold	No effect	No side effects reported in humans as long as phosphorus does not exceed calcium intake greatly; can lead to brittle bones
Sodium Bicarbonate	Used to increase the buffer capacity of the blood, reducing the effect of lactate on fatigue	Earlier studies show increased duration of high-intensity exercise; many studies show unfavorable results	Acute GI distress, nausea, bloating, diarrhea, reduced by increased water intake; prolonged use reduces serum potassium — cardiac arrhythmias
Vanadyl Sulfate	Theorized to improve protein retention and protein anabolism	No effect	No side effects reported in humans

REFERENCES

1. *Dietary Guidelines for Americans*, U.S. Department of Agriculture and Health & Human Services, Washington, D.C., 1990.
2. U.S. Department of Agriculture, *Food Guide Pyramid*, U.S. Government Printing Office, Washington, D.C., 1992.
3. *National Health and Nutrition Examination Survey III, 1988–1994*, National Center for Health Statistics, Washington, D.C., 1997.
4. Peterkin, B.B., Rizek, R.L., and Tippett, K.S., Nationwide food consumption survey, *Nutr. Today*, January/February 1988, p. 18+.
5. Wotechi, C.E., Hitchcock, D.C., and Winn, D.M., National Health and Nutrition Examination Survey — NHANES, *Nutr. Today*, January/February 1988, p. 25.
6. The National Research Council, *Recommended Daily Allowances*, 10th ed., National Academy Press, Washington, D.C., 1989.
7. Beck, M. and Hager, M., An epidemic of obesity, *Newsweek*, August 1, 1994, pp. 62-63.
8. Wardlaw, G.M., Insel, P.M., and Seyler, M.F., *Contemporary Nutrition: Issues and Insights*, Mosby Year Book Inc., St. Louis, 1992.
9. McArdle, W.D., Katch, F.I., and Katch, V.L., *Exercise Physiology: Energy, Nutrition, and Human Performance*, Lea & Febiger, Philadelphia, 1986.
10. Williams, M.H., *Nutrition for Fitness and Sport*, Wm. C. Brown Publishers, Dubuque, 1995.
11. Public Health Service, *The Surgeon General's Report on Nutrition & Health*, DHHS(PHS) #88-50210, Washington, D.C., 1988.
12. Block, G., Dresser, C.M., Hartman, A.M., and Carroll, M.D., Nutrient sources in the American diet: Quantitative data from the NHANES II survey: II. Macronutrients and fats, *Am. J. Epidemiol.*, 122, 27-40, 1985.
13. Jenkins, D.J.A., Taylor, R.H., and Wolever, T.M.S., The diabetic diet, dietary carbohydrate and differences in digestibility, *Diabetologia*, 23, 477-484, 1982.
14. Bray, G.A., Obesity, a disorder of nutrient partitioning: the MONA LISA hypothesis, *J. Nutr.*, 121, 1146-1162, 1991.
15. Foster-Powell, K. and Miller, J.B., International tables of glycemic index, *Am. J. Clin. Nutr.*, 62, 871S-893S, 1995.
16. Schulte, L., Faster Food and Drink: Do you need carbo supplements? *Outside*, July 1992.
17. Coleman, E., Sports drink update, *Sport Sci. Exch.*, Vol.1, August 1988.
18. Nadel, E.R., New ideas for rehydration during and after exercise in hot weather, *Sports Sci. Exch.*, Vol. 1, June 1988.
19. Special report: What the new food labels will (and won't) dish up, *Tufts University Diet and Nutrition Letter*, Vol. 10, February 1993.
20. Pellett, P.L., Protein requirements in humans, *Am. J. Clin. Nutr.*, 51, 723-737, 1990.
21. Block, G., Dresser, C.M., Hartman, A.M., and Carroll, M.D., Nutrient sources in the American diet: Quantitative data from the NHANES II survey: I. Vitamins and minerals, *Am. J. Epidemiol.*, 122, 13-26, 1985.
22. Pollock, M.L. and Wilmore, J.H., *Exercise in Disease and Health: Evaluation and Prescription for Prevention and Rehabilitation*, W.B. Saunders Co., Philadelphia, 1990.
23. Brody, J.E., *Jane Brody's Good Food Book: Living the High-Carbohydrate Way*, Bantam Books, New York, 1987.

24. Hoeger, W.W.K., *Lifetime Physical Fitness and Wellness: A Personalized Program*, Morton Publishing Co., Denver, 1989.

25. Nutrition and exercise: What your body needs, *University of California at Berkeley Wellness Letter*, Vol. 9, May 1993.

26. Marmot, M. and Brunner, E., Alcohol and cardiovascular disease: The status of the U shaped curve, *Br. Med. J.*, 303, 565-568, 1991.

18 Principles of Weight Management

Purpose: To identify and explain the principles of weight management.

Objectives:

1. Know the definitions of overweight and obese.
2. Know the definition of and be able to estimate ideal body weight using height/weight tables or body composition.
3. Know the components of total energy expenditure.
4. Estimate energy need based on body weight and activity level.
5. Understand and be able to explain why short-term dieting seldom leads to permanent loss of fat weight; be aware of the potential dangers of ketogenic, high-protein, and very low-calorie diets.
6. Know the definition of weight cycling or yo-yo dieting and potential problems.
7. Explain why a low-fat high-carbohydrate diet combined with exercise is the safest and most effective method for losing fat weight.

INTRODUCTION

Obesity and overweight have become widespread health problems contributing to disease and injury. Recent studies have indicated that about one-third of the adult population could be considered obese.[1] Obesity is associated with higher risk for certain cancers, hypertension, high cholesterol, and noninsulin-dependent diabetes mellitus (adult onset or Type II diabetes). Hypertension, high cholesterol, and diabetes are risk factors for heart disease. The close association of the major risk factors for heart disease with obesity has made it difficult to determine the independent contribution of being overweight/obese to heart disease.[2] However, severe obesity has been considered a risk factor for heart disease by the National Cholesterol Education Program Adult Treatment Guidelines and the Framingham Study.[3]

Many factors are involved in weight control. They include habitual physical activity, food intake, and genetics.[4] The human body is very efficient at storing fat. During the majority of time that humans have been alive, food has been scarce and the ability to store extra energy (fat) was an important "advantage" for survival. Today, access to food is relatively unlimited, and the "advantage" has become somewhat of a disadvantage. The content of the modern diet also contributes to being overweight. Americans eat more fat per capita than any other nation in the world and are among the most inactive people in the world.[4] Low levels of physical activity coupled with a high-fat diet will result in weight gain. We also know that a

---

TABLE 18.1
**Body Composition Classifications Based
on Body Fat Content and Body Mass Index**

		Desirable	Mild Obesity	Severe Obesity
Men	(% Fat)	15–20%	>25%	>30%
	BMI	<25	25–30	>30
Women	(% Fat)	19–25%	>30%	>35%
	BMI	<25	25–30	>30

---

small portion of the population can attribute their obesity to genetically related hormonal imbalances and low resting metabolism. Losing weight is a multibillion dollar business in America today. There is regularly at least one diet book on the best-seller list. Multiple for-profit weight loss programs are evident in all communities. Everyone is looking for the "quick fix." However, research has demonstrated that there is no quick fix for being overfat! "Weight management is accomplished through a lifetime commitment to physical activity and adequate food selection."[5] Thus, there appears to be considerable importance placed on life-long weight control. Because exercise has become an important part of weight control, those involved with exercise programs should have some basic knowledge of the principles of weight management.

CONCEPTS OF OBESITY AND OVERWEIGHT

Ideal body weight: Ideal body weight refers to the weight that is considered healthy for an individual based on averages determined by weighing large numbers of people. Ideal weight usually takes into account gender, height, frame size, and age. It is better to think of ideal weight as a range rather than one absolute number. Ideal weights are based on averages. Due to individual variation, many people may have "actual" ideal weights that are higher or lower than the population norms. There are several methods for estimating ideal weight.[6,7] The most accepted are the height/weight tables and body mass index (BMI). Body mass index is a ratio of weight to height. It is computed by taking the weight in kilograms and dividing it by the height in meters, squared. Table 18.1 presents the ideal ranges in both BMI and percent body fat.

Overweight: This is a condition in which an individual's weight exceeds their ideal body weight, as determined on the basis of gender, height, and frame size, by 10%.[2]

Obesity: In general, when a person exceeds their "ideal weight" by 20% or greater, they are considered moderately obese. Severe obesity is classified as being 30% above ideal weight.[2]

Rather than measuring body fat, many studies have examined BMI to determine the prevalence of overweight and obesity. The second (1976–80) National Health and Nutrition Examination Survey (NHANES II) using height/weight measures

---

TABLE 18.2
Theoretical Computation of Ideal Body Weight

Ideal Weight = Lean Weight/(1 − Desired %Body Fat)
Example: 175-lb male with 25% fat would like to be 17% fat
  Current Weight × Actual % Body Fat (as a decimal) = Fat Weight
    175 lb × .25 = 43.75 lb Fat Weight
  Total Body Weight − Fat Weight = Lean Weight (LW)
    175 lb − 43.75 lb = 131.25 lb
  Ideal Weight = LW × (1 + Desired % Body Fat (in decimal form))
    131.25 lb/(1 − .17)
  131.25 lb/.83 = 158 lb
To reach his desired body composition, this person would have to lose 21.5 lb (9.75
  kg) of fat without losing lean body mass.

---

estimated that 24.2% of men and 27.1% of women were overweight, and 8% of men and 10.8% of women were severely overweight.[2] The more recent National Health Survey study has shown that about 33% of the population is overweight, and the incidence of severe obesity is increasing.[1] The actual number of people who are obese is probably higher because it is possible to be at one's "ideal weight" and have low muscle mass and excess body fat. As people age, the problem of weight gain becomes more severe. The percentage of the population that is overweight or obese increases by 5% or more for every five years of age older. Over 50% of women over age 55 and about 60% of men over age 55 are overweight.[2]

DETERMINING IDEAL BODY WEIGHT

A common and simple method for determining ideal body weight uses gender, frame size and height/weight charts developed by the Metropolitan Life Insurance Co.[5] Frame size is estimated using wrist circumference and height. The wrist circumference is measured at the base of the hand just above the styloid process (the bone that sticks out a little on the outside of the wrist). Frame size can then be determined from tables based on wrist circumference and height (see Appendix B; Tables B-1, B-2, and B-3). Gender, frame size, and height are used to find the range of ideal weights. The tables are based on heights for men wearing 1-in. shoes and for women wearing 2-in. shoes.

The major problem with the height and weight charts is that they do not take into account body composition, the proportion of fat and lean in the body. Total body weight is made up of lean body weight and fat weight. Lean body weight includes muscle, bone, organs, blood, and other bodily fluids and tissues. Fat weight is simply fat. It is possible to be overweight and not be overfat, such as in the case of a football player or weight lifter with a large muscle mass and very low body fat.[7] On the other hand, it is possible to be at your ideal weight according to height and weight charts and be overfat.[7] The formula in Table 18.2 uses lean body weight and desirable percent body fat to estimate ideal weight. This is a theoretical method, and in reality may not be completely accurate. However, the method does give an individual a logical goal.

PHYSIOLOGY OF WEIGHT CONTROL

Fat has many important functions in the body.[7] It helps to regulate body temperature. North American natives (Eskimos) living near the Arctic Circle have a fairly high percent of body fat, which insulates the body against the cold and also helps the body retain heat. Conversely, members of the Masai Tribe living in the heat of Africa are very tall and have very low levels of body fat, thus facilitating the release of heat from the body. Fat in the abdominal area helps to cushion the internal organs. Fat is also important in the production of hormones that are necessary in reproductive and other physiological processes.

Fat is stored in adipose tissue, which is composed of fat cells or adipocytes. Fat accumulates by the filling of existing adipocytes (hypertrophy) and by the formation of new adipocytes (hyperplasia). Studies of fat cell number and size in obese and nonobese subjects show that obese subjects have on the average three times as many adipocytes as the nonobese participants. The fat cells were also at least twice as large in the obese subjects compared to the nonobese subjects. It is believed that when fat cells reach a certain size, events are triggered that result in an increase in the number of fat cells. Unfortunately, even though fat cells decrease in size with weight loss, the number of fat cells does not decrease.[2] That may be one reason why adults who were fat children are much more likely to be fat than adults who were normal weight children. Also, the number of fat cells can increase throughout life but usually after childhood fat cell numbers increase very slowly. That can contribute to "creeping obesity."

There is evidence that suggests that obesity may be an inheritable trait like eye or hair color. Studies of identical twins separated at birth have found that if one twin was obese, the other twin tended to be obese, even if one or both of the twins lived with parents who were normal weight. Part of the genetic difference may be related to the number of fat cells that are formed during the early growth stage. Some studies have suggested that fat cell numbers may stabilize after the first decade in life. Thus, weight gain for adults is related to increased fat deposition in the existing cells and not an increase in the number of fat cells.[2] Studies of extremely obese people suggest that at some point the existing fat cells can no longer hypertrophy, so new fat cells are formed.[2]

SET POINT THEORY OF WEIGHT CONTROL

The Set Point Theory attempts to explain how the body regulates weight and why some people gain weight very easily and others do not.[2,5] This theory suggests that the brain regulates the metabolic rate to keep the body at a set weight.[8] For example, if a person eats more than the usual amount of food, the body increases the metabolic rate to burn off the extra calories, thus body weight is maintained. Alternately, if a person reduces the amount of food eaten, the body slows the metabolic rate and fewer calories are required to maintain body weight. That may be a coping mechanism that evolved in humans to improve the odds of survival during famine; however, it is just a theory.[4] According to the Set Point Theory, certain people may be at higher risk of obesity because their set point weight is elevated or their regulatory mechanism is blunted. In addition, it appears that once the body gains fat, it "protects" these stores. The Set Point Theory says that dieting is perceived by the body as a period of starvation, so the body lowers metabolic rate to preserve fat stores. Regular exercise seems to lower the "set point" weight over a long period of time. Drugs and substances such as nicotine also modify the "set point."[5] That may be one reason why smokers tend to weigh less than nonsmokers.

THE FAT CELL HORMONE LEPTIN

Leptin is a hormone secreted from the adipose tissue that can reduce appetite and potentially increase energy expenditure. As the fat cells become larger, there is a greater output of leptin, which then is transported by the blood back to the brain where it suppresses the appetite center.[9] Conversely, as fat deposits are reduced, leptin decreases. And that enhances the appetite. This hormone has been considered to be one of the signals for the Set Point Theory. This feedback system works fairly effectively in normal weight individuals. In obese persons leptin is elevated, and appetite does not appear to be suppressed nor is energy expenditure elevated. The reason for the lack of effect of leptin in obese individuals is not well understood; however, there is some belief that the cells lose their responsiveness to leptin.[9] Clearly, more research is needed to clarify the role of leptin.

ENERGY BALANCE

The energy in food is measured in kilocalories (kcal). A kilocalorie is the amount of energy it takes to heat 1 kg (2.2 lb) of water 1° Celsius (1.8° Fahrenheit). Kilocalories are the same as calories that are listed on labels and in tables of foods that give calorie and nutrient content of food. Energy balance occurs when energy intake equals energy used. Positive energy balance occurs when more calories are taken in than are used. Negative energy balance happens when energy intake is less than energy output. You may also see the terms negative calorie balance or positive calorie balance. Unfortunately, it does not take a very large excess of calories to result in weight gain, especially when the excess intake is maintained over a long period of time. An additional 115 calories a day (less than a 12-oz. soda) amount to a weight gain of about a pound a month.

$$115 \text{ cal} \times 30 \text{ days} = 3450 \text{ calories } (3500 \text{ calories} = 1 \text{ lb fat})$$

For most of history, the majority of the human diet consisted of plant foods, which are lower in calories, higher in carbohydrates and fiber, and lower in fat than animal-based foods. In fact, many present-day primitive tribes and "peasant societies" still eat diets composed of 60 to 80% of carbohydrates.[10] Those tribes have very low rates of heart disease and do not have the age-related increases in body fat, blood pressure, and cholesterol that we see in Western societies.

Today, meat and dairy products account for almost half of the calorie intake.[11] Typically, those foods obtain more than 40% of the calories from fat. Also, fat has more than twice the calories that carbohydrates have for the same weight of food. Thus, excess consumption of fat means that many people eat more calories than they need and are in positive energy balance. Consuming extra fat has other disadvantages besides the fact that it is high in calories. Dietary fat is effortlessly converted to body fat. The large amount of sweets and desserts consumed by Americans also contributes to positive energy balance. As little as 10 extra calories per day could potentially add up to a little over 1 lb of fat gained per year. Although extra carbohydrate calories can be converted to fat, the conversion process uses about 23% of the total food energy in the conversion. Thus, about one-fourth of the calories of carbohydrates is used to make the conversion rather than being stored. That process may occur to some extent in individuals with very high calorie intake, but in reality it does not happen very frequently.

The modern sedentary human has evolved from hunter/gatherer, a lifestyle that requires high energy expenditure including bouts of strenuous activity. Until recently, humans spent most of their time being physically active, looking for or producing food, farming, and herding. The development of machines in the 20th century, mainly since World War II, has drastically reduced required daily physical activity. Today, very few jobs require physical activity.[11] People get up in the morning and sit in cars to drive to work. When they arrive at work, they sit at desks (or in a car) to do their work. After work they sit in cars to drive home. At home they sit down to dinner, then sit on the couch and watch television or read a book. Today, only about 20% of the American population exercises three times per week.[2] Another 20% of Americans are moderately active, and 60% of Americans can be classified as sedentary. Low levels of physical activity can lead to positive energy balance, which contributes as much to the development of obesity as increased food and fat intake. The key to weight control over time is consistency in caloric intake and physical activity level.[5]

ESTIMATING CALORIC NEED

The number of calories expended each day depends on several factors, including total body weight, muscle mass, and activity level. Total calorie expenditure is made up of the following components:

- Basal Metabolic Rate (BMR): The number of calories burned to keep the body functioning at its lowest level.[7] It is dependent upon weight and muscle mass. A person with a high proportion of muscle mass will burn more calories than a person of the same weight with less muscle mass. BMR is also affected by hormones. BMR is highly variable between individuals.
- Thermogenesis: The number of calories burned to digest meals.
- Physical and daily activity: The number of calories burned to do all activities above the basal level (talking, sitting, shivering, fidgeting, walking, running, etc.).

ESTIMATING CALORIC EXPENDITURE

To determine directly the exact number of calories an individual uses per day is difficult, time-consuming, and expensive. The gold standard for measuring calorie expenditure is to measure heat produced while a person is inside a calorimeter.[7] There are several indirect methods that can provide a fairly close estimate.

1. *Activity factor*: One very simple way to estimate caloric need (to maintain current weight) is to take the person's weight and multiply it by an activity factor.[12] The activity factors are 15 to 18 for men and 12 to 15 for women; the low numbers in the range indicate an inactive lifestyle, and the high numbers indicate a very active lifestyle. Designating the activity level is not easy or exact. A person who has an active job such as construction or landscaping would be considered very active as would a person with a relatively inactive job who worked out at least four times per week.

> Example: A male runs 3 miles a day and weighs 175 lb
> Activity factor would be: 17
> Weight × Activity Factor = Caloric Expenditure per Day
> 175 × 17 = 2975 calories/day

2. *BMR + activity factor + exercise*: This method is often used in computer programs that estimate caloric need. In this method, BMR is calculated and then work and other activities are added in to come up with total caloric expenditure.

> BMR = 1 calorie per kg per hour for a man
> 0.9 calorie per kg per hour for a woman

Activity factor expressed as percentage of basal metabolism as a function of work activity:

> Sedentary lifestyle — 20% (mostly sitting)
> Light activity — 30% (a teacher)
> Moderately active — 40% (a nurse or law enforcement officer)
> Very active — 50% (a roofer or landscaper)

Exercise factor: Tables 18.5 and 18.6 at the end of this chapter indicate the number of calories burned doing specific activities.

> Example: Same male runs 3 miles twice a week and weighs 175 lb
> Weight lb/2.2 kg = Weight kg
> 175/2.2 = 79.5 kg
> Weight kg. × 1 kcal = BMR/hour
> 79.5 kg × 1 kcal/kg/hr = 79.5 kcal/hour
> BMR/hour × 24 = BMR/day
> 79.5 kcal/hour × 24 hours = 1908 kcal/day
> Add work activity for a police officer
> BMR + (40% × BMR)
> 1908 kcal/day + 763 kcal = 2671 kcal/day
> Add exercise program
> 3 mile run = 400 kcal (calculated from Table 18.5)
> 2671 kcal/day + 400 kcal = 3071 kcal

In those examples of the same person, the caloric expenditure calculated in two different ways was fairly consistent. The first example may have underestimated the person's daily expenditure, but it could be the other way around. The second method gives an idea of how much work and other activities contribute to total calories burned per day. Both of those methods are general estimates.

The two methods were designed to provide an estimate of the number of calories needed to maintain weight. If a person is overweight, then obviously that person does not want to maintain current weight. To determine the ideal number of calories a person needs to maintain his desired weight, the person would simply substitute desired weight for their actual weight in the above formulas.

Example: Same male who runs 3 miles twice a week has an ideal weight of 165 lb
65/2.2 = 74.8 kg
74.8 kg × 1 kcal/kg/hr = 74.8 kcal/hour
74.89.5 kcal/hour × 24 hours = 1796 kcal/day
1796 kcal/day + 718 kcal = 2514 kcal/day
3 mile run = 400 kcal
2514 kcal/day + 400 kcal = 2914 kcal
3072 kcal − 2914 = 158 kcal/day decrease to maintain 165 lb

METHODS FOR LOSING WEIGHT

It is important that a person who wants to lose weight choose a weight that is appropriate for them. Someone who would like to lose a great deal of weight should choose intermediate weight loss goals as well as a final goal weight. Total weight loss per week should be no more than 1 to 2 lbs. Table 18.3 gives an example of how to calculate the total time needed for weight loss. The information given above and in the chapter on body composition (Chapter 4) should provide sufficient information to determine an appropriate goal weight for a program participant. The desired weight can then be used to estimate the number of calories required to maintain the new weight. Setting unrealistic (too low) weight goals usually leads to frustration, decreased motivation, and ultimate noncompliance on the part of the person trying to lose weight. Although many people lose weight each year, more than half of them will gain the weight back within a year.[2] Maintenance of weight loss appears to be more difficult than losing weight.

DIETING

Dieting is reducing food or calorie intake to create a negative energy balance. Ideally, more calories are burned than taken in, and the body must use fat stores to supply the extra energy. In general, dieting causes significant weight loss in the first few weeks; however, most of the loss is due to water loss.[7] When few calories are eaten, the body first uses its glycogen stores, which results in loss of stored water. For each unit of glycogen used, approximately 3 units of water are released.[7] As the glycogen stores deplete, the body will start to metabolize protein. Protein metabolism causes

TABLE 18.3
Estimating Amount and Time for Weight Loss

Man: 190 lb & 25% body fat	Woman: 150 lb & 30% body fat
Desired body fat = 18%	Desired body fat = 25%
190 × .25 = 47.5 lb fat mass	150 × .3 = 45 lb fat mass
190 – 47.5 = 142.5 lb LBM	150 – 45 = 105 lb LBM
142.5/(1–.18) = 174 lb	105/(1–.25) = 140 lb
190 – 174 = 16 lb weight loss	150 – 140 = 10 lb weight loss
16 lb/1.5 lb per week = about 11 weeks	10 lb/2 lb per week = 5 weeks

considerable water loss; each unit of protein used for energy causes the release of 15 units of water.[7]

After about two weeks of dieting, weight loss slows considerably. That is because the body starts to use considerable fats. Fat has more than twice the calories of protein or glycogen and very little water. Thus, it takes over twice the amount of work to burn off the same amount of fat weight as compared to protein and carbohydrate weight (9 kcal/g vs. 4 kcal/g), and in addition, little water weight is lost. Another disadvantage of dieting is that it lowers BMR by as much as 40%![7] Thus, the body requires fewer calories to maintain current weight, and weight loss is further slowed. Those occurrences slow weight loss and often lead to frustration, disappointment, and discontinuation of the weight-loss program. There is also some evidence that the reduction in BMR remains for some time after the diet is discontinued.[13] Therefore, if the dieter resumes his prediet eating pattern, he will regain the weight that was lost more quickly. However, it appears that the effect on BMR is not maintained for long periods of time, as research shows that years of on-again/off-again dieting does not result in more weight gain than would occur without the dieting.[14]

Many diets have been designed and marketed. Some of those diets are healthy, recommending reductions in fat and refined sugar combined with increases in fruits, vegetables, low-fat meat and dairy, and whole grain products. Other diets, often those promising quick results, are unbalanced nutritionally and can be very dangerous to one's health. Some of the more questionable diets are discussed below.

Single food diets: These diets are based on one food, such as grapefruit or eggs. There is usually a claim that the food has weight-reducing benefits. In general, these diets are low in calories and do produce weight loss. However, due to lack of food variety, they are not balanced nutritionally and can lead to micronutrient deficiencies. These diets should be avoided.[5,7]

Ketogenic diets: These diets are usually high in protein, high in fat, and low in carbohydrate.[5,7] They are based on the concept that if there are no carbohydrates, the body must burn fat. This type of diet is usually advertised as allowing the dieter to eat as much of whatever they want as long as they stay away from carbohydrates. Without carbohydrates, fat cannot be completely metabolized. The incomplete metabolism of fat causes ketone bodies to be formed. Proponents of ketogenic diets maintain that the presence of these ketone bodies reduces appetite and causes loss of unused calories in urine. Actually, the number of calories lost this way is about 100 to 150 per day. This loss would, at best, result in a loss of about 1 lb. per month. The majority of weight lost is due to loss of water and muscle. The water loss is related to the use of glycogen (3 oz. water/1 oz. CHO burned) and protein (15 oz. water/1 oz. protein burned). Some individuals using ketogenic diets may actually gain body fat because of the high intake of fatty foods. Moreover, the high fat intake can increase cholesterol. Research has shown that ketogenic diets are potentially dangerous because of the accumulation of the ketones which disturb the body's acid-base balance and can lead to cardiac arrhythmia's, acidosis, kidney problems, dehydration, and electrolyte imbalance.[5,7] In summary, these types of diets are ineffective, dangerous, and should be avoided.

High protein/low carbohydrate diets: These diets are very similar to ketogenic diets except that they are low in calorie and fat intake. Proponents of these diets claim that high protein/low carbohydrate diets increase fat use and cause the formation of ketone bodies that suppress appetite.[5,7] A further claim is that the negative calorie balance is enhanced because the body uses more calories to digest protein foods than carbohydrates. This type of diet causes dramatic water loss, loss of muscle tissue, and lowered resting metabolic rate.[5,7] This type of diet has the same problems as the ketogenic diets and is risky.

Very low calorie diets and protein-sparing fasts: These diets use low caloric intake to create a large negative energy balance. Protein and carbohydrate are consumed to reduce metabolism of lean body mass and promote metabolism of fat tissue. These diets were designed to bring about rapid weight loss in individuals with life-threatening obesity.[7] This kind of diet should be attempted only under physician supervision. It is hoped that the break from prior dietary habits will give the dieter a chance to establish new dietary habits conducive to maintaining weight loss. The dieter typically gets fewer than 1,000 calories per day, including 15 to 24 g of protein, about 45 g of carbohydrate, and vitamin and mineral supplements.[5,7] Supposedly, this combination of nutrients spares lean tissue. These diets do lead to rapid weight loss, but a large part of the weight loss will be lean body mass and water. Optifast® and Slimfast® are popular versions of these diets. One of the major drawbacks of these diets is that the excessively low caloric intake greatly reduces BMR. Physical activity is also reduced because of feelings of low energy and lethargy. Reductions in physical activity level increase the loss of lean tissue (use it or lose it!) and also decrease the number of calories burned per day. Although the very low calorie diets are effective in reducing weight, the weight is typically regained rapidly after the diet is discontinued.

Yo-Yo Dieting

Over half of the people who lose weight by dieting will regain the weight lost, plus some extra within one year.[2] That is believed to be due to the lower metabolic rate as a result of the diet, making it easier to regain weight. The weight gained back is typically fat with a small proportion of muscle mass. Thus, dieters often end up "fatter" than before they began to diet. That will cause the person to repeat the diet cycle again to lose the additional weight. The repeated cycle will again have an effect on resting metabolic rate, causing the same sequence of events to occur as did after the first weight-loss cycle. This cyclic or yo-yo dietary pattern can happen over and over, leaving the person fatter each time. There is evidence that yo-yo dieting can make it increasingly difficult for the person to lose weight due to permanent reduction in BMR.[5,6] Although recent research has suggested that yo-yo dieters may not be fatter than normal, weight cycling may be even more harmful to health than being overfat.[14] The phenomenon of weight cycling is one of the best reasons to make gradual lifelong changes in diet and exercise and to lose weight very slowly.

EXERCISE

Physical activity has been recognized as an important part of weight control.[15] Until a few years ago, obesity was thought to be a problem of eating too much. Today, we realize that the total picture is much more complicated. Exercise, either alone or in combination with diet, can be used to lose weight. In fact, those weight loss programs that include exercise seem to be the most successful in the long term.[16] Exercise burns calories, and if caloric intake stays the same or is decreased, exercise can create a negative energy balance. Compared to dieting, exercise causes more fat to be used for energy and at the same time causes proteins to be conserved. However, the number of calories burned in a typical exercise session is only about 300 to 400, which if completed four days a week would result in the loss of 1 to 2 lb per month.[17] The energy deficiency due to exercise may be small, but if exercise is maintained, over time gradual weight loss will occur.

A long-term exercise program does have other benefits. During all exercise, the body burns a combination of carbohydrates and fats. Studies of trained and untrained individuals have shown differences in their metabolisms.[13] Aerobically trained individuals begin to burn fat earlier in the exercise session and can burn fats at higher exercise intensities than untrained people.[7] The changes that occur in the muscle increase the capacity for burning fat at all work loads.[13] Exercise also raises metabolic rate for a short time after exercise, causing additional caloric usage.[2,7] However, the postexercise calorie burn is small, ranging from 20 to 30 kcal after a 20 to 30 minute walk to only 150 kcal after three hours of moderate-intensity exercise. In addition, regular exercise leads to an increase in muscle mass, which increases resting metabolic rate.[5] Finally, exercise helps improve self-image, which can help motivate those trying to change to stay with their programs.[5] Those changes seem small, but they are favorable with regard to weight loss and weight maintenance.

A pitfall of exercise is that too much exercise can increase appetite to the point where it may overcompensate for the calories burned during exercise.[17] That is why it is best to avoid high-intensity exercise of long duration and stick with moderate-intensity exercise (50 to 70% of maximal intensity) for 30 to 40 minutes four to five times per week. It is especially important to understand that extra body weight places an additional load on the heart and body in general. Anyone who has been inactive and is extremely overweight should see their physician before starting an exercise program. The exercise program should be instituted gradually to give the heart and muscles a chance to adapt to new activity requirements. That will also help prevent injury and exercise burnout.

There is accumulating evidence that a strength-training program (weight training) should be a part of an exercise program to lose weight.[18] The strength training conserves muscle mass more than aerobic exercise. At the same time, strength training increases muscle mass, which contributes to a higher BMR; thus, more calories are utilized at rest. Strength training for two to three days a week appears to be all that is necessary to have a positive effect.[19] Thus, an aerobic program combined with weight training may provide the optimal exercise program for weight loss.

DIET AND EXERCISE

The safest, healthiest and most effective way to lose weight is to combine a low-fat, high-carbohydrate diet with regular moderate exercise.[2] By reducing calorie intake and increasing energy use, a negative energy balance is created and weight is lost. Most people can cut the calories in their diets by cutting out the fat. The key to reducing fat seems to be an awareness of which foods contain fat. Thus, food labels become a key to increasing awareness. For example, switching from whole milk (8 g of fat per cup) to skim milk (less than 1 g fat per cup) saves 72 calories per cup. Eating 1 oz. of pretzels (1 or 2 g of fat) as a snack instead of 1 oz. of potato chips (9 to 10 g of fat) saves 63 to 81 calories. Consuming fruit as a snack instead of a candy bar increases carbohydrates, vitamins, and minerals intake and eliminates the fat (9 to 12 g) found in candy bars. Also, one apple has about 70 calories, whereas the typical candy bar has 200 to 230 calories. Three apples could replace one candy bar! Even switching from using cream or half and half in coffee to plain milk reduces fat calories, especially over a period of time.

The other important items in the diet to reduce calories are simple sugars. Dietary sources of simple sugars typically contain limited amounts of other nutrients; they are only calories. Once in the system, sugars elevate insulin, which causes cells to absorb the sugar. If the cellular stores of sugar are full, the blood sugar will be absorbed by the fat cells and converted to fat for storage. Thus, high-sugar diets can contribute to weight gain.

Combining changes in diet with exercise to create a negative energy balance reduces the amount of exercise as compared to the use of exercise alone. That is beneficial because many people who need to lose weight have been inactive for a long time and cannot tolerate high doses of exercise. It is much safer for overweight individuals to start out with an exercise program of moderate intensity and moderate duration. Exercises such as brisk walking, cycling, low-impact aerobic dance, or a walk/jog program are good activities for beginners. As fitness increases, the duration and intensity of the activity can also be increased. Thus, new and more strenuous activities can be added. Weight training in addition to aerobic training is now recommended for those trying to lose fat.[18] However, that type of exercise does not burn fat, so if time is limited, priority should go to aerobic exercise which does burn fat. You can also increase activity and calorie use in your life by doing the following:

- Walking a greater part of the way to your destination (park a block away from where you are going, and walk the rest).
- Taking the stairs instead of the elevator or escalator.
- Using a hand mower and manual clippers when working in the yard.
- Carrying or pulling your golf clubs instead of riding in a cart.
- Walking to an associate's office instead of calling on the phone.
- Getting rid of the remote control for the TV.

Another way to increase activity is to take an active vacation. National and state parks offer a variety of scenic hiking trails. Walking tours of historical districts can be educational as well as helpful with weight loss. Bicycling at the beach or taking extra long walks can be fun. Cycling tours are available for all levels of fitness. Ads in the back of cycling and travel magazines promote a multitude of those tours. For the more adventurous, backpacking and mountain bike camping might be an alternative. In addition, most major hotels now offer on-site workout facilities for guests.

BEHAVIOR MODIFICATION

An important component of weight loss strategies is behavior modification.[2,5] Behavior modification techniques try to change eating habits by teaching awareness behaviors and alternative, better habits. Awareness behavior helps in understanding where behavioral changes can be made and can help in understanding feelings about dietary change. Behavior modification is often a component of formal weight loss programs such as Weight Watchers.®

Human beings eat to satisfy emotional as well as physiological needs. People also respond to certain external cues by eating. For example, many people eat lunch at noon even if they just had a large snack at 11:00 a.m. and are not physically hungry. The first step in behavior modification is to determine the eating behaviors of the person who wants to lose weight. The person is asked to document what and how much he eats, where it is eaten, how he felt when he ate, how much time was spent, what activities (such as television watching) he did, and with whom he ate. Examination of that information helps to identify patterns of behavior associated with eating. For example, a person who has problems with weight may find out that he eats most of his calories while watching television, or may eat when angry. Once the person is aware of those patterns, the next step is to replace existing eating behavior patterns with alternative behaviors. For example, if someone eats after an argument, he could replace eating with a relaxation technique such as taking a walk. Other techniques that may help improve eating and activity behaviors are listed in Table 18.4.

DANGEROUS AND INEFFECTIVE WEIGHT-LOSS TECHNIQUES

Besides diets, many other gadgets and substances have been promoted to accomplish weight loss. Spot reduction is often promoted to remove fat from specific areas. This does not work.[7] Repetitive exercise will tone muscle in a certain area, but it will not

TABLE 18.4
Common Behavioral Modifications Used for Weight Loss Programs[5]

1. Make a commitment to change.
2. Set reasonable goals for weight loss, dietary change, and physical activity.
3. Avoid automatic eating.
4. Stay busy.
5. Plan meals and exercise sessions ahead of time, and stick to the plan.
6. Keep meals as low in fat as possible.
7. Avoid putting extra food on the table (family style), as this may encourage overeating.
8. Serve meals on smaller plates.
9. Eat slowly, give the body time to register as full.
10. Make the act of eating a ritual; restrict eating to one place in the house.
11. Avoid social binges and using holidays or special occasions as rationalization for overeating.
12. Avoid making or buying high-calorie foods.
13. Use stress management techniques to deal with problems rather than eating.
14. Monitor changes in dietary change, physical activity, and weight and reward yourself
    (but not with food).
15. Be gentle on yourself and keep a positive attitude.
16. Make gradual changes so that the process does not become overwhelming.

burn just the local fat stores. The body loses fat from all stores in the body no matter what area is exercising. Electric muscle stimulators, vibrating belts, and elastic belts are all ineffective in causing weight loss.[18] Rubber and plastic suits worn during exercise simply increase the amount of water lost from sweating.[18] They do not increase the amount of fat lost during exercise and can be very dangerous because they limit the body's ability to cool itself. Diet pills are generally ineffective and may be harmful to your health as well as addictive. In general, any plan that promises quick results is probably not safe, healthy, or scientifically correct.

CONCLUSION

The American College of Sports Medicine[15] states in its Position Statement on the components of a desirable weight loss program that a desirable weight loss program does the following:

1. For normal adults, it provides a caloric intake not lower than 1,200 kcal/day so that the proper blend of foods to meet nutritional requirements can be obtained.
2. Includes foods acceptable to the dieter from the viewpoints of sociocultural background, usual habits, taste, cost, and ease in acquisition and preparation.
3. Provides a negative caloric balance (not to exceed 500 to 1,000 kcal/day lower than recommended), resulting in gradual weight loss without metabolic problems. Maximal weight loss should be 1 kg (2.2 lb) per week.

4. Includes the use of behavior modification techniques to identify and eliminate dieting habits that contribute to improper nutrition.
5. Includes an endurance exercise program of at least three days per week, 20 to 30 minutes in duration, at a minimum intensity of 60% of maximal heart rate.
6. Provides that the new eating and physical activity habits can be continued for life to maintain the achieved lower body weight.

Obesity and overweight are increasingly common conditions in the U.S. today.[12] There are supposedly quick routes to weight loss available. However, the success rate of those quick routes is dismal. The safest and most effective way to lose and maintain weight is to adopt a healthy diet (low fat/high carbohydrate) and make exercise a permanent part of life.

TABLE 18.5
Calories Used per Pound of Body Weight per Minute for Selected Activities. Based on Reference 7

Activity	Cal/lb/min	Activity	Cal/lb/min
Archery	0.030	Rowing vigorous	0.090
Badminton rec	0.038	Running 11.0 min/mile	0.070
Badminton comp	0.065	Running 8.5 min/mile	0.090
Basketball mod	0.046	Running 7.0 min/mile	0.102
Basketball comp	0.063	Running 6.0 min/mile	0.114
Cycling 5.5 mph*	0.033	Deep water running	0.100
Cycling 10.0 mph*	0.050	Skating mod	0.038
Cycling 13.0 mph*	0.071	Downhill skiing	0.060
Bowling	0.030	Skiing X-country 5.0 mph	0.078
Calisthenics	0.033	Strength training	0.050
Dance mod	0.030	Swimming crawl 20 yd/min	0.031
Dance vigorous	0.055	Swimming crawl 25 yd/min	0.040
Golf	0.030	Swimming crawl 45 yd/min	0.057
Gymnastics light	0.030	Swimming crawl 50 yd/min	0.070
Gymnastics hard	0.056	Table tennis	0.030
Handball	0.064	Tennis rec	0.045
Hiking	0.040	Tennis comp	0.064
Judo/Karate	0.086	Volleyball	0.030
Racquetball	0.065	Walking 4.5 mph	0.045
Rope jumping	0.060	Walking in shallow pool	0.090
		Wrestling	0.085

* rec = recreational; comp = competition; mod = moderate
* Cycling taken from a level surface

TABLE 18.6
Approximate Caloric Cost of Various Household and Yard Activities[6]

Activity	Cal/hour
Riding lawn mower, typing on manual typewriter	150–240
Cleaning windows, mopping floors, vacuuming, pushing light-power mower	240–300
Scrubbing floors, raking leaves, hoeing	300–360
Digging garden	360–420
Hand lawn mowing, splitting wood, snow shoveling	420–480
Sawing hardwood, digging ditches	480–600

REFERENCES

1. *National Health and Nutrition Examination Survey III, 1988–1994*, National Center for Health Statistics, Washington, D.C., 1997.
2. Pollock, M.L. and Wilmore, J.H., *Exercise in Disease and Health: Evaluation and Prescription for Prevention and Rehabilitation*, W.B. Saunders Company, Philadelphia, 1990.
3. Bray, G.A., Exercise and Obesity, in *Exercise, Fitness, and Health: A Consensus of Current Knowledge*, Bouchard, C., Shepard, R.J., Stephens, T., Sutton, J.R., and McPherson, B.D., eds., Human Kinetics Books, Champaign, 1990.
4. Blackburn, H. and Prineas, R., Diet and hypertension: anthropology, epidemiology, and public health implications, *Prog. Biochem. Pharmacol.*, 19, 31-79, 1983.
5. Hoeger, W.W.K., *Lifetime Physical Fitness and Wellness: A Personalized Program*, Morton Publishing Co., Denver, 1989.
6. Katch, F.I. and McArdle, W.D., *Introduction to Nutrition, Exercise, and Health*, Lea & Febiger, Philadelphia, 1993.
7. McArdle, W.D., Katch, F.I., and Katch, V.L., *Exercise Physiology: Energy, Nutrition, and Human Performance*, Lea & Febiger, Philadelphia, 1991.
8. Ornish, D. Dr., *Dean Ornish's Program for Reversing Heart Disease*, Random House, New York, 1990.
9. Friedman, J.M., Leptin, leptin receptors and the control of body weight, *Eur. J. Med. Res.*, 2, 7-13, 1997.
10. Brody, J.E., *Jane Brody's Good Food Book: Living the High-Carbohydrate Way*, Bantam Books, New York, 1987.
11. Block, G., Dresser, C.M., Hartman, A.M., and Carroll, M.D., Nutrient sources in the American diet: Quantitative data from the NHANES II survey: II. Macronutrients and fats, *Am. J. Epidemiol.*, 122, 27-40, 1985.
12. Schaefer, P.M., *NCJA Physical Fitness Instructors Training Manual*. NCJA Press, Salemburg, 1988.
13. Newsholme, E.A., Effects of exercise on aspects of carbohydrate, fat, and amino acid metabolism, in *Exercise, Fitness, and Health: A Consensus of Current Knowledge*, Bouchard, C., Shepard, R.J., Stephens, T., Sutton, J.R., and McPherson, B.D., eds., Human Kinetics Books, Champaign, 1990.
14. National Task Force on the Prevention and Treatment of Obesity, Weight cycling, *J. Am. Med. Assoc.*, 272, 1196-1202, 1994.

15. American College of Sports Medicine, Proper and improper weight loss programs: Position stand, *Med. Sci. Sports Exer.*, 15, 9-13, 1983.

16. Miller, W.C., Koceja, D.M., and Hamilton, E. J., A meta-analysis of the past 25 years of weight loss research using diet, exercise or diet plus exercise intervention, *Int. J. Obesity*, 21, 941-947, 1997.

17. Stefanik, M.L., Exercise and weight control, in *Exercise Science and Sport Reviews*. Hollozsy, J.O., Ed., Williams & Wilkins, Baltimore, 1993.

18. Williams, M.H., *Nutrition for Fitness and Sport*, Wm.C. Brown Publishers, Dubuque, 1988.

19. Westcott, W., Weight gain and weight loss, *Nautilus,* p. 8-9, 1991.

19 Stress Management

Purpose: To introduce the reader to the basic concepts of stress management.

Objectives: At the end of this session, the reader should be able to do the
following:

1. Recognize the symptoms of stress and distress.
2. Understand the sources of stress and some of the coping mechanisms.
3. Understand how to practice stress management skills.
4. Understand the basics of long-range stress reduction techniques and the need for professional referrals.

INTRODUCTION

The typical model to describe stress starts with a mental or physical stimulus causing a real or perceived strain on the body. This causes the stress response: increased activity in the sympathetic nervous system resulting in vasoconstriction, an elevation of heart rate, blood pressure, ventilation and possibly a release of catecholamines (adrenaline). If the stress response is used to provide a beneficial outcome, the stress is considered eustress.[1] However, if the stress is too great and/or the organism cannot adapt to the stress, physiological and/or psychological damage can occur. That is called distress.[1] Distress also increases anxiety levels, which can further increase stress levels. Distress commonly occurs when the demands of a situation outweigh the perceived abilities to cope with or handle those demands.[2,3] It is prolonged occurrences of distress that need to be brought under control to reduce stress-related maladies.

THE STRESS RESPONSE

There are three phases to the response to stress.[3] The first is the acute *alarm response*. The alarm response increases the sympathetic nervous system and the adrenal glands activity resulting in the following:

1. Vasoconstriction, which results in an increase in blood pressure.
2. Increased heart rate. The increase in blood pressure and heart rate combine to increase the work load on the heart.
3. Reduction in gastric motility. The reduced activity in the stomach will dramatically slow digestion and increase the possibility of gas formation.

4. Increased activation of blood clotting factors, which enhances the risk of thrombosis or clotting.
5. Increased blood lipids. This effect could lead to an increased risk of cardiovascular disease.
6. Increased metabolic rate.
7. The release of catecholamines (adrenaline), which intensifies the sympathetic nervous effects.

If the stress continues over a long period of time, the body responds by adapting or learning to cope with the stress. This is the second, or *resistance, phase*. If the body cannot adapt to or cope with the stress, it enters the third phase, *failing adaptation*. During failing adaptations, there is a greater susceptibility to many diseases and an increased risk of many lifestyle diseases because the body has lost its ability to counter the stress.

Some stress is thought to be necessary. An organism does not grow, learn, or develop without some eustress. However, too much stress, distress, is what leads to problems. The difficulty is determining how much stress a person can handle. In addition, not all people respond to the same stress the same way. Thus, comparisons of adaptive abilities between individuals is not appropriate: "One man's distress is another's stimulus."[1] Furthermore, the symptoms of distress may take 20 years to be evident. Thus, it may be difficult to determine when someone is experiencing distress.

An individual needs to know when the body is distressed so that attempts can be made to reduce stress. Furthermore, there is a need to know the signs and symptoms of prolonged distress so that attempts can be made to reduce it. The following are typical indicators of stress or distress.

Acute signs and symptoms of stress include the following:[4]

Clenched teeth or muscle tension	Migraine headaches
Biting fingernails or pen tops	Irritability
Cold skin	Sudden accident proneness
Frequent urination	

Signs and symptoms of prolonged stress include the following:[3,4]

Insomnia, continuous fatigue — waking up each morning still tired
Back and neck aches
Morning nausea or heartburn and potentially irritable bowel syndrome — diarrhea or constipation
Increased frequency of minor illness

Because signs and symptoms of prolonged stress may not be obvious to an individual, the following 10 questions are actually used as common signs of distress.[4] These questions are answered with a yes or no. If the person answering these questions finds that the majority of responses are yes, then there is a good possibility

---

TABLE 19.1
Job Related Sources of Stress

1. *Intrinsic to Job*
   Poor physical working conditions
   Work overload
   Time pressures
   Physical danger
3. *Relationships at Work*
   Poor relations with boss
   Poor relations with subordinates
   Poor relations with colleagues
   Difficulty delegating responsibilities
5. *Career Development*
   Over promotion
   Under promotion
   Lack of job security
   Thwarted ambition

2. *Role in the Organization*
   Role ambiguity
   Role conflict
   Responsibility for people
   Conflicts on boundaries
4. *Organizational Structure*
   Office politics
   Restrictions on behavior
   No effective consultation
   Limited participation in decision making

---

that distress is occurring and that something needs to be done to reduce stress levels. Experience has shown that having an observer who knows the person responding to the questionnaire also respond to the questions can be revealing because those under stress may not want to admit it.

1. Are you restless and unable to relax?
2. Do you get angry if things do not go your way?
3. Do you seem excessively fatigued?
4. Do you have concentration difficulties?
5. Have you lost interest in recreational activities?
6. Do you worry about things that cannot be changed?
7. Are you working excessively but not effectively?
8. Do you take more and more work home?
9. Are you smoking or drinking more?
10. Do you have the perception of "losing what's important?"

TYPE A BEHAVIOR PATTERN

Type A behavior pattern has been implicated as one cause of a stressful lifestyle. Type A people are characterized by a chronic struggle to do more and more in less and less time.[3] These types of people usually are praised by society as hard workers. However, as time progresses they become "pencil pushers" because they lose creativity, and numbers and deadlines control their lives. Because they cannot keep up, they become very aggressive. There is a need to become aggressive to achieve in our society, but not overaggressive! Perhaps the most damaging part of the behavior pattern is free-floating hostility that many Type A's exhibit. Recent evidence suggests that as long as the hostility can be controlled and adequate coping mechanisms exist, Type A behavior may not be as big a health problem as once suspected.

SOURCES OF WORK-RELATED STRESS

Table 19.1 is a list of the typical job stressors.[3] The list is quite long. Add to this list other personal stresses such as family problems, midlife crises, financial difficulties, and even commuting, and it is easy to see how the modern world creates overstress.

APPROACHES TO STRESS REDUCTION

Drugs: Prescription drugs, street drugs, or alcohol all reduce the stress response but do not remove the stressor.[3] Thus, there becomes a dependency on these drugs to reduce the feelings of stress in all stressful situations — possibly for life. The following is a list of drugs commonly used to reduce stress, along with their side effects.

Prescription drugs typically include the following:

Diuretics (Thiazides, Furosemides): considerable potassium loss, muscle weakness, calf pains, cardiac arrhythmias

Tranquilizers (Valium, phenothiazines, lithium): drowsiness, stupor, slurred speech, cardiac arrhythmias

Beta blockers (Inderal, Pindolol, Atenolol, Timolol): fatigue, forgetfulness, depression, impotence

Street drugs:

Marijuana: lethargy, apathy, deterioration of mental and physical performance

Cocaine: heart failure, euphoria replaced with depression, hallucinations, malnutrition, sexual impotence

Alcohol: depressant effects (even crying jags), loss of mental and physical capacity to perform, DTs, malnutrition, liver and brain damage

Opiates: lethargy, drowsiness, nausea, itching, loss of appetite, constipation, depression, loss of sex drive

Behavior modification: Behavior modification works better than drugs in the long run because it removes or reduces the stressor.[3,4] This is probably the most difficult route and it will increase stress levels in the short run but ultimately improves the life of the individual in the long run. The first step is to determine the stressors. The second step is to determine if the stressor is modifiable. If a change is possible, then behavior modification should be applied. There is no single best behavioral technique to reduce stress. Many approaches might need to be taken before one will work. The following are some suggestions that others have used successfully.[3,4]

Set goals or priorities and evaluate from two perspectives: Career goals: Where do you want to be in the future? Are you happy in your present job? Private life priorities: 1st family, 2nd church, 3rd friends? Those goals and priorities will allow the individual to make decisions concerning incorporating additional responsibilities into his life. To reduce stress, the individual needs to keep "the straight and narrow." Goals and priorities will need to be reviewed frequently as life changes.

The person should set aside a portion of the day for himself. At first this must be deliberate — "each day at ___." To many individuals it will seem like a waste of time, an unpleasurable experience, but as time progresses the person will look forward to this period. This time can be used to organize life, read a book, go fishing, or even exercise.

Remove the clutter from life. Clutter can be evident in the form of schedule, miscellaneous tasks, or messy desks. The stressed individual needs to schedule hard work at the optimal times of day whenever possible. Some people are morning people; others are at their best in the afternoon. Also, people should schedule time to prepare for each client: role play. Cubby holes or an improved filing system can be used to get rid of clutter on desks. Subordinates can be used to do unimportant tasks.

Improve physical surroundings to promote peace. Pastel colors on the office walls and comfortable furniture promote relaxation. Personalized areas with pictures, plants, or other memorabilia also promote relaxation. Interruptions can be reduced by turning the desk away from others or away from the door. With regard to doors, they were designed close as well as open. Busy people cannot feel obligated to be available at all times. They should try to predict busy and slow times and close the door during the slow times. Experience has shown that co-workers will only be annoyed a couple of times, and then they will adjust. Noise level can also cause stress. Radios and white noise can be used to tune in or out others.

Activities can be added to life that are considered "humane," such as art, music, drama, nature, and fishing. Participation in those activities increases contact with others in a noncompetitive atmosphere, thus reducing stress.

Good nutrition can reduce stress. Hypoglycemia (low blood sugar) increases anxiety and stress. Meals should not be skipped, as this practice leads to hypoglycemia. Coffee and doughnuts breakfasts or midafternoon candy pick-me-ups should be avoided for the same reason. The donuts and candy elevate insulin, which can result in a rebound hypoglycemia, increasing irritability and anxiety. Fruit or fruit juices, which provide some sugar but do not "load" the system, are better choices of snacks than high-sugar snacks.

Alcohol intake should be reduced. Individuals at cocktail parties should stop early or schedule something toward the end of the evening that forces early "regrets." Alternating alcoholic and nonalcohol drinks can also help, as will diluting alcoholic drinks by adding soda or water. Waiters carrying drinks should be avoided. Instead, the person should go to the bar to get the drinks. Chances are they will meet people along the way and engage in conversations, which slows down the drinking. Some people will sip drinks slowly; the longer it takes, the poorer it tastes. (Think about warm beer or a diluted Bloody Mary!) When a person is eating out, the food should be ordered first and the drinks second. Fine wine with dinner is preferable to drinks before dinner. Some people will arrive at a restaurant early and order nonalcoholic beverages, then they keep ordering "the same." Other people will schedule to be back at the office.

Some traditions should be kept, such as enjoyed events and fond memories. These are not the Christmases at the homestead with all the children and grandchildren. These are small events that bring pleasure to life and can bring back fond memories.

Exercise can be used to reduce stress, tension, anxiety, and depression. Exercise training improves the ability to manage stress. Research has shown that trained individuals have a reduced response to a given amount of stress. Exercise creates a sense of confidence and control, which reduces stress. Exercise can be useful for bridging two stressful situations (job vs. home). Exercise promotes relaxation. In general, the body responds the same to psychological and physiological stress. However, the stress response was intended for physical stress. Thus, exercise benefits from the stress. In contrast, mental stress causes the same responses but those responses are not beneficially used. The best form of exercise to reduce stress is aerobic and noncompetitive in nature, of moderate intensity, lasting 10 minutes or longer.

Reduce uncertainty on the job. A specific job description, regular performance review sessions with some form of self-evaluation will reduce feelings of uncertainty regarding employment.

For time-pressure deadlines, be clear in what is required of you. The person that will be completing the task should explain his position, being clear regarding what he needs to meet the demand (Help? Personnel? Time? Money?). At the same time, the person making the demands should help determine how other duties or priorities should be shifted.

Compartmentalizing job and home life is difficult for many high stress individuals. There are three misconceptions that enhance stress levels at home: 1) "My family and friends will understand." Family and friends understand when this happens sporadically, but they will not understand if it happens regularly. 2) "At home I can be myself." (A mean, grouchy, inconsiderate person?) 3) "This is only temporary." It is *not*! In this modern world, pressure is a way of life. Here are some possible solutions.

- End the day smoothly. Easier projects finished in the afternoon before going home give a feeling of accomplishment. Also, listening to relaxing music on the way home helps some individuals reduce stress.
- Leave unfinished business on the desk. Some individuals find that making a list of tomorrow's priorities before leaving work helps them feel organized for tomorrow.
- Exercise between work and home can be used to bridge two stressful situations. Professional women who also have family responsibilities find this useful.

- Everyone should ask for a few minutes when first arriving at home in an attempt to refocus from work to home life. The family or friends should not be rejected, but that time could be obtained by simply changing clothes or even taking a shower.
- The dinner conversation should be directed away from work. This helps some people start to put the job into perspective. For others, discussing the job at dinner may reduce stress.
- Schedules should not be planned too far in advance. It is easier to keep track of schedules and reduces family, social, and job-related conflicts. Conversely, procrastination simply increases stress levels. We all need to keep in mind a successful life is unfinished.

Everyone needs to learn to say "no" nicely.

A. The art of saying no tries to minimize the negative and emphasize the positive. "Our sincere thanks for your input. We were impressed by your efforts, but unfortunately..."
B. Bridges should not "be burned," and hard work should be praised. In other words, a door should be left open for future contact: "You're on the right track, but we need to go further."
C. Responsibilities should be shared. "Thanks for sending me the sample. I will try to use it when I get a chance."
D. A graceful "no" also conveys gratitude without commitment. "Thanks for your invitation, but I cannot attend. Perhaps another time?"
E. An elegant "no" gets the point across in a firm, but in a friendly manner. "I hope you don't take offense, but I really dislike cigarette smoke. Could we move to a more vented area?"
F. In many cases a "no" should be followed up with offers of alternative solutions.

To reduce stress, on-the-job petty anger should be resolved without blowing up or brooding. The angry person should first make a list of things that are causing the anger. Then the situation should be reappraised based on that list. The appraisal should include a look for any environmental factors that could have caused the anger (hot weather, hunger, noise). This a situation in which rudeness will not help. The person should try to remember that laughter can be used to break down anger.

People should try to avoid no-win situations to reduce stress. "Social war games" and job or social-related "treadmills" greatly enhance feelings of stress.

CRITICISM

One of the biggest causes of stress both in the workplace and in nonwork-related settings is receiving and getting criticism. Criticism can be a no-win situation. Therefore, the criticizer needs to think through the criticism before making it. Psychologists have suggested several key points when giving or receiving criticism:

A. Pinpoint the specific behavior causing the problem.
B. Once the problem is determined, there needs to be some consideration as to whether or not a change is possible or if criticism will help. If a change is not possible or the criticism will not improve the situation, then another approach to the problem may be necessary.
C. Emotions should be avoided during the exchange between the individuals. In some cases, it may be best to wait to respond. This way the criticizer can think through the situation and decide possible solutions
D. The criticizer should consider role play before giving the criticism. This way the possible scenarios can be worked out. Further, the stress level of the criticizer will be reduced during the actual confrontation (they are in control).
E. In all cases, the specific criticism should be completely understood by the person receiving the criticism.
F. Both parties should listen to each other.
G. In general, "there are three solutions: mine, yours, and the correct one."

As an employee of an irrational boss, the best thing to do is to learn to cope (or quit!). Attempts should be made to get all directives put in writing to reduce ambiguity. Persistence pays on this point. A boss kept up-to-date on occurrences tends to be less irrational. Thus, the boss should be kept abreast of work proceedings. For best results, the employee should always approach problems from the positive side: "Let's try this new system" rather than "the old one won't work."

A mastery or pleasure log of life events can be used to "put life into perspective." This can visually demonstrate that there has been success and enjoyment in life. At the same time, it could point out where changes need to be made.

Finally, a person must be aware of the stressor via thoughts or feelings. Psychologists suggest taking six deep breaths, during which things can be put into perspective. Then the person should react or, if not ready, set an appointment to respond.

LONG-RANGE STRESS-REDUCTION TECHNIQUES

The following is a compilation of several methods used to reduce stress.[3,4] Some take practice to master; others are easy to use. The techniques should be used as needed. Keep in mind these techniques will reduce the stress response. However, ultimately to reduce the stress, the stressor needs to be removed or the behavior needs to be modified. New skills will be needed to deal with the stress.

Deep breathing: Breathe in through the nose. Hold the breath for a count of seven. Breathe out slowly through the mouth. Repeat three to six times. This technique should be used for extended periods of time (no more than six to eight breaths at a time) because the hyperventilation can cause dizziness and even fainting.

Mental imagery "Mind Trip": This technique is based on the concept that the body's nervous system cannot tell the difference between real and imagined experiences. The person chooses a favorite enjoyable past place or setting. (A picture or memorabilia can be used to jog the memory.) He then closes the eyes and concentrates on the experience, putting himself into the memory. The mind may wander, but if the experience was pleasurable, it will come back to the thoughts. This technique is not easy for some people to learn. It will take practice, one to two minutes, twice a day, to develop the technique. As a child, teachers used to reprimand us for "day dreaming;" now it is a stress-reduction technique.

Thought stopping: People have tried to use this particularly when they cannot sleep. The individual first tries to identify the problem that is causing the stress. Then he asks himself if there is anything that can be done about it right now? If not, mentally say, "stop." The process is repeated until thought is under control. This technique takes practice to use it effectively.

Self-coaching or preprogramming: During preparation for a scheduled stressful encounter, the person tries to generate his own instructions: "If this ... then this ...." The attempt is to try to identify the other person's weaknesses. In doing so self-confidence will increase, and stress will be reduced.

Muscle relaxation: Alternately tighten and relax muscles: tension for 5 seconds, then go limp (relax the muscle). The person starts at the end of the appendages and works toward the torso, adding muscle groups each time (1st fingers, 2nd fingers and forearm, 3rd fingers, forearm and upper arm). Finally, ending with all the muscles of the body being tightened and relaxed. The person should try to feel the relaxation of specific muscles between each contraction. The idea is to learn to recognize the muscle tension. Deep breathing may also help. This may be a good aid for sleeping.

Meditation: To accomplish this, a quiet environment with few distractions is needed. The person sits in a supported comfortable position, wearing loose clothing. The person should bring to the session a positive attitude, as a response cannot be forced. A mental device is needed, a simple sound/word — "one."

Sit, close eyes, and relax muscles. Breathe through the nose; be aware of it. Say, "oonnneeee," during a more prolonged expiration. Practice for 20 minutes. When finished, open eyes and sit quietly for a couple minutes.

Biofeedback: This takes special equipment that measures heart rate, blood pressure, skin temperature or EEG (brain wave) activity. The idea is to concentrate on these physiological markers and try to lower the response. It takes some time to learn, but it will reduce stress. Once learned, this technique can be used without equipment during any stressful event.

CONCLUSION

Stress is a way of life. Some stress is necessary to bring about change and is good. Too much stress can lead to physiological or psychological damage. The problem is that everyone's ability to cope with stress is different. Thus, people should not compare themselves to one another. Stress reduction works only when the individual prioritizes himself before the group; "I comes before we or you." The individual also must dig back into their memory of their early childhood to remember the word "no" and start using it to limit involvement. People must remember that no-one is indispensable or irreplaceable.[2] Also, no single way will reduce stress for all individuals.[3] Problems need to be put into perspective, support needs to be secured, and diversions or means to release tension need to be found. Many methods will need to be tried; some will work, and others will fail. Stress management does take time and effort, but the individual will be better off.

REFERENCES

1. McCauley, C.D., Stress and the eye of the beholder, *Iss. Obs.*, 7:1-8, 1987.
2. Kofodimos, J.R., To love or to work: must we choose?, *Iss. Obs.*, 6:1-8, 1986.
3. Winter, R.E., *Coping with Executive Stress*, McGraw-Hill Book Co., New York, 1983.
4. *Executive Fitness Newsletter*, Rodale Press Inc., Emmaus, PA, January 1982, April 1982, November 1982, June 1983, August 1983, September 1983, January 1984, March 1985, July 1985, October 1985, May 1986, February 1987, December 1987, July 1988.

Appendices

APPENDIX A:
Fitness Testing and General Exercise Guidelines

TABLE A-1
Heart Rate Conversion Chart

Beats per 10 Seconds	Beats per Minute	Beats per 15 Seconds	Beats per Minute
15	90	23	92
16	96	24	96
17	102	25	100
18	108	26	104
19	114	27	108
20	120	28	112
21	126	29	116
22	132	30	120
23	138	31	124
24	144	32	128
25	150	33	132
26	156	34	136
27	162	35	140
28	168	36	144
29	174	37	148
30	180	38	152
31	186	39	156
32	192	40	160
33	198	41	164
34	204	42	168
		43	172
		44	176
		45	180
		46	184
		47	188
		48	192
		49	196
		50	200
		51	204

TABLE A-2
Cycle Ergometer Test Form

Name _____ Date _____
Sex ___ Age ____ Weight _____ lb _____ kg
Pre-Exercise Heart Rate _____ bt/min
Seat Height ____

Exercise Minute	Work Rate (kgm)	Heart Rate (bt/min)	RPE	BP Sys/Dia
1	_____	_____	___	_____
2	_____	_____	___	_____
3	_____	_____	___	_____
4	_____	_____	___	_____
5	_____	_____	___	_____
6	_____	_____	___	_____
7	_____	_____	___	_____

Active Recovery

1	_____	_____	___	_____
2	_____	_____	___	_____

Resting Recovery

1	_____	_____	___	_____
2	_____	_____	___	_____

Men: $VO_2max = 6.98 + (WKLD_{kg} \times 0.0035) - (HR \times 0.046)$
Women: $VO_2max = 7.01 + (WKLD_{kg} \times 0.0038) - (HR \times 0.045)$

Estimated VO_2max _____ ml/kg/min

TABLE A-3

Age Correction Factors for Astrand and Rhyming Cycle Ergometer Test

Age	Factor	Age	Factor
15	1.10	35	0.870
16	1.09	36	0.862
17	1.08	37	0.854
18	1.07	38	0.846
19	1.06	39	0.838
20	1.05	40	0.830
21	1.04	41	0.820
22	1.03	42	0.810
23	1.02	43	0.800
24	1.01	44	0.790
25	1.00	45	0.780
26	0.987	46	0.774
27	0.974	47	0.768
28	0.961	48	0.762
29	0.948	49	0.756
30	0.935	50	0.750
31	0.922	55	0.710
32	0.909	60	0.680
33	0.896	65	0.650
34	0.883		

TABLE A-4

Example Calculation for the Astrand and Rhyming Cycle Ergometer Test

Example: 27-year-old male subject who weighs 197.5 lb has a heart rate of 139 for his final minute of work at 900 kpm/min.

1. Convert weight to kilograms: $197.5 \times 0.4536 = 89.586$ kg.
2. Using the formula for males for an HR of 139 bt/min at a final work load of 900 kpm/min,
   VO_2max (l/min) $= 6.98 + (WKLD_{kgm} \times 0.0035) - (HR \times 0.046)$
   $3.73 = 6.98 + (900 \times 0.0035) - (139 \times 0.046)$.
3. Convert l/min to ml/min by multiplying by 1,000: $3.73 \times 1,000 = 3730$ ml/min.
4. Obtain the ml/kg/min (this is maximum oxygen uptake expressed relative to body weight) by dividing the absolute oxygen uptake expressed in ml/min. by the body weight in kg:
   3,730 ml/min, divided by 89.59 kg = 41.6 ml/kg/min.
5. Correct for age by multiplying by the appropriate age correction factor, which is 0.974 for a 27-year-old: 41.6 ml/kg/min $\times$ 0.974 = 40.6 ml/kg/min.
6. Refer to Table A-6 for norms.

TABLE A-5
The Rating of Perceived Exertion (RPE) Scale

6
7 Very, very light
8
9 Very light
10
11 Fairly light
12
13 Somewhat hard
14
15 Hard
16
17 Very hard
18
19 Very, very hard
20

Source: From Borg, G., Subjective effort in relation to physical performance and working capacity, in *Psychology: From Research to Practice*, Pick, H.L., Ed., Plenum Publishing, New York, 1978, pp. 333-361.

TABLE A-6
Fitness Norms for Men and Women from 20 to 60+ Years of Age by Decade of Life

Rating	3-min Step Test Heart Rate	12-min Run Distance (miles)	1.5-mile Run (time)	VO$_2$max (ml/kg/min)	Body Fat (%)	Sit & Reach (inches)	Sit-ups (#/min)	Push-ups (#/min)	Bench Press lbs. lifted Body Weight	Leg Press lbs. pushed Body Weight
Part I. Men										
20–29 years										
Excellent	<78	>1.74	<9:09	>51	7	>21.8	>52	>41	>1.48	>2.27
Good	78–91	1.74–1.61	9:09–10:47	50–47	8–12	21.8–19.5	52–45	41–30	1.48–1.22	>2.27–2.05
Average	92–107	1.60–1.46	10:47–12:52	46–41	13–17	19.4–16.5	44–38	29–21	1.21–0.99	2.04–1.83
Fair	108–121	1.45–1.34	12:51–14:13	40–37	18–22	16.4–14.4	37–33	20–16	0.98–0.88	1.82–1.63
Poor	>121	<1.34	>14:13	<37	>22	<14.4	<33	<16	<0.88	<1.63
30–39 years										
Excellent	<80	>1.71	<9:30	>50	11	>21.0	>48	>32	>1.24	>2.07
Good	81–94	1.70–1.55	9:30–11:34	50–45	11–16	21.0–18.5	48–41	32–24	1.24–1.04	2.07–1.85
Average	95–111	1.54–1.39	11:35–13:36	44–39	17–21	18.4–15.5	40–35	23–16	1.03–0.88	1.84–1.65
Fair	112–122	1.38–1.29	13:37–14:52	38–35	22–24	15.4–13.0	34–30	15–11	0.88–0.78	1.64–1.52
Poor	>122	<1.29	>14:52	<35	>24	<13.0	<30	<11	<0.78	<1.52
40–49 years										
Excellent	<86	>1.65	<10:16	>48	14	>20.0	>43	>25	>1.10	>1.92
Good	86–99	1.65–1.47	10:16–12:34	47–42	15–18	20.0–17.5	43–36	25–19	1.10–0.93	1.92–1.74
Average	100–115	1.46–1.33	12:35–14:29	41–37	19–23	17.4–14.3	35–29	18–12	0.92–0.80	1.73–1.57
Fair	116–125	1.32–1.23	14:30–15:41	36–33	24–26	14.2–12.0	28–24	11–8	.79–0.72	1.56–1.44
Poor	>125	<1.23	>15:41	<33	>26	<12.0	<24	<8	<0.72	<1.44

TABLE A-6 (continued)
Fitness Norms for Men and Women from 20 to 60+ Years of Age by Decade of Life

Rating	3-min Step Test Heart Rate	12-min Run Distance (miles)	1.5-mile Run (time)	VO₂max (ml/kg/min)	Body Fat (%)	Sit & Reach (inches)	Sit-ups (#/min)	Push-ups (#/min)	Bench Press lbs. lifted Body Weight	Leg Press lbs. pushed Body Weight
50–59 years										
Excellent	<82	>1.57	<11:18	>45	15	>19.0	>39	>24	>0.97	>1.80
Good	82–99	1.57–1.38	11:18–13:45	45–38	16–20	19.0–16.5	39–31	24–14	0.97–0.84	1.80–1.64
Average	100–115	1.37–1.25	13:46–15:26	37–34	21–24	16.4–13.3	30–24	13–9	0.83–0.71	1.63–1.46
Fair	116–125	1.24–1.15	15:27–16:43	33–30	25–28	13.2–10.5	23–19	8–5	0.70–0.63	1.45–1.32
Poor	>125	<1.15	>16:43	<30	>28	<10.5	<19	<5	<0.63	<1.32
60+ years										
Excellent	<86	>1.49	<9:30	>41	15	>19.0	>35	>24	>0.89	>1.73
Good	86–97	1.49–1.29	9:30–11:34	41–35	16–20	19.0–15.5	35–26	24–11	0.89–0.77	1.73–1.56
Average	98–114	1.28–1.15	11:35–13:36	34–29	21–25	15.4–12.5	25–19	10–7	0.76–0.65	1.55–1.38
Fair	115–126	1.14–1.05	13:37–14:52	28–25	26–29	12.4–10.0	18–15	6–4	0.64–0.57	1.37–1.25
Poor	>126	<1.05	>14:52	<25	>29	<10.0	<15	<4	<0.57	<1.25
Part II. Women										
20–29 years										
Excellent	<84	>1.54	<11:43	>44	15	>23.8	>49	>32	>0.90	>1.82
Good	84–101	1.54–1.37	11:43–13:53	44–38	16–19	23.8–21.5	49–41	32–22	0.90–0.74	1.82–1.58
Average	102–120	1.36–1.25	13:54–15:26	37–34	20–24	21.4–19.3	40–32	21–14	0.73–0.59	1.57–1.37
Fair	121–132	1.24–1.16	15:27–16:33	33–31	25–28	19.2–17.0	31–27	13–9	0.58–0.51	1.36–1.22
Poor	>132	<1.16	>16:33	<31	>28	<17.0	<27	<9	<0.51	<1.22

30–39 years

Excellent	<86	>1.45	<12:51	>41	16	>22.5	>40	>31	>0.76	>1.61
Good	86–103	1.44–1.33	12:51–14:24	41–37	17–20	22.5–20.5	40–32	31–21	0.76–0.63	1.61–1.39
Average	104–121	1.32–1.21	14:25–15:57	36–32	21–25	20.4–18.3	31–25	20–12	0.62–0.53	1.38–1.21
Fair	122–133	1.20–1.11	15:58–17:14	31–29	26–29	18.2–16.5	24–20	11–7	0.52–0.47	1.20–1.09
Poor	>133	<1.11	>17:14	<29	>29	<16.5	<20	<7	<0.47	<1.09

40–49 years

Excellent	<90	>1.41	<13:22	>40	19	>21.5	>34	>28	>0.71	>1.48
Good	90–105	1.41–1.25	13:22–15:26	40–34	20–24	21.5–19.8	34–27	28–18	0.71–0.57	1.48–1.29
Average	106–121	1.24–1.13	15:27–16:58	33–29	25–28	19.7–17.3	26–20	17–10	0.56–0.50	1.28–1.13
Fair	122–133	1.12–1.05	16:59–18:00	28–27	29–32	17.2–15.0	19–14	9–4	0.49–0.43	1.12–1.02
Poor	>133	<1.05	>18:00	<27	>32	<15.0	<14	<4	<0.43	<1.02

50–59 years

Excellent	<93	>1.29	<14:55	>35	22	>21.5	>29	>23	>0.61	>1.37
Good	93–106	1.29–1.17	14:55–16:27	35–31	23–27	21.5–19.3	29–22	23–13	0.61–052	1.37–1.17
Average	105–120	1.16–1.06	16:28–17:55	30–27	28–32	19.2–16.8	21–14	12–5	0.51–0.44	1.16–0.99
Fair	119–132	1.05–0.98	17:56–18:49	26–24	33–36	16.7–14.8	13–10	4–1	0.43–0.39	0.98–0.88
Poor	<132	<0.98	>18:49	<24	>36	<14.8	<10	<1	<0.39	<0.88

60+ years

Excellent	<93	>1.29	<14:55	>35	21	>21.8	>26	>25	>0.64	>1.32
Good	99–106	1.29–1.13	14:55–16:58	35–29	22–28	21.8–17.5	26–12	25–12	0.64–0.51	1.31–1.13
Average	107–120	1.12–0.99	16:59–18:44	28–24	29–33	17.4–15.5	11–6	11–3	0.50–0.43	1.12–0.93
Fair	121–132	0.98–0.94	18:45–19:21	23	34–37	15.4–13.0	5–3	2–1	0.42–0.39	0.92–0.85
Poor	>132	<0.94	>19:21	<23	>37	<13.0	<3	<1	<0.39	<0.85

Norms based on Golding, L.A., Myers, C.R.., and Sinning, W.E., *Y's Way to Physical Fitness: The Complete Guide to Fitness Testing and Instruction*, Human Kinetics Inc., Champaign, 1989.

Canadian Standardized Test of Fitness (CSTF) Operations Manual, Fitness Canada, Ottawa, 1986.

Nieman, D.C., *Fitness and Sports Medicine: An Introduction*, Bull Publishing Co., Palo Alto, CA, 1990.

GENERAL EXERCISE PROGRAM GUIDELINES

EXERCISE PROGRAMMING FOR ADULTS

1. Aerobic Exercise
   Intensity: 60 to 90% of maximal heart rate (50 to 80% of maximal metabolic rate)
   Duration: 20 to 60 minutes per session
   Frequency: 3 to 5 days a week
2. Strength (Resistance) Exercise
   1 to 3 sets of 8 to 12 repetitions
   2 to 3 days per week, separated by at least one day of rest
   Include all major muscle groups
   Use each muscle through its full range of motion
3. Flexibility Exercises
   Intensity: Stretch to the point of feeling the tension
   Duration: Each exercise should be held 6 to 30 seconds
   Frequency: Daily
   Include: Legs, hips, back, and shoulders

EXERCISE PROGRAMMING FOR SENIORS

1. Aerobic Exercise
   Intensity: Moderate intensity or modified based on conditions
   Duration: 20 to 40 minutes per session
   Frequency: 5 to 7 days a week
2. Strength (Resistance) Exercise
   1 to 3 sets of 8 to 12 repetitions
   Two days per week, separated by at least two days of rest
   Include all major muscle groups
   Use each muscle through its full range of motion
   When possible, use machines rather than free weights
3. Flexibility Exercises
   Intensity: Stretch to the point of feeling the tension
   Duration: Each exercise should be held 6 to 30 seconds
   Frequency: Daily
   Include: Legs, hips, back, and shoulders

Summarized from: American College of Sports Medicine, *ACSM's Resource Manual for Guidelines for Exercise Testing and Prescription (3rd edit.),* Williams & Wilkins, Baltimore, 1998.

APPENDIX B:
Body Composition

TABLE B-1
Estimating Body Frame Size Using Height and Wrist Circumference

Frame Size	Height	Wrist Circumference
Small	4'7"–6'	4¾"–5½"
	5'2"–6'	5½"–6"
	5'5"–6'	6"–6¼"
Medium	4'7"–6'	5½"–5¾"
	5'2"–6'	6"–6¼"
	5'5"–6'	6¼"–6½"
Large	4'7"–6'	5¾"–6¼"
	5'2"–6'	6¼"–6½"
	5'5"–6'	6½"–7"

TABLE B-2
Alternative Method of Approximating Frame Size

Method: Bend the dominant forearm upward at a 90° angle, keeping fingers straight and palm of the hand toward body. Measure the distance between the two prominent bones at the elbow by placing the thumb and index finger of the other hand at each protrusion. Then measure the space between the fingers using a ruler. Look in the table below for appropriate gender and height. If the elbow breadth measure is within the limits listed below, then the person has a medium frame. If below the limit, the frame size is small. Conversely, if it is above the limit, the person has a large frame.

Elbow Measurements for Medium Frame Size

Men Height	Elbow Breadth	Women Height	Elbow Breadth
5'2"–5'3"	2½"–2⅞"	4'10"–4'11"	2¼"–2½"
5'4"–5'7"	2⅝"–2⅞"	5'0"–5'3"	2¼"–2½"
5'8"–5'11"	2¾"–3"	5'4"–5'7"	2⅜"–2⅝"
6'0"–6'3"	2¾"–3⅛"	5'8"–5'11"	2⅜"–2⅝"
6'4"	2⅞"–3¼"	6'0"	2½"–2¾"

Reprinted courtesy of Metropolitan Life Insurance Co., *Statistical Bulletin*, New York, NY.

TABLE B-3
Body Weight Ranges Related to the Best Mortality for Men Age 25 and Over for Height and Frame Size

Feet	Inches	Small Frame	Medium Frame	Large Frame
5	2	128–134	131–141	138–150
5	3	130–136	133–143	140–153
5	4	132–138	135–145	142–156
5	5	134–140	137–148	144–160
5	6	136–142	139–151	146–164
5	7	138–145	142–154	149–168
5	8	140–148	145–157	152–172
5	9	142–151	148–160	155–176
5	10	144–154	151–163	158–180
5	11	146–157	154–166	161–184
6	0	149–160	157–170	164–188
6	1	152–164	160–174	168–192
6	2	155–168	164–178	172–197
6	3	158–172	167–182	176–202
6	4	162–176	171–187	181–207

For nude weight, deduct 5 lb
Height measured with shoes that have 1-in. heels
(in indoor clothing).
Reprinted courtesy of Metropolitan Life Insurance Co.,
Statistical Bulletin, New York, NY.

TABLE B-4
Body Weight Ranges Related to the Best Mortality for Women Age 25 and Over for Height and Frame Size

Feet	Inches	Small Frame	Medium Frame	Large Frame
4	10	102–111	109–121	118–131
4	11	103–113	111–123	120–134
5	0	104–115	113–126	122–137
5	1	106–118	115–129	125–140
5	2	108–121	118–132	128–143
5	3	111–124	121–135	131–147
5	4	114–127	124–138	134–151
5	5	117–130	127–141	137–155
5	6	120–133	130–144	140–159
5	7	123–136	133–147	143–163
5	8	126–139	136–150	146–167
5	9	129–142	139–153	149–170
5	10	132–145	142–156	152–173
5	11	135–148	145–159	155–176
6	0	138–151	148–162	158–179

For nude weight, deduct 3 lb
Height measured with shoes that have 1-in. heels
(in indoor clothing).
Reprinted courtesy of Metropolitan Life Insurance Co.,
Statistical Bulletin, New York, NY.

TABLE B-5
Percent Fat for Women Estimated from Skinfolds Using the Sum of Triceps, Abdomen, and Suprailium Skinfolds and Age

Sum of Skinfolds (mm)	Age to Last Year								
	18–22	23–27	28–32	33–37	38–42	43–47	48–52	53–57	>57
8–12	8.8	9.0	9.2	9.4	9.5	9.7	9.9	10.1	10.3
13–17	10.8	10.9	11.1	11.3	11.5	11.7	11.8	12.0	12.2
18–22	12.6	12.8	13.0	13.2	13.4	13.5	13.7	13.9	14.1
23–27	14.5	14.6	14.8	15.0	15.2	15.4	15.6	15.7	15.9
28–32	16.2	16.4	16.6	16.8	17.0	17.1	17.3	17.5	17.7
33–37	17.9	18.1	18.3	18.5	18.7	18.9	19.0	19.2	19.4
38–42	19.6	19.8	20.0	20.2	20.3	20.5	20.7	20.9	21.1
43–47	21.2	21.4	21.6	21.8	21.9	22.1	22.3	22.5	22.7
48–52	22.8	22.9	23.1	23.3	23.5	23.7	23.8	24.0	24.2
53–57	24.2	24.4	24.6	24.8	25.0	25.2	25.3	25.5	25.7
58–62	25.7	25.9	26.0	26.2	26.4	26.6	26.8	27.0	27.1
63–67	27.1	27.2	27.4	27.6	27.8	28.0	28.2	28.3	28.5
68–72	28.4	28.6	28.7	28.9	29.1	30.6	30.7	30.9	31.1
78–82	30.9	31.0	31.2	31.4	31.6	31.8	31.9	32.1	32.3
83–87	32.0	32.2	32.4	32.6	32.7	32.9	33.1	33.3	33.5
88–92	33.1	33.3	33.5	33.7	33.8	34.0	34.2	34.4	34.6
93–97	34.1	34.3	34.5	34.7	34.9	35.1	35.2	35.4	35.6
98–102	35.1	35.3	35.5	35.7	35.9	36.0	36.2	36.4	36.6
103–107	36.1	36.2	36.4	36.6	36.8	37.0	37.2	37.3	37.5
108–112	36.9	37.1	37.3	37.5	37.7	37.9	38.0	38.2	38.4
113–117	37.8	37.9	38.1	38.3	39.2	39.4	39.6	39.8	39.2
118–122	38.5	38.7	38.9	39.1	39.4	39.6	39.8	40.0	40.0
123–127	39.2	39.4	39.6	39.8	40.0	40.1	40.3	40.5	40.7
128–132	39.9	40.1	40.2	40.4	40.6	40.8	41.0	41.2	41.3
133–137	40.5	40.7	40.8	41.0	41.2	41.4	41.6	41.7	41.9
138–142	41.0	41.2	41.4	41.6	41.7	41.9	42.1	42.3	42.5
143–147	41.5	41.7	41.9	42.0	42.2	42.4	42.6	42.8	43.0
148–152	41.9	42.1	42.3	42.8	42.6	42.8	43.0	43.2	43.4
153–157	42.3	42.5	42.6	42.8	43.0	43.2	43.4	43.6	43.7
158–162	42.6	42.8	43.0	43.1	43.3	43.5	43.7	43.9	44.1
163–167	42.9	43.0	43.2	43.4	43.6	43.8	44.0	44.1	44.3
168–172	43.1	43.2	43.4	43.6	43.8	44.0	44.2	44.3	44.5
173–177	43.2	43.4	43.6	43.8	43.9	44.1	44.3	44.5	44.7
178–182	43.3	43.5	43.7	43.8	44.0	44.2	44.4	44.6	44.8

From: Hoeger, W.W.K. and Hoeger, S.A., *Principles & Labs for Fitness and Wellness,* 5th edit., Morton Publishing Co., Englewood, CO, 1995.

TABLE B-6
Percent Fat for Men Age 40 and Younger Estimated From Skinfolds Using the Sum of the Chest, Abdomen, and Thigh Skinfolds and Age

Sum of Skinfolds (mm)	Age to Last Year							
	<19	20–22	23–25	26–29	30–31	32–34	35–37	38–40
8–10	0.9	1.3	1.6	2.0	2.3	2.7	3.0	3.3
11–13	1.9	2.3	2.6	3.0	3.3	3.7	4.0	4.3
14–16	2.9	3.3	3.6	3.9	4.3	4.6	5.0	5.3
17–19	3.9	4.2	4.6	4.9	5.3	5.6	6.0	6.3
20–22	4.8	5.2	5.5	5.9	6.2	6.6	6.9	7.3
23–25	5.8	6.2	6.5	6.8	7.2	7.5	7.9	8.2
26–28	6.8	7.1	7.5	7.8	8.1	8.5	8.8	9.2
29–31	7.7	8.0	8.4	8.7	9.1	9.4	9.8	10.1
32–34	8.6	9.0	9.3	9.7	10.0	10.4	10.7	11.1
35–37	9.5	9.9	10.2	10.6	10.9	11.3	11.6	12.0
38–40	10.5	10.8	11.2	11.5	11.8	12.2	12.5	12.9
41–43	11.4	11.7	12.1	12.4	12.7	13.1	13.4	13.8
44–46	12.2	12.6	12.9	13.3	13.6	14.0	14.3	14.7
47–49	13.1	13.5	13.8	14.2	14.5	14.9	15.2	15.5
50–52	14.0	14.3	14.7	15.0	15.4	15.7	16.1	16.4
53–55	14.8	15.2	15.5	15.9	16.2	16.6	16.9	17.3
56–58	15.7	16.0	16.4	16.7	17.1	17.4	17.8	18.1
59–61	16.5	16.9	17.2	17.6	17.9	18.3	18.6	19.0
62–64	17.4	17.7	18.1	18.4	18.8	19.1	19.4	19.8
65–67	18.2	18.5	18.9	19.2	19.6	19.9	20.3	20.6
68–70	19.0	19.3	19.7	20.0	20.4	20.7	21.1	21.4
71–73	19.8	20.1	20.5	20.8	21.2	21.5	21.9	22.2
74–76	20.6	20.9	21.3	21.6	22.0	22.2	22.7	23.0
77–79	21.4	21.7	22.1	22.4	22.8	23.1	23.4	23.8
80–82	22.1	22.5	22.8	23.2	23.5	23.9	24.2	24.6
83–85	22.9	23.2	23.6	23.9	24.3	24.6	25.0	25.3
86–88	23.6	24.0	24.3	24.7	25.0	25.4	25.7	26.1
89–91	24.4	24.7	25.1	25.4	25.8	26.1	26.5	26.8
92–94	25.1	25.5	25.8	26.2	26.5	26.9	27.2	27.5
95–97	25.8	26.2	26.5	26.9	27.2	27.6	27.9	28.3
98–100	26.6	26.9	27.3	27.6	27.9	28.3	28.6	29.0
101–103	27.3	27.6	28.0	28.3	28.6	29.0	29.3	29.7
104–106	27.9	28.3	28.6	29.0	29.3	29.7	30.0	30.4
107–109	28.6	29.0	29.3	29.7	30.0	30.4	30.7	31.1
110–112	29.3	29.6	30.0	30.3	30.7	31.0	31.4	31.7
113–115	30.0	30.3	30.7	31.0	31.3	31.7	32.0	32.4
116–118	30.6	31.0	31.3	31.6	32.0	32.3	32.7	33.0
119–121	31.3	31.6	32.0	32.3	33.3	33.6	34.0	34.3
122–124	31.9	32.2	32.6	32.9	33.3	33.6	34.0	34.3
125–127	32.5	32.9	33.2	33.5	33.9	34.2	34.6	34.9
128–130	33.1	33.5	33.8	34.2	34.5	34.9	35.2	35.5

From: Hoeger, W.W.K. and Hoeger, S.A., *Principles & Labs for Fitness and Wellness,* 5th edit. Morton Publishing Co., Englewood, CO, 1995.

TABLE B-7
Percent Fat for Men Over Age 40 Estimated From Skinfolds Using the Sum of Chest, Abdomen, and Thigh Skinfolds and Age

Sum of Skinfolds (mm)	Age to Last Year							
	41–43	44–46	47–49	50–52	53–55	56–58	59–61	>61
8–10	3.7	4.0	4.4	4.7	5.1	5.4	5.8	6.1
11–13	4.7	5.0	5.4	5.7	6.1	6.4	6.8	7.1
14–16	5.7	6.0	6.4	6.7	7.1	7.4	7.8	8.1
17–19	6.7	7.0	7.4	7.7	8.1	8.4	8.7	9.1
20–22	7.6	8.0	8.3	8.7	9.0	9.4	9.7	10.1
23–25	8.6	8.9	9.3	9.6	10.0	10.3	10.7	11.0
26–28	9.5	9.9	10.2	10.6	10.9	11.3	11.6	12.0
29–31	10.5	10.8	11.2	11.5	11.9	12.2	12.6	12.9
32–34	11.4	11.8	12.1	12.4	12.8	13.1	13.5	13.8
35–37	12.3	12.7	13.0	13.4	13.7	14.1	14.4	14.8
38–40	13.2	13.6	13.9	14.3	14.6	15.0	15.3	15.7
41–43	14.1	14.5	14.8	15.2	15.5	15.9	16.2	16.6
44–46	15.0	15.4	15.7	16.1	16.4	16.8	17.1	17.5
47–49	15.9	16.2	16.6	16.9	17.3	17.6	18.0	18.3
50–52	16.8	17.1	17.5	17.8	18.2	18.5	18.8	19.2
53–55	17.6	18.0	18.3	18.7	19.0	19.4	19.7	20.1
56–58	18.5	18.8	19.2	19.5	19.9	20.2	20.6	20.9
59–61	19.3	19.7	20.0	20.4	20.7	21.0	21.4	21.7
62–64	20.1	20.5	20.8	21.2	21.5	21.9	22.2	22.6
65–67	21.0	21.3	21.7	22.0	22.4	22.7	23.0	23.4
68–70	21.8	22.1	22.5	22.8	23.2	23.5	23.9	24.2
71–73	22.6	22.9	23.3	23.6	24.0	24.3	24.7	25.0
74–76	23.4	23.7	24.1	24.4	24.8	25.1	25.4	25.8
77–79	24.1	24.5	24.8	25.2	25.5	25.9	26.2	26.6
80–82	24.9	25.3	25.6	26.0	26.3	26.6	27.0	27.3
83–85	25.7	26.0	26.4	26.7	27.1	27.4	27.8	28.1
86–88	26.4	26.8	27.1	27.5	27.8	28.2	28.5	28.9
89–91	27.2	27.5	27.9	28.2	28.6	28.9	29.2	29.6
92–94	27.9	28.2	28.6	28.9	29.3	29.6	30.0	30.3
95–97	28.6	29.0	29.3	29.7	30.0	30.4	30.7	31.1
98–100	29.3	29.7	30.0	30.4	30.7	31.1	31.4	31.8
101–103	30.0	30.4	30.7	31.1	31.4	31.8	32.1	32.5
104–106	30.7	31.1	31.4	31.8	32.1	32.5	32.8	33.2
107–109	31.4	31.8	32.1	32.4	32.8	33.1	33.5	33.8
110–112	32.1	32.4	32.8	33.1	33.5	33.8	34.2	34.5
113–115	32.7	33.1	33.4	33.8	34.1	34.5	34.8	35.2
116–118	33.4	33.7	34.1	34.4	34.8	35.1	35.5	35.8
119–121	34.0	34.4	34.7	35.1	35.4	35.8	36.1	36.5
122–124	34.7	35.0	35.4	35.7	36.1	36.4	36.7	37.1
125–127	35.3	35.6	36.0	36.3	36.7	37.0	37.4	37.7
128–130	35.9	36.2	36.6	36.9	37.3	37.6	38.0	38.4

From: Hoeger, W.W.K. and Hoeger, S.A., *Principles & Labs for Fitness and Wellness,* 5th edit. Morton Publishing Co., Englewood, CO, 1995.

TABLE B-8
Percent Body Fat Based on Specific Gravity Obtained from Underwater Weighing or Skinfold Measurements

Specific Gravity	Percent Body Fat
1.002	49.3
1.004	48.2
1.005	47.1
1.008	46.0
1.010	44.9
1.012	43.8
1.014	42.7
1.016	41.7
1.018	40.6
1.020	39.5
1.022	38.5
1.024	37.4
1.026	36.3
1.028	35.3
1.030	34.2
1.032	33.2
1.034	32.2
1.036	31.2
1.038	30.1
1.040	29.1
1.042	28.0
1.044	27.0
1.046	26.0
1.048	25.0
1.050	24.0
1.052	23.0
1.054	22.0
1.056	21.0
1.058	20.0
1.060	19.0
1.062	18.0
1.064	17.0
1.068	16.1
1.070	14.1
1.072	13.1
1.074	12.2
1.076	11.2
1.078	10.3
1.080	9.3
1.082	8.4
1.084	7.4
1.086	6.5
1.088	5.5
1.090	4.6
1.092	3.7

Based on Rathbun, E.N. and Pace, N., Studies of body composition: the determination of total body fat by means of the body specific gravity, *J. Biol. Chem.*, 158, 667–676, 1945.

APPENDIX C:
Exercise Circuit

INSTRUCTIONS FOR CALISTHENIC/AEROBIC CIRCUIT

The calisthenic/aerobic circuit was designed to develop both dynamic muscle strength and aerobic fitness. Using upper body weight or the assistance of a partner to provide resistance, the following exercises will strengthen the muscles. By interspersing short bouts of jogging, jumping jacks, and rope skipping, an aerobic conditioning component is provided.

Prior to performing the circuit, subjects must be assessed to determine their maximal 1-minute performance capability for each exercise. An easy way for an instructor to do this is to demonstrate the exercises to the class, divide into several small groups (two to three individuals), and proceed through each station. Someone will need to monitor the 1-minute time intervals. One person counts the number of repetitions completed by the exerciser. It is important that the subject correctly perform as many repetitions as possible within the minute (only correctly executed repetitions are counted). As long as subjects are given a sufficient warm-up to prepare their bodies for the upcoming exercise, it does not matter at which station they begin (see diagram for example of circuit flow chart). Use the Calisthenic/Aerobic Circuit Assessment sheet for recording assessment results and the training level for each exercise.

During a workout session, the subject should pair up with a partner, go through the circuit and perform the appropriate number of repetitions for each station. Following one completion of the circuit, subjects should run, cycle, or perform some other aerobic conditioning activity at their target heart rate for 10 minutes. Then they should complete the circuit a second time.

Because the number of repetitions for most of the exercises in the circuit is based on 75% of the maximum number performed during the evaluation, improvements resulting from training necessitate reevaluations on four week intervals so that adjustments in work loads can be made.

SPECIAL EQUIPMENT REQUIRED

1. 12–16-in. high benches (at least two are needed)
2. Saw horse and a bar, or edge of table that can be gripped and can support body weight
3. Three sturdy chairs

DESCRIPTION OF EXCERCISES

1. *Half squat jumps*: 75% maximal number
   Purpose: To strengthen the muscles of the upper leg.
   Starting position: Stand erect with feet shoulder-width apart.
   Movement: Lower the body to a semisquatting position by bending the knees.
   Keeping the back straight, jump about a foot off the floor.

2. *Elevated push-ups*: 75% maximal number
   Purpose: To strengthen the muscles of the chest, back of the arm, and front of the shoulder.
   Starting position: Lay on stomach with hands flat on the floor and positioned beneath the shoulders with fingers pointing forward. Feet are elevated about a foot off the floor (cinder blocks, stairs, or bleacher seats can be used).
   Movement: Keeping the back as straight as possible, push the body off the floor until the arms are straight; lower the body until the chin comes within 4 in. off the floor.

3. *Low-bar pull-ups*: 75% maximal number
   Purpose: To strengthen muscles of the front of the arm, upper back, and shoulder.
   Starting position: Lay on back with legs together and extended; grip the "bar" (edge of the table, crossbeam of a saw horse) using a palm-forward grip at shoulder-width apart. Arms should be straight.
   Movement: Keeping the feet stationary and the back as straight as possible, pull the body up so that the chin touches the bar.

4. *Single leg step-ups*: 75% maximal number
   Purpose: To strengthen muscles of the front of the legs and calves.
   Starting position: Stand erect with feet slightly apart.
   Movement: Step up onto a 12- to 16-in. high block (steps, cinder blocks, bleacher seats) with one leg. Bring up the other leg. Fully straighten both legs. Step off using the initial leg. Repeat, but use the other leg to begin the step on and off the block.

5. *Hamstring curl with two people**: 20 repetitions each leg
   Purpose: To strengthen muscle on the back of the thigh.
   Starting position: Lay on stomach with hands folded under chin. Partner kneels to the side of outstretched legs.
   Movement: As one leg at a time is drawn toward the buttocks, the partner provides moderate resistance to the movement by pushing gently against the back of the lower leg. The leg is then straightened and the other leg is drawn toward the buttocks.

6. *Chair dips*: 75% maximal number
   Purpose: To strengthen muscles on the back of the arm and shoulder.
   Starting position: Three chairs are placed, one just to the side of each shoulder and one to support the feet when the legs are extended. Support oneself between the chairs in a "seated" position by straightening the arms and placing the palms of each hand in a chair. Fingers are pointing toward the feet. With legs straightened, the heels are placed in the third chair.
   Movement: While keeping the legs and back as straight as possible, raise and lower oneself by bending and straightening the arms. When done correctly, the elbows should be bent at right angles. Care should be taken to prevent the chairs from sliding.

7. *Sit-ups*: 20 repetitions
   Purpose: To strengthen muscles of the abdomen and hip.
   Starting position: Lay on back with knees bent and arms folded on chest.
   Movement: Raise head and trunk to an upright position and touch elbows to knees. Hold the position for one count, and slowly return to the starting position.

8. *Lower body leg-ups*: 20 repetitions
   Purpose: To strengthen muscles of the abdomen.
   Starting position: Lay on back with legs straight. Place hands on thighs.
   Movement: Draw both legs toward the abdomen by bending the knees while pressing against the thighs with the hands to offer resistance to the movement. Slowly return to the starting position. Be sure to keep the back in contact with the floor.

9. *Low-back butterflies*: 10 repetitions
   Purpose: To strengthen the muscles of the back and hip.
   Starting position: Lay on stomach with arms extended over the head and legs extended.
   Movement: Raise the right arm and left leg simultaneously, and keep them extended for several seconds. Return to the starting position. Repeat the movements using the left arm and right leg. Perform the exercise slowly without jerking legs and arms.

EXAMPLE FLOW CHART OF THE CALISTHENIC/AEROBIC CIRCUIT

To facilitate flow of the circuit, stations with appropriate signs can be set up. Jump ropes and mats should be placed at the appropriate stations. Following is an example of a flow chart of the circuit:

1. Half squat jumps
   30 seconds of jumping jacks
2. Elevated push-ups
   30 seconds of rope skipping

3. Low bar pull-ups
   30 seconds of jogging
4. Single leg step-ups
   30 seconds of jogging
5. Hamstring curls
   30 seconds of rope skipping
6. Low bar pull-ups
   30 seconds of jumping jacks
7. Chair dips
   30 seconds of rope skipping
8. Sit-ups
9. Lower body leg-ups
10. Low-back butterflies
11. Run, cycle, or perform other aerobic activity for 10 minutes at target heart rate

CALISTHENIC/AEROBIC CIRCUIT   NAME:_____

Program Steps:

1. Determine the number of repetitions that can be performed in 1 minute.
2. Multiply the 1-minute maximal number by 3/4 to determine the training level.
3. Exercises with * will be performed at the set number of repetitions.
4. Go through the circuit one time.
5. Jog, cycle, or perform other aerobic activity for 10 minutes at target heart rate.
6. Go through the circuit a second time.
7. Jog, cycle, or perform other aerobic activity for 10 minutes at target heart rate.
8. Retest every four weeks and adjust as needed.

Exercise	Max Number in 1 Minute	Training Level	
Half Squat Jumps	_____	_____	(75%)
Elevated Push-ups	_____	_____	(75%)
Low-bar Pull-ups	_____	_____	(75%)
Single Leg Step-ups	_____	_____	(75%)
Hamstring Curls*	20 repetitions (each leg)		
Chair Dips	_____	_____	(75%)
Sit-ups	_____	_____	(75%)
Lower Body Leg-ups	_____	_____	(75%)
Low-back Butterflies*	10 repetitions		

Index of Key Terms